The GLUTEN-FREE Pantry

How to Save **Time**, **Money**, and **Effort** in the Kitchen

LAURA HUFFMAN

Available at special pricing for quantity discounts to organizations.
Contact Laura Huffman at www.viviansliveagain.com for inquiries.
Vivian's Live Again
PO Box 6731
Logan, UT 84341

Huffman, Laura W.
The Gluten-Free Pantry: How to Save Time, Money, and Effort in the Kitchen.
First edition. North Logan: April 6, 2024.
ISBN 979-8-9888706-0-9 (paperback)
Subjects: Gluten-free diet— Handbooks, manuals, etc. | Gluten-free diet—Recipes.
BISAC: COOKING / Health & Healing / Gluten-Free. | COOKING / Health & Healing / Allergy | COOKING / Reference.
641.56/3 – dc23

LOOKING TO LIVE AND EAT GLUTEN-FREE?

Come and visit Vivian's Live Again

VIVIANSLIVEAGAIN.COM

This book is dedicated to my mother, Vivian Willardson, for teaching me to think scientifically about cooking and instilling in me the belief that food should taste good and bring people together.

INTRODUCTION

FRUSTRATING IS PROBABLY THE BEST WORD to sum up going gluten free cold turkey. Have you recently learned you're gluten-free and don't know where to start your new diet? Do you cringe every time you look at the price of the gluten-free food you're buying and wish for a more economical and budget-friendly way to create your favorite gluten-free baked goods and dishes? Could there be a way to save time cooking? Have you ever wondered about stocking up on food for saving and preparing for a rainy day? Do you feel like you lost your cooking skills overnight?

No matter where you are in your gluten free journey, beginner to veteran, *The Gluten-Free Pantry* will empower you to make gluten free living easier, cheaper and more nutritious.

What you can expect to learn in this book:

- Converting your favorite recipes to gluten free
- Saving money on food
- Convenient and time saving home cooking methods
- Storing food for savings and emergency preparedness
- What to eat to boost nutrients commonly missing in gluten free diets
- Secrets of gluten free flour and baking along with a troubleshooting guide

Until now, no one has assembled in one place all the right information to buy and store bulk foods, convert recipes, and save time and money while eating gluten-free. If any diet needs to be less costly, more convenient, more nutritious, and more prepared for the unexpected, it's the gluten-free diet. The best thing about *The Gluten-Free Pantry* is that in addition to teaching how, it teaches why. Understanding the underlying principles of gluten free living and cooking allows you to adapt the ideas to your own situation. No matter where you are in your food journey, start with my book, *The Gluten-Free Pantry*, to discover new food skills to improve cooking, baking and food storage practices inside your home.

My entrance into the world of gluten free did not come in a doctor's office, but rather in the kitchen of my friend Helene, who had celiac disease. I was troubled that her food was isolating, expensive and poor tasting. I kept asking questions and researching. I was sure there were answers to the struggles she encountered.

At a gluten free cooking class, I shared a gluten-free cream of chicken soup recipe with the woman who sat next to me. Later that year, I made that recipe dairy free to accommodate a dairy allergic girl at a church girls camp. It was then I decided to go into business selling soup mixes that were dairy and gluten free. I named the company Wheat Free Nutrition and later changed the brand name to Vivian's Live Again in honor of my mother. Like my mom, I believe food should taste good and bring people together.

Through the last 12 years in my business, my team and I have experimented and learned what makes gluten free recipes succeed and fail. Knowledge I can't wait to share with you in this book.

The skills and ideas for cooking conveniently, were honed in my own kitchen. With 5 closely spaced children (including a set of twins) I had to find efficient ways to cook. Gluten free living means cooking more at home and I offer effective strategies. No matter why you are short on time, ideas in the book can help.

In 2017, I purchased Tree Street Grains, a small milling company that focused on stone milled, 100% whole grain products including a 9-grain gluten-free flour. I was disillusioned with the nutritional content of gluten-free foods and wanted the secrets of making whole grain flour perform well in gluten-free baking. Knowledge gained about whole grain flours, commercial or home milled, is included in our whole grain and flour chapters.

I grew up in a culture that stores food for financial savings and emergencies but realized later that traditional recommendations won't work for the gluten free. Section 4 Food Storage explains short term storage plans which work for anyone's needs and provides helpful information to build and implement a long term home storage plan which is gluten free.

I hope you will take advantage of my years of hard work and research summarized in *The Gluten-Free Pantry* to allow you to enjoy gluten-free eating and living like never before.

How to Use This Book

The most important way to live a better gluten free life is to begin now. With that in mind, I created stand-alone chapters with easy to implement ideas. Skip to the chapter you need most or start reading in chapter one. As you read *The Gluten-Free Pantry*, consider which concepts fit into your time, budget, lifestyle preference, and current skills. Next, experiment with one or two new skills and incorporate these new food related skills into your routine.

A few of the methods mentioned in this book, particularly the food storage section, describe ideal conditions which may not be feasible with available resources. Fortunately, the principles taught allow you to adapt to your own circumstances.

Even though there are gluten free living and emergency preparedness resources, different bloggers, and food influencers on the internet, no one has time in their busy lives to look at even a fraction of the available content. The information you need to successfully organize and establish an easier, more nutritious and prepared gluten-free food life is found in the pages of *The Gluten-Free Pantry: How to Save Time, Money, and Effort in the Kitchen.*

ACKNOWLEDGMENTS

THIS BOOK HAS BEEN YEARS IN THE MAKING. A long series of experiments, research and answering gluten free cooking questions inspired me to write. Along the way many have encouraged, supported, prodded, reviewed and edited, without whose help I never would have completed the book. To mention just a few:

Thanks to Lynn Smargis, creator of the *Travel Gluten Free* Podcast. I met her at a gluten free expo where she encouraged me to write this book. Without her convincing me I was capable of writing a book, I would not have even tried. She also mentored me through the process of writing and publishing and was especially helpful in the content creation of the Finding Resources section.

This would be a much lesser book without the talents of Christina Hartman, my main editor. I was amazed by her ability to drastically improve the readability, flow, and clarity of the text with only a few changes. With fresh, non-gluten free eyes she brought the perspective of someone new to gluten-free living. She also suggested and created the wonderfully useful resource and reference list at the end of the book.

Kelly Brown curated and tested most of the recipe collection. Her experience as a food scientist and healthy home cook were invaluable. Jaylee Bastian, my on staff food scientist, ran tests of whole grain flour and formulated a very tasty whole grain flour blend.

Candace Rowley is the incredible designer whose artistic ability and book formatting skills transformed my manuscript into a beautiful and user-friendly book. Her beautiful design allows readers to fully access the information in easy-to-find and remember ways.

I also wish to thank Dave Cobia of Tree Street Grains who figured out the secrets of 100% whole grain gluten free flour then taught me. He shared his flour recipe and tips for milling gluten free grains. He also reviewed the whole grain and milling sections and gave valuable suggestions.

Last but not least, I wish to thank my husband, Mark Huffman, for his willingness to put up with my business and endless experimenting with love and encouragement.

CONTENTS

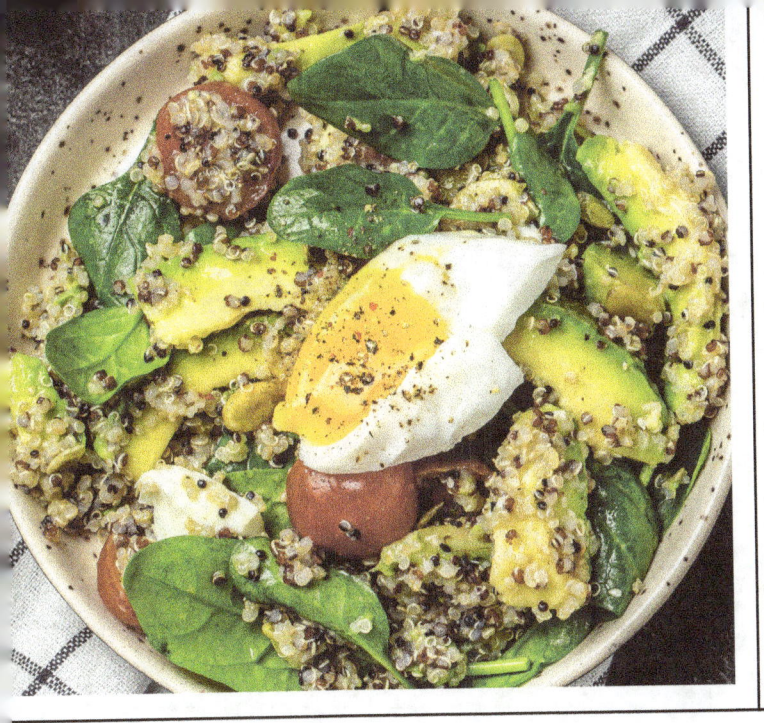

For **BEGINNERS**

1 FINDING RESOURCES

2 UNDERSTANDING FOOD LABELS

3 SHOPPING AND EATING STRATEGIES

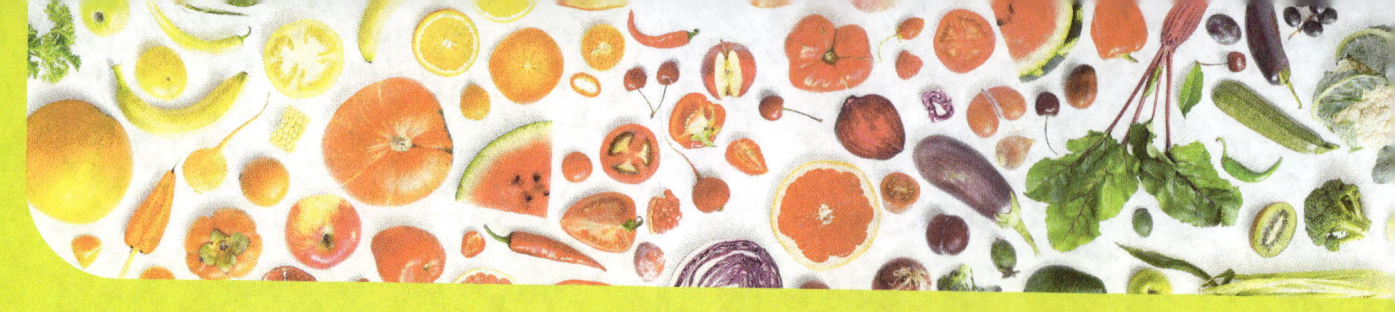

CHAPTER ONE
Finding RESOURCES

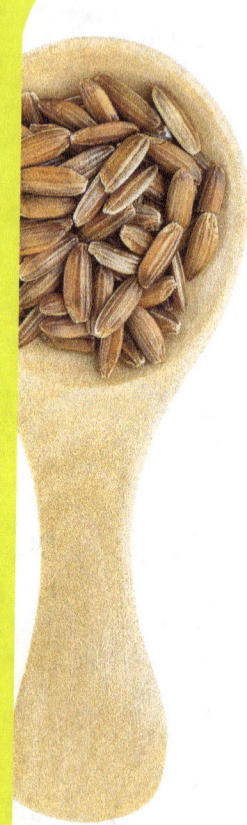

WHEN I FIRST TRIED GOING GLUTEN FREE, I FELT LIKE I WAS STARVING. Do you? I started cooking gluten free to help my friends and it grew into a gluten-free mix company. Several years into the business, I realized I didn't truly understand my customers' pain. I could already cook gluten free, but had never HAD to live that way. I went gluten and dairy free cold turkey on a Monday morning determined to not eat anything with gluten or dairy for one month. I made it, but it wasn't easy.

It was a drag to always wonder if I would be able to find something safe to eat. I underestimated the required planning to have the right ingredients on-hand, not to mention how many convenience foods wouldn't work anymore. Since I already knew how to read labels and cook gluten free, I thought I was ready, but breakfast the first day brought a big surprise. I think I ended up eating grits (very bland, no butter) and some fruit. I was hungry—a theme that continued for several weeks until I got the hang of it.

If you have just been diagnosed with gluten intolerance, allergy or celiac disease, you may have a lot of the same feelings. Don't worry! Things will get better as you find resources and practice living gluten free. Begin your new diet by consulting a registered dietician. A dietician can look at what you currently eat and assist in creating new food choices, suggestions, and resources of which you may not be aware. Each person requiring a gluten-free diet has unique needs that can be addressed explicitly with a dietician. She or he can suggest foods you may like based on what you are currently eating and help you find local resources.

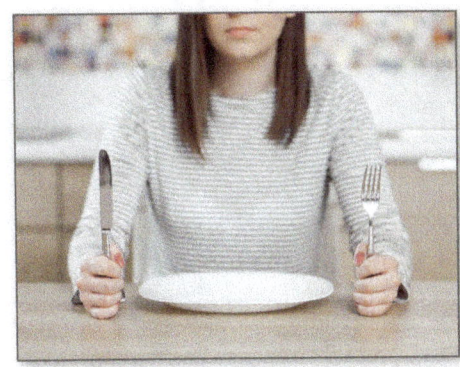

Find Your Tribe

Once you have consulted a dietician, the next step is to find people and organizations who understand what you are going through and can point you to the best local sources of help, education, and food. Join gluten-free Facebook groups in your state. Locals know where the safe restaurants are located, the best professional help can be found, and good gluten-free brands are sold. There might even be local groups that meet together! Some national groups like Gluten Intolerance Group have local chapters that can be found through their websites.

Transition Your Kitchen

Now that you are diagnosed, and have started your gluten-free learning, your kitchen will need a remodel. Not the kind we traditionally think of, rather a change of which foods are there and where they are kept and prepared. Setting up rules and zones can help you automatically avoid cross contamination.

The first step is to go through all the food in the kitchen and determine if it is gluten free. Use the guide in the following chapter to help read labels. Separate the gluten-free foods from the glutinous. Use colored stickers to indicate which foods are gluten free. Different colored stickers help the family in several ways. It is a no-nag approach to teaching the entire family to be conscious of foods that contain gluten, a simple way for young children to know what is safe for them to eat at a glance, and prevents accidental gluten exposure due to poor memory.

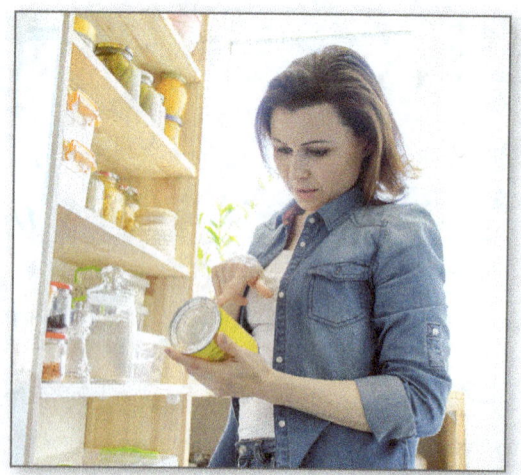

Next, decide where gluten-free foods will be kept and how the kitchen will be run. These decisions will be highly influenced by the ages of children, the percentage of family members needing to eat gluten free, and so forth. Is there a special cupboard that is strictly gluten free? Is the whole kitchen gluten free? Will the kitchen have a small area where gluten is allowed?

Some families choose to have the whole family go gluten free because it is easier to avoid cross contamination or because of an extreme sensitivity. Others designate gluten-free and glutenous zones. One family I know does a hybrid of a glutenous zone which allows bread and a separate toaster plus sandwich making ingredients in one area, but maintains a strict no wheat flour kitchen policy due to spreading dust. Try what you think will work best for your household and adjust as needed.

Empower Yourself with Knowledge

There is a lot to learn to navigate your new world. Fortunately, there is more easily-accessible, reliable information than ever before. Below are descriptions of some favorite organizations with loads of great information.

Beyond Celiac

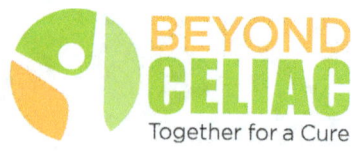

Mission Statement: Beyond Celiac unites with patients and partners to drive diagnosis, advance research and accelerate the discovery of new treatments and a cure.

This is our favorite celiac site because of its broad scope and scientific under-pinnings. The information presented is strongly research-based. It also covers pre-and post-diagnoses, cooking challenges, negotiating the social interactions surrounding food, how to shop, and a host of other topics.

Web: BeyondCeliac.org
Facebook: Facebook.com/beyondeliac
Twitter: @beyondceliac

Celiac Canada

Mission Statement: To provide information on sources of gluten-free food, to fos-ter research and to encourage mutual support among people with celiac disease. Today the association serves people with celiac disease, non-celiac gluten sen-sitivity, and dermatitis herpetiformis through affiliated chapters across Canada. The CCA is here to help individuals regain power over every aspect of their lives.

This is a reliable source of information and has lists of local support groups throughout Canada.

Web: www.Celiac.ca

Celiac Community Foundation of Northern California

Mission Statement: The Celiac Community Foundation of Northern California pro-vides evidence-based support to those with celiac disease and other gluten-relat-ed disorders. We carry out this mission by heightening awareness; educating the medical community, food purveyors and the general public; administering Camp Celiac; facilitating medical research; advocating on federal issues; and by offering group and individual support.

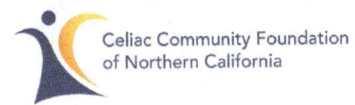

This site has good general information as well as strong regional resource listings.

Web: https://celiaccommunity.org/

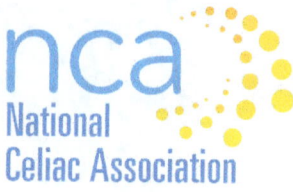

The National Celiac Association

Mission Statement: We educate, advocate and raise awareness of celiac disease and gluten intolerance. We foster a sense of community, belonging and camaraderie. We keep a close affiliation with a core of expert gastroenterologists and nutritionists.

Made up of six regions with chapters and resource units across the United States, this site helps find local support and information about programs for food assistance. It is also the sponsor of **Raising Our Celiac Kids group (R.O.C.K.).**

The R.O.C.K program provides education and support along with age-appropriate educational tools and advocacy training. Some features of the ROCK program include:

- Local support groups and meet-up events
- Phone helpline available each weekday
- A course for caregivers that explains celiac disease, the gluten-free diet and the gluten-free lifestyle in three easy steps (coming soon)
- A teen blog about living gluten free (coming soon)
- Downloadable educational materials for families and clinicians
- An educational website covering many relevant topics, including: managing at school, parties and holidays; finding gluten-free camps; and meeting challenges specific to dating and attending college

Web: https://nationalceliac.org/
Facebook: Facebook.com/nationalceliac

Gluten Intolerance Group of North America (GIG)

Mission Statement: Making life easier for everyone living gluten free is the mission of the Gluten Intolerance Group of North America.

The organization focuses on support groups, help for parents of gluten-free children, education for individuals, schools and the food industry, as well as certifications for food manufacturers and restaurants. GIG also has a great program for children which includes a magazine subscription called Generation GF and a mentoring program.

Web: https://gluten.org

For Generation GF

Web: https://gluten.org/community/kids/#:~:text=What%20is%20Generation%20GF%3F,your%20kids%20covered%20from%20A%2DZ!

Facebook: Facebook.com/glutenintolerancegroup

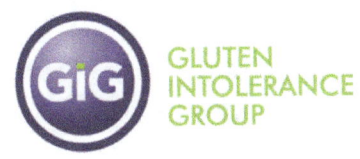

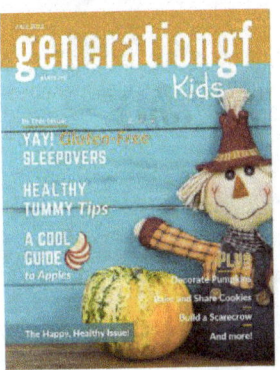
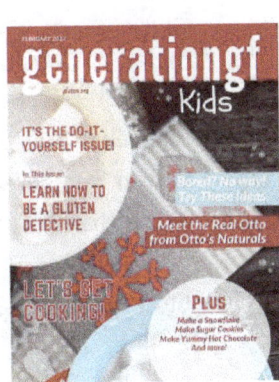
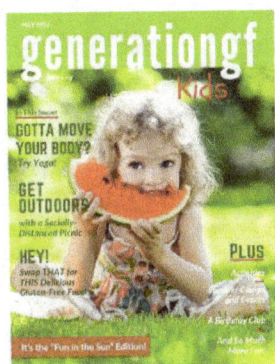

Other Helpful Resources

Below is a chart of our favorite gluten-free resources for everything from label reading apps to gluten-free communities and recipes. Complete web addresses are in our resource section.

Gluten-Free Support Groups	Beyond Celiac Canadian Celiac Association Celiac Disease Foundation National Celiac Foundation American Celiac Society
Gluten-Free Recipes	Gluten Free On a Shoestring Food Allergy Recipes from Spokin GFF Magazine Iowa Girl Eats GF Jules Gluten-Free Living
Gluten-Free Podcasts	The Gluten Free Baking Show The Celiac Project Podcast Gluten Free News Podcast A Canadian Celiac Podcast Oh Crumbs! Gluten Free You & Me
Gluten-Free Apps	Spoonful Find Me Gluten Free mySymptoms Food and Dairy Tracker
Gluten-Free Magazines	Simply Gluten Free Gluten Free Living GenerationGF

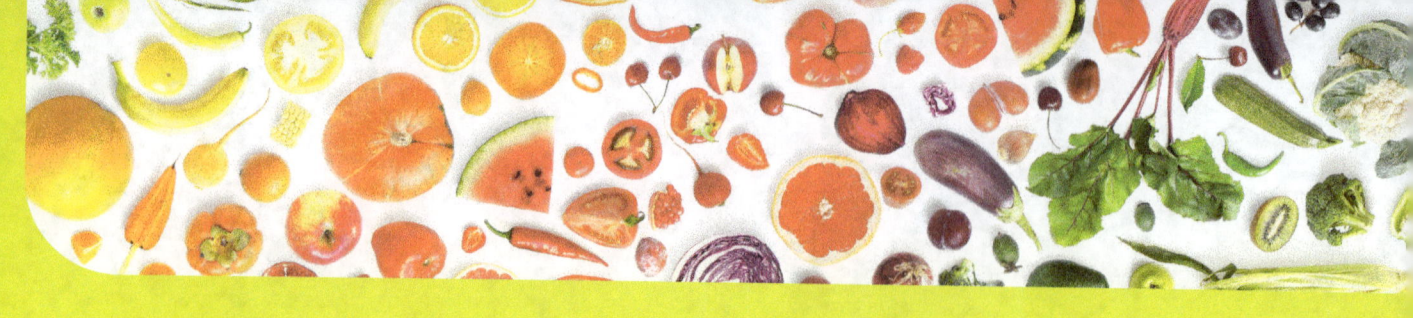

CHAPTER TWO
Understanding
FOOD LABELS

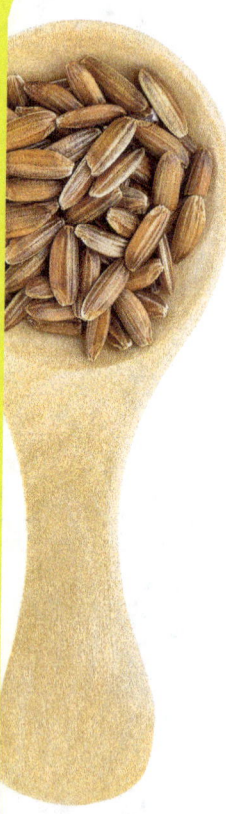

LABEL READING IS AN ESSENTIAL SKILL TO LIVING GLUTEN FREE, and the first one to learn and practice. Never just assume your food is gluten free. Some foods with gluten are surprising, like licorice and imitation crab. The following rules for determining gluten status from labels will give you the tools you need to confidently understand labels. Apps like The Gluten Free Scanner, Is That Gluten Free?, or Shopwell Diet Allergy Scanner can also help.

The Beginner's Guide to Reading Labels

Reading labels to determine if a food is gluten free can be overwhelming at first, especially if you do not know what to look for. To help, we put together some basic information about labels and spotting ingredients that contain gluten. With these skills, you will soon be reading labels like a pro!

Which Grains Naturally Contain Gluten?

Gluten is a protein found in wheat, barley, rye and triticale. Some mistakenly believe that Kamut, einkorn and spelt (varieties of wheat) are gluten free. Though they have reduced levels of gluten, they still contain gluten and are therefore unsafe for those with Celiac disease. Titicale is a cross of wheat and rye and is unsafe as well, fortunately it is rarely in foods.

Five Words to Look for on Labels

The words **wheat**, **barley**, **rye**, **malt** and **brewers yeast** will indicate 99% of gluten-containing products. If you see any of these words on a label, don't eat it.

Malt is the most challenging ingredient in this list. Malt is made from barley and may turn up on labels as **malt**, **malt flavoring**, **malt syrup**, and/or **malt vinegar**. Traditional vinegar is gluten free, but not malt vinegar. A good example of finding malt in unexpected places is in crispy rice cereal. This product seems like it should be gluten free, but some brands have gluten because malt is used as a flavoring ingredient.

Brewer's yeast is a byproduct of beer brewing and contains traces of barley. A few brands come from sugar beets or other sources and are specifically labeled as gluten free.

What about oats? Oats do not contain gluten, but they are often cross contaminated, so it is better to eat oats labeled as gluten free. A small percentage of celiacs cross react with a protein in oats called avenin. If you are reacting with certified gluten-free oats, also called "purity protocol oats," you may not tolerate avenin.

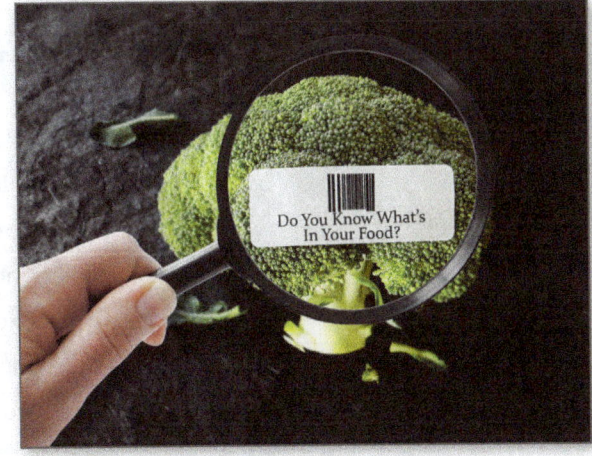

Do You Know What's In Your Food?

FDA Rules on Allergen Labeling

Ingredients: Creamer (sunflower oil, corn syrup solids, sodium caseinate, dipotassium phosphate, mono & triglycerides, sodium stearoyl laclate, algin) (milk) modifed food starch, white rice flour, natural and artificial flavor, chicken fat, salt, dried milk, corn flour, hydrolyzed corn protein (soy) silicon dioxide, sugar, onion powder, disodium inosinate & guanylate, & spice extracts. **Contains:** Milk and Soy.

The FDA requires that packaged food give allergen information for the nine major allergens which are: milk, egg, fish, crustacean shellfish, tree nuts, wheat, peanuts, sesame and soybeans. Beginning in 2023, sesame was added to the allergens required by law to be listed on labels. The presence of sulfites is required on the label if it is added as an ingredient as with dried fruit or naturally present in food at 10 ppm or more such as in wine.

The 9 major allergens may be called out in ingredient lists in several ways:

1. **If the allergen appears in the ingredient list itself, no additional notation is required.**

2. **If an ingredient contains the allergen but it is not named as such, the allergen can be placed in parentheses after the ingredient.** For instance, a list might say flour followed by (wheat).

3. **Allergens may also be listed in a "Contains" statement following the ingredient list with all the allergens listed.** Note that malt, rye, etc., which contain gluten, are not required to be in the contains statement so read the whole list of ingredients even if it has a contains statement.

What about Natural Flavors and Colors?

If a natural flavor or color contains any of the nine major allergens listed above it must be on the label in one of the forms described in the previous paragraph. Suppose you see nothing suspicious for gluten on the ingredient list, yet there is a "Contains" statement that lists wheat or other allergens. The allergen may be in the natural flavors or colors, but there is no need to worry if nothing is listed. The nine major allergens must be labeled in one of the above forms no matter which ingredient they are in.

Should I be Concerned about "May Contain" Statements?

"May Contain" statements on labels are a company's way to tell you that foods with allergens are handled in the same factory. Although those allergens are not ingredients in that particular food, they may be present as a cross contaminant. This type of statement is not required by the FDA, so you cannot assume that no cross contamination is possible if you don't see this mentioned on the label. Individual companies decide whether to include this information or not. Each consumer must make their own decision as to whether to eat food with a "May Contain" statement. Food companies make efforts to keep cross-contaminating allergens out—the risk is low, but still exists.

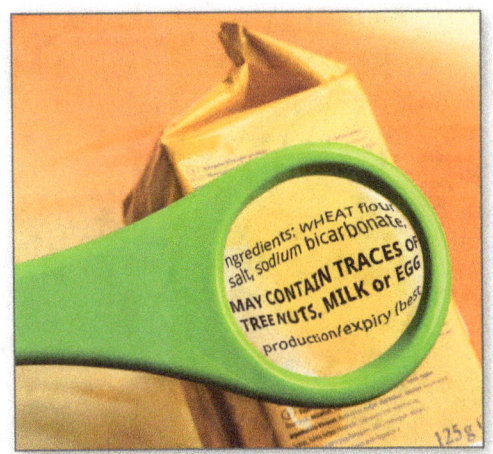

Ingredients that Confuse People

Even with the rules above there are often questions about several ingredients.

Maltodextrin is not a malt product and therefore not made from barley. Maltodextrin is starch, usually from corn that has been partially converted to sugars. It is free from gluten.

Caramel Color is often listed in older literature as possibly containing gluten. Modern caramel color is NOT made from wheat. Also, with changes made to food labeling laws, products must list any of the nine major allergens even if they are found in coloring agents.

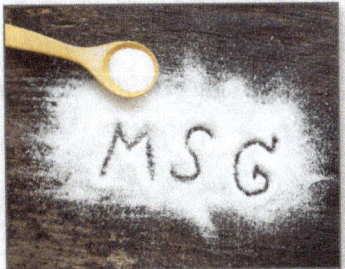

MSG or monosodium glutamate does not contain gluten. Glutamate sounds like gluten but is really an amino acid.

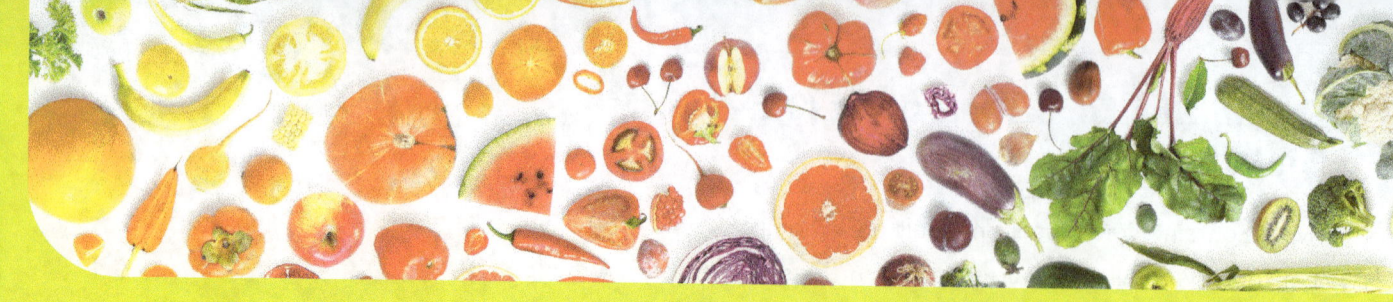

CHAPTER THREE
SHOPPING and
Eating Strategies

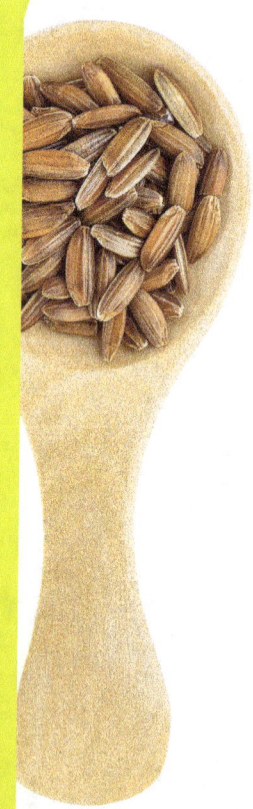

WHAT ARE YOU GOING TO EAT NOW? A new diagnosis thrusts you into the foreign world of gluten-free foods without speaking the language or knowing how to get around. Even the familiar grocery store seems foreign until you realize you understand more of the dialect than you thought. A conscious effort to notice how many things are not off-limits to you in your store is the first step to fluency.

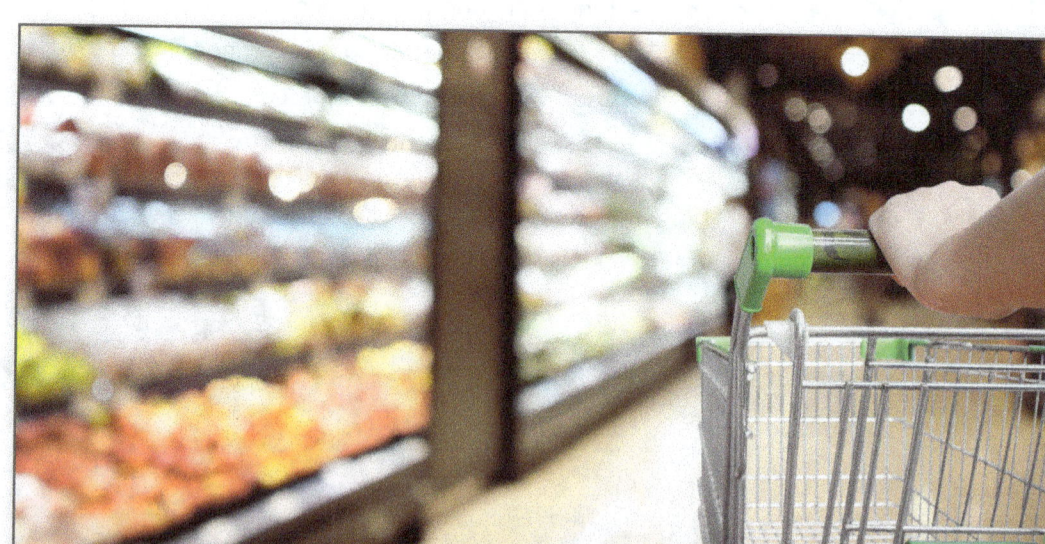

Many items you know and love are naturally gluten free, and the beautiful thing about these foods is that they are almost always cheaper than food designed as gluten free replacements for traditionally glutenous food.

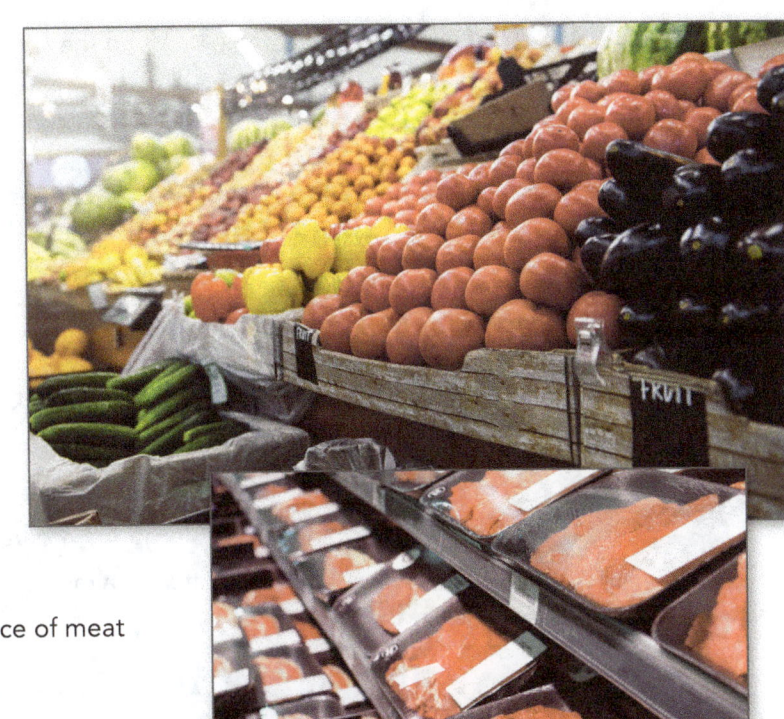

- You can eat any fresh produce or any plain canned or frozen fruit or vegetable
- You can eat nearly anything in the store section of bagged rice, beans, quinoa, and lentils
- You can eat any whole, unseasoned piece of meat without even reading a label

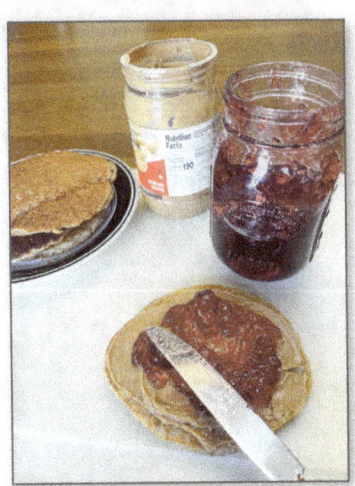

Notice how many of the naturally gluten-free foods are things you already knew you should be eating more of anyway!

Six Gluten-Free Eating Quick Start Ideas

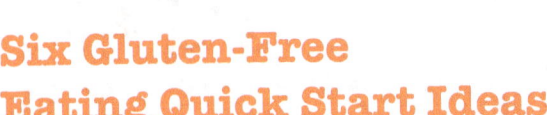

Here are a few gluten-free ideas that you can adopt quickly while you're learning the lifestyle. With any food you purchase, ALWAYS check the label to see the complete list of ingredients in addition to using the following suggestions.

Idea #1: Use Gluten-Free Pancakes Instead of Bread

For most, bread is a long quest, but delicious pancake mixes and recipes abound. Find one you like, let it cool after cooking, and use it for sandwiches—think of it as an Uncrustable®. Wrap the sandwich in plastic wrap, then place inside a sandwich zip bag and freeze. Put it in your lunch box in the morning and it's perfectly thawed by lunch.

Idea #2: Discover New Carbs

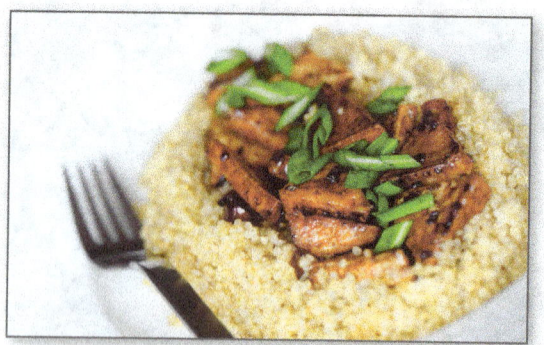

Add potatoes, rice, or quinoa for the carbohydrate portion of meals rather than bread, rolls, or pasta. They can be made into tasty side dishes like salads and pilafs, and you may be surprised how good your favorite sauces and gravies (remember to read labels) are on carbs other than pasta. If you just can't do without a roll, go for a gluten-free muffin. They are easy to make from scratch or a mix.

Idea #3: Eat Your Fruits and Vegetables!

Fruits and vegetables are naturally gluten free, fresh, frozen, or canned. The produce aisle can be your new gluten-free haven with a multitude of choices readily available.

Idea #4: Use Individual Herbs and Spices Instead of Blends

Individual spices, such as oregano, sage, and turmeric are all gluten free, but seasoning blends may not be. Fortunately, many spice companies have eliminated gluten, but read labels carefully and never assume. Gluten-free should not mean taste-free, so season to your heart's content. Don't be afraid to experiment with seasonings and try the combinations that appeal to you. Make sure to season little by little when making a new recipe, and taste frequently as you concoct your culinary creation.

Fresh herbs are always gluten free and taste better than dried herbs. Find them in the produce section or your store, local farmers markets, or grow them yourself.

Idea #5: Meat Lovers Rejoice

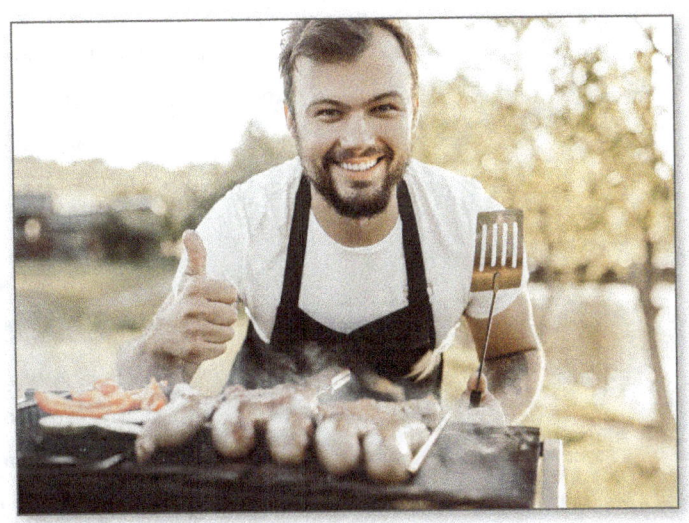

Unprocessed meat is gluten free and a good source of complete protein. Buying plain cuts of meat and cooking them yourself is always gluten free. Processed and pre-seasoned meat may contain gluten. Beware of included gravy packets and read labels on all processed meats carefully. From a nutrition and health perspective, meat should be eaten sparingly, but it is gluten free.

If you are vegetarian and eat meat substitutes you must be particularly vigilant reading labels. Seitan, or wheat meat, is made almost entirely of gluten.

Idea #6: Choose a Gluten-Free Dessert

Desserts can be a challenge, but you do have options. There are good pre-made gluten-free desserts which will be labeled as such. Also, pudding and ice cream are usually gluten free (read the label- obviously cookies and cream ice cream is not gluten free, but many flavors are). Fruit is naturally gluten free. Pies are a simple make-at-home dessert if you buy a gluten-free crust. You can make a greater variety of desserts as your gluten-free baking skills progress.

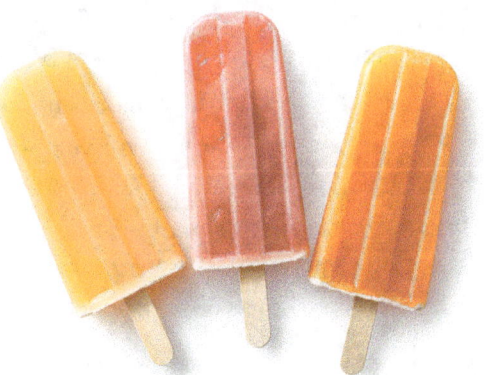

Where Can I Buy Gluten-Free Foods?

Many gluten-free foods can be found in places you already shop. Learn how the stores you frequent indicate these items. Some stores have a special section that features products unique to gluten-free living, usually items traditionally made of flour. Other retailers place gluten-free items among non-gluten-free foods in the same category and label them on the shelf. There are now chains that staff registered dieticians who know where foods for special diets are located throughout the store. Such programs are tremendously valuable while you learn. Ask at your local grocery store if they have such a program.

Traditional grocery stores tend to carry fewer gluten-free brands that have broad appeal and move quickly while specialty stores like Whole Foods, Trader Joes, and Natural Grocers have a larger selection.

Use the large and diverse selection of gluten-free products in online gluten-free stores or Amazon to discover what is available on the market. Save time when you aren't sure what you need by looking first at online shops. Usually, no one outlet has everything you need so you may end up using a patchwork of sources. Shopping online can eliminate this stress, but compare prices if the same product is available locally.

Online Gluten-Free Stores

The Gluten Free Mall specializes in offering new and unique items that you might not find at your local market or grocery. They have hundreds of brands and items to choose from, such as baking mixes, frozen meals, tasty snacks, and wholesome cereals. You can browse vitamins, personal care items, and household cleaners. All items on the site are guaranteed gluten free! https://glutenfreemall.com/

Gluten Free Palace (GFP) where their slogan is: "It's not about us; it's about you." GFP provides you with specialty gluten-free products. They regularly improve and update their product line to bring the finest-quality products at the lowest prices. https://www.glutenfreepalace.com/

Find Me Gluten Free is a popular app that provides a storefront for folks looking to shop for gluten-free food items. You can type in the brand you are looking to shop, and they will send you to their website to purchase from their company directly. https://www.findmeglutenfree.com/products/brands/shipping-now

The Gluten Free Shoppe has over 900 gluten-free items to choose from. The website is laid out in easy-to-find categories and includes many products that cater to other special diets like egg, nut, and soy free. https://theglutenfreeshoppe.com/

Sticker Shock

Gluten-free diets are notoriously expensive, but there are legitimate reasons why they are more costly. First, the market for gluten-free foods is much smaller. With only about 3% of the population eating a gluten-free diet, the consumer pool is small. As a result, sales volumes are low, and a higher price must be charged to make the product profitable.

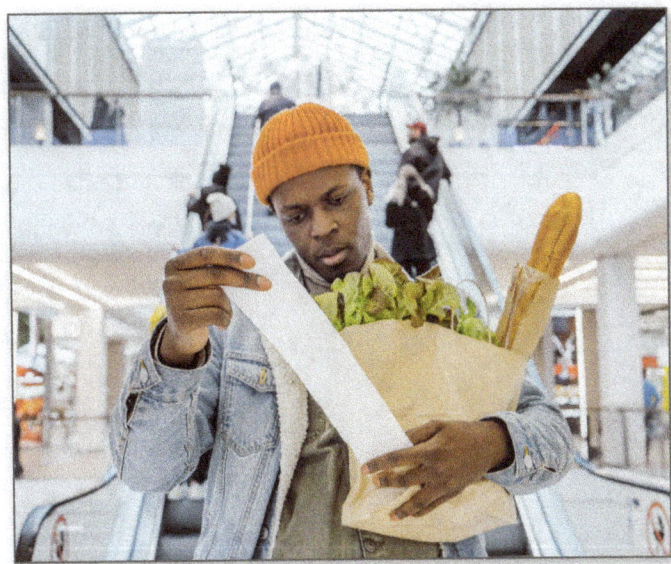

Secondly, more ingredients are needed to produce these foods. For instance, a combination of starches and gums is required to create gluten-free bread. In contrast, wheat bread has only three essential ingredients: wheat flour, water, and yeast.

Third, gluten-free ingredients cost more because they are not produced and priced as commodities like flour and sugar. Consider the difference between the cultivation and production of wheat flour and tapioca flour. Tapioca flour is a by-product of cassava flour production. This is a

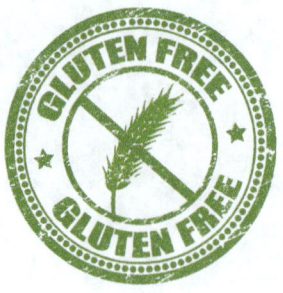

second manufacturing process with many labor intensive steps, making tapioca flour more expensive than wheat flour.

Fourth, avoiding cross-contamination requires special handling of ingredients and extra processing, which is more costly.

Fifth, gluten-free testing and certifications add an additional cost.

What is a budget-minded gluten-free person to do? Here are a few suggestions to eat gluten free without breaking the bank.

Economical Eating Tips at a Glance

- Learn when local stores run gluten-free promotions. Stores often run specials during May in honor of Celiac Awareness Month. Stock up on your favorite products during these times.
- Buy gluten-free ingredients such as flour in bulk. Bulk is often cheaper, but check per-unit costs to be sure.
- Use coupons. Coupons are a good way to try new products for less or save on products you purchase regularly. More on coupons below.
- Cook and bake more at home. See chapter 7: Five Strategies to Make Cooking Convenient.
- Grow your own garden or purchase fresh, local food from your neighborhood farmer's market.
- Change your diet focus to include more naturally gluten-free foods.

Using Coupons for Saving Money

You can easily find e-coupons or printable coupons either on your local supermarket's mobile app or online at the manufacturer's website. You can also find coupons on coupon code websites to get the best deals on the products and stores you like to shop.

Manufacturer's Coupons

As the name implies, manufacturers will create their own coupons for consumers. To use these coupons, go directly to the company website and search for coupons in their search bar. Some companies will have a tab for coupons, while others give you a coupon when signing up for their newsletter. Still other companies will have an email sign-up specifically for sending you deals. If you use a product consistently, this is a great way to save big on the items you buy for your daily needs.

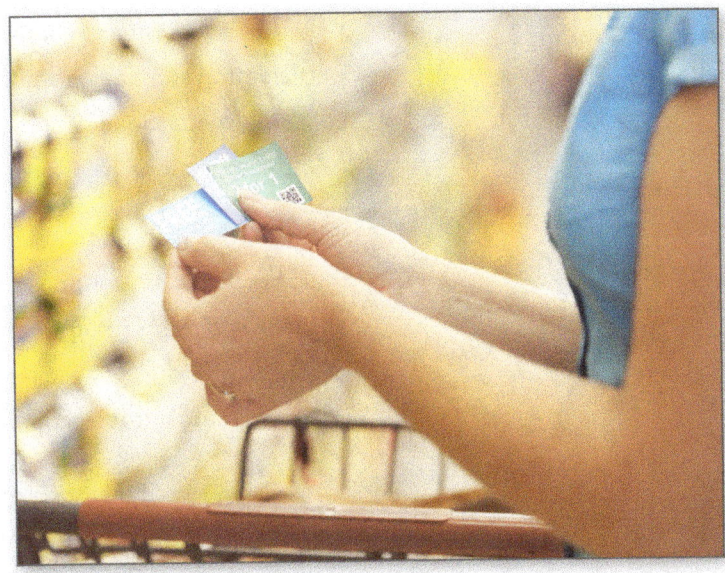

Coupon Websites

In addition to finding coupons on your favorite brand websites, you can find coupons on dedicated websites. There are also online tools to help you find specialty dietary items you may be looking for. The following are a few of the popular websites you can use to find discount codes for shopping online and e-coupons. Each company has its own redemption limitations. Make sure to read about the discount to understand how you can save money online before purchasing a product.

The Krazy Coupon Lady[1] is a searchable site that finds coupons based on brand or popular category. Some coupons require you to sign up on Ibotta, so be aware of what coupons you can download and which ones you can print without signing up.

Gluten Free Coupon Blog[2] by Jenny Finke from Good For You Gluten Free keeps her blog post "Where to Find Gluten-Free Coupons and Deals" updated regularly. You can find out what deals she has found by visiting her online. The website also contains other helpful gluten-free resources.

Coupon Birds[3] offers real-time coupons online. In addition to offering codes at participating stores, this website also shows online deals that are going on to save you even more money. Some companies will accept coupon codes in addition to sale prices, so look for those huge money-savers online!

Honey Gold[4] is an app or browser extension (Chrome or Firefox) that searches their database for coupons and online discounts for the store you are shopping and delivers them straight to your cart! Choose if you would like to get coupons, or if you would like the extension to find deals for you while you are shopping online. Create a free account through their website and start finding deals today.

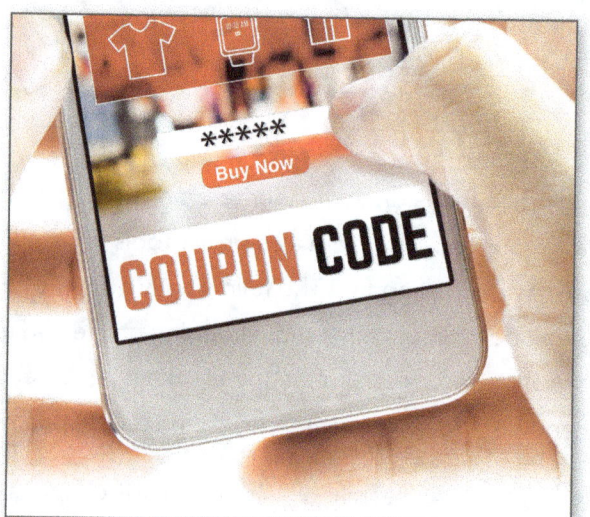

[1]The Krazy Coupon Lady. (n.d.). Retrieved May 3, 2023, from https://thekrazycouponlady.com

[2]Finke, J. (n.d.). Find Gluten-Free Coupons & Deals. Good For You Gluten Free. Retrieved May 3, 2023, from https://www.goodforyouglutenfree.com/find-gluten-free-coupons-deals/

[3]CouponBirds. (n.d.). Retrieved May 3, 2023, from https://www.couponbirds.com/

[4]Join Honey. (n.d.). Retrieved May 3, 2023, from https://www.joinhoney.com/

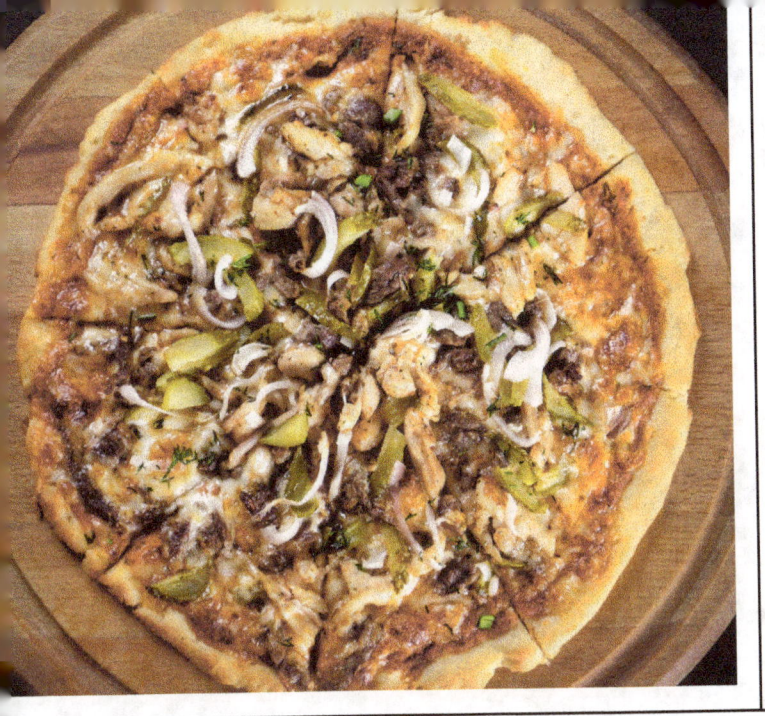

section

two

WHAT to Eat

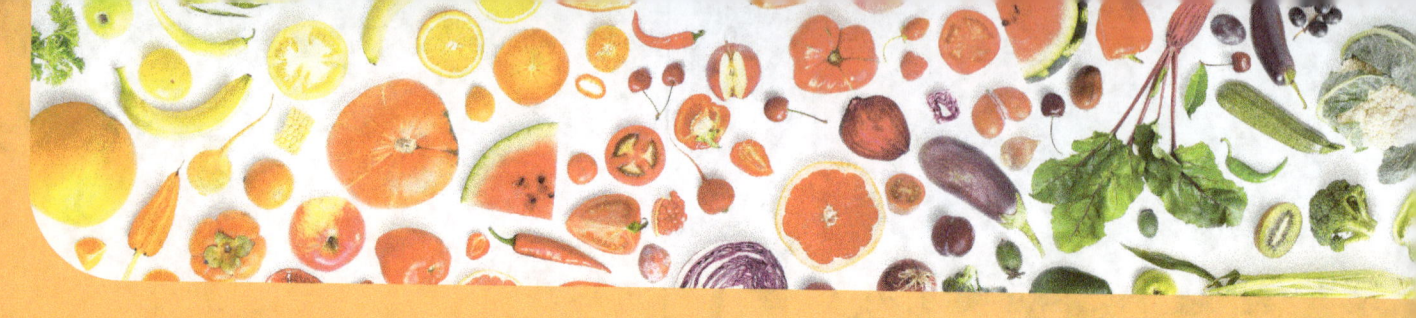

CHAPTER FOUR
Gluten Free Nutrition
MADE EASY

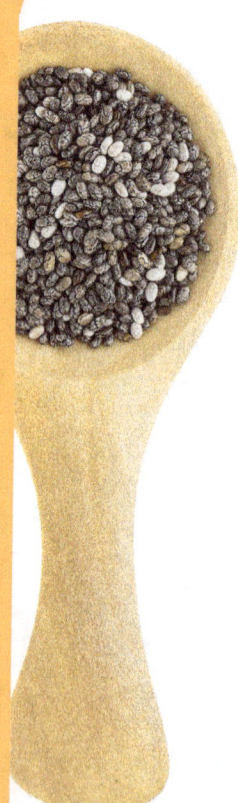

GOING GLUTEN FREE CHANGES YOUR LIFE IN AMAZING WAYS, some good and some bad. You probably feel much better without the assault on your body gluten has been inflicting, but there is more to feeling good than just avoiding the bad stuff. Nutrition has a powerful impact on energy, mental acuity, and overall well being. Many symptoms caused by gluten arise slowly over time, so you don't realize how awful you felt until things improve. This chapter is all about restoring nutritional health in easy ways.

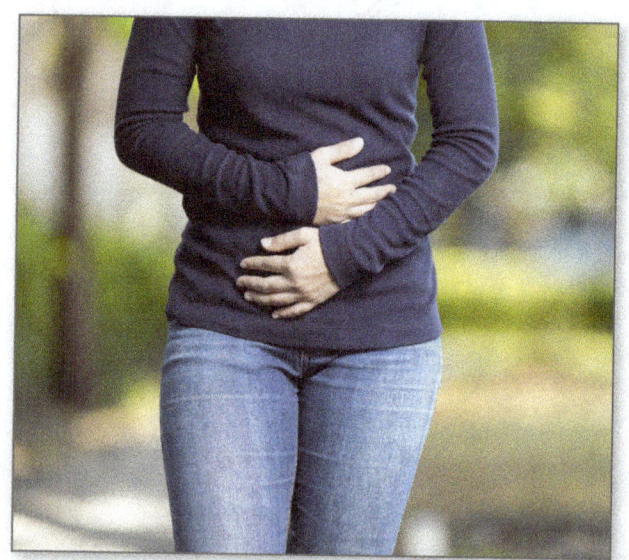

What You're Missing

Celiac disease causes autoimmune destruction of villi of the small intestines in the presence of gluten. Villi are small, fingerlike projections which manage the bulk of your nutrient absorption. As they flatten and decrease in number, you lose the ability to absorb nutrients. Deficiencies of iron, calcium, zinc, copper, and vitamin B12 are common among people who have lived with undiagnosed celiac disease. In fact, iron deficiency is the most common symptom driving the diagnosis of celiac disease in older patients.

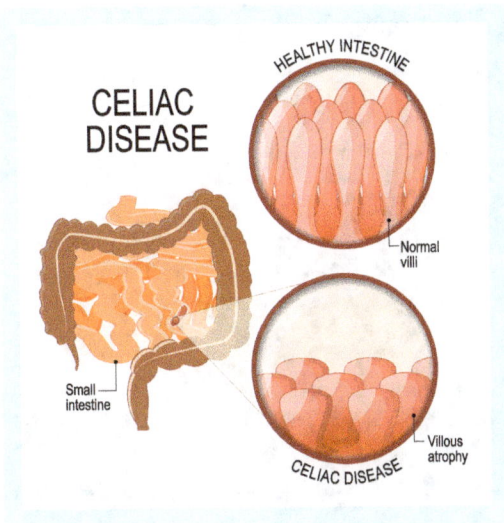

Taking a daily multivitamin will help restore the nutrients your body has been missing due to malabsorption. As your intestines heal over time, your body will begin to absorb more and more from the food you eat. How long this takes depends on severity and length of time damage has been occurring and the quality of your diet.

In addition to missing nutrients by not absorbing them, gluten-free diets are often limited in fiber and B vitamins because gluten-free flour is not typically enriched and most are not made from whole grains. In the late 1930s the government determined that people in America were suffering from nutrient deficiencies and encouraged food companies to enrich white flour and bread, pasta, and rice. White flour from wheat is currently enriched with iron and four B vitamins:

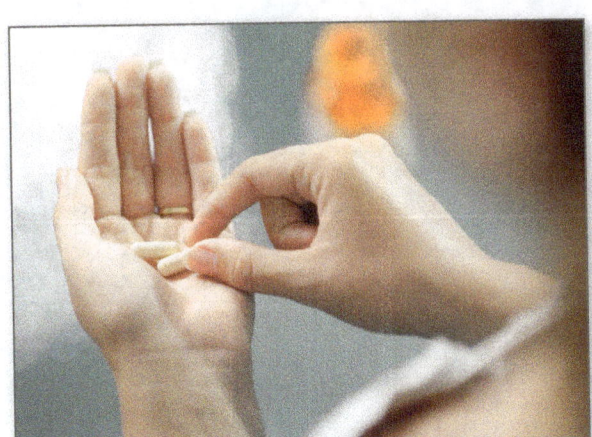

riboflavin, niacin, thiamine, and folate. The flour-based foods you ate prior to going gluten free contained these important B vitamins and iron through enrichment, but their gluten-free counterparts usually do not.

Restoring the Balance

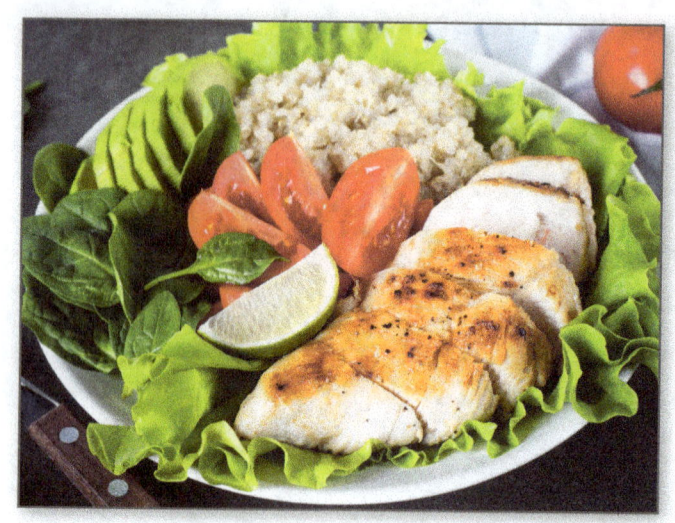

Returning to optimum health requires two things of your diet: removing gluten and eating well. If you already have a healthy diet, keep up the good work. If you know you should eat better but have not succeeded yet, here is an easy way to set things right.

Each day make sure you get **ONE** serving each of a whole grain, fruit, vegetable, and lean protein, along with 1 tsp of plant oils.

What?! One serving? That's all? Yes, focus on one serving a day.

Review your day's food as you approach dinner time. Are you missing one of the above categories in your daily menu? Make sure you pick up the missing category at dinner. No fruit so far? Add a banana or apple. No veggies? Add a salad. No protein? Add some meat, beans, or nuts to that salad. The plant oils are probably already in your ingredients or salad dressing.

What does one serving look like? Cup your hands together as if you're going to drink from your hands. One serving of most foods is what would fit in your cupped hands.

Easy! You've got this. By the way, it's ok if you get more than one serving of these great foods.

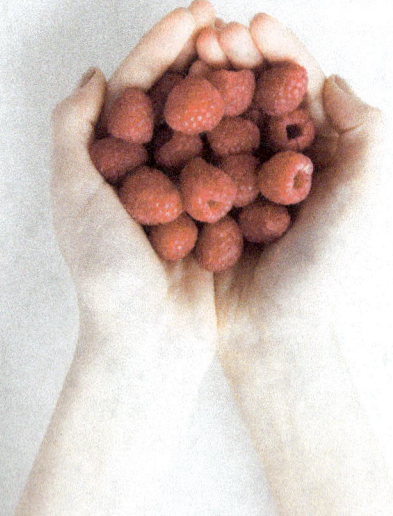

Power Foods for Gluten-Free Nutrition

Whole grains are a power food for anyone, but especially for people who don't eat gluten. Gluten-free grains include:

- Brown rice
- Corn
- Millet
- Quinoa
- Teff
- Buckwheat (no relation to wheat)
- Amaranth
- Sorghum
- Oats

Grains contain fiber, protein, B vitamins, and minerals—just what the doctor ordered! See chapter 5—Grains, Nuts and Seeds—for more information about each grain.

Beans and lentils are packed with protein, fiber, iron, phosphorus, potassium, complex carbohydrates, and B vitamins including folate. Beans have been shown to decrease appetite and lower insulin resistance. Along with amazing nutrition, beans are incredibly inexpensive. It is cheapest to cook your own, but even canned beans are inexpensive. Try sneaking beans into dishes you already make or experiment with new recipes made with beans.

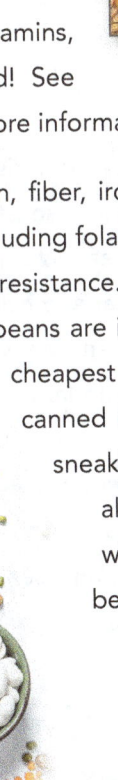

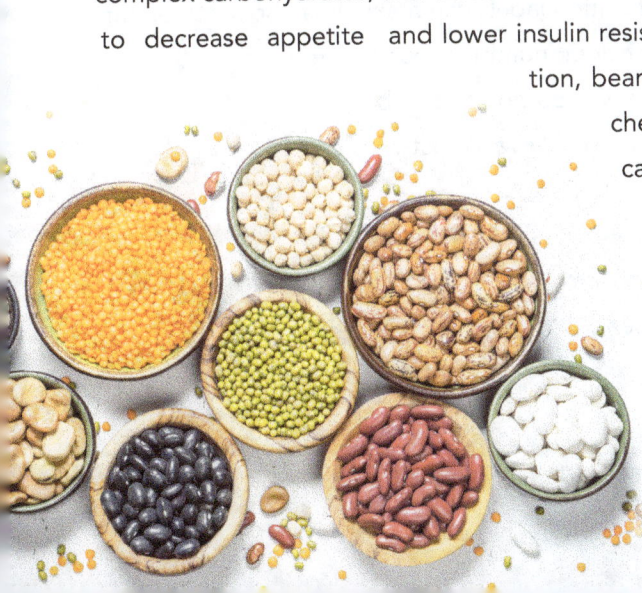

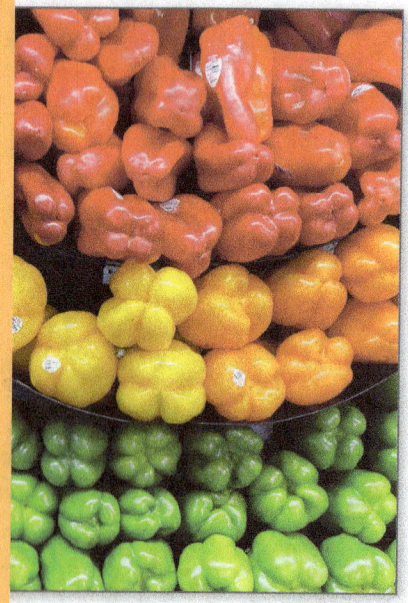

Fruits and Vegetables have been shown to have anti-inflammatory and antioxidant properties as well as high vitamin and mineral contents. They are nutrient-dense and calorie-light while still being filling. Eat to your heart's content! They are always gluten free and almost impossible to overdo.

It is hard to make general statements on the nutrient content of fruits and vegetables because of the broad range among different varieties. In addition to the vitamins and minerals we often think of as nutrients, plants also make phytochemicals which help plants protect themselves from bacteria, fungi, and predators. Some of these compounds turn out to be incredibly good for us, too, like carotenoids (carrots, squash) and anthocyanins (blueberries, purple cabbage) and are usually produced in the colorful parts of plants. You can maximize the benefit of your produce by adding a variety of different colors to your diet. Eat the rainbow and let your body reap the benefits of biodiversity.

Nuts & Seeds have been important in our diets since hunter gatherer times. Though each nut or seed has its own specific nutritional benefits, these foods contain heart healthy fats, protein, fiber, vitamins and minerals, and antioxidants. The evidence is so good that nuts are good for your heart that the FDA allows food producers to make health claims on packaging. The FDA allows the health claim "may reduce the risk of heart disease" for a 1.5 oz serving per day of nuts.

Nuts are especially hunger satisfying. A snack of nuts even reduces calorie intake at your subsequent meal. Nutrition labels can make nuts appear to be fattening because of the high fat and calorie numbers, but our bodies absorb the calories in nuts inefficiently. You don't absorb all the calories that are on the label. However, most of the calories in highly-processed nuts (like nut butters) can be absorbed easily because they are ground into highly digestible particle sizes. The moral of the nut and seed story is to eat a variety of types and eat them whole.

The Importance of Gluten-Free Snacks and Treats

Not all our needs surrounding food are physical. We also have emotional and social needs associated with eating. Removing gluten is a necessary part of your diet but not addressing the emotional functions of food increases the odds that you will cheat on being strictly gluten free.

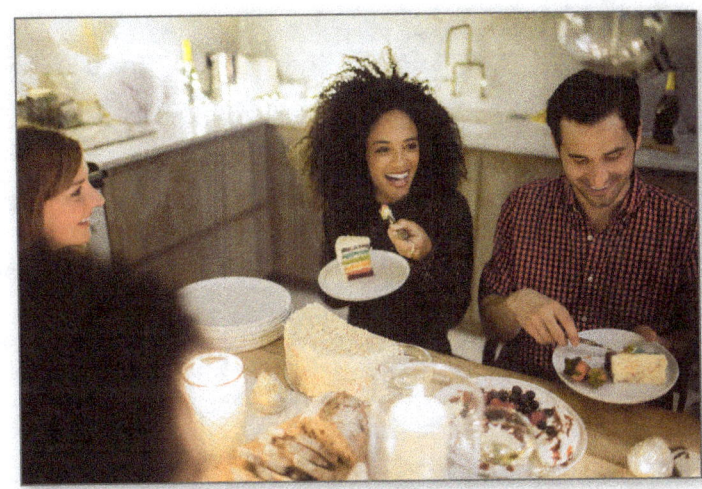

There is nothing like a satisfying dessert or treat to help you feel normal. Find several treats and snacks that really hit the spot for you like the gluten-free version of your former snacks and desserts and keep them on hand. I suggest not leaving these snacks in visible places so the gluten eaters in your house won't eat them. Also, you might be tempted to eat the whole package if you can always see them.

Safe snacks which are easy to take along with you are an important strategy for staying gluten free as well. This was brought home to me when a local college marketing class used my business for a project. One of the students assigned to work on my business had celiac disease. I asked her what she usually did for lunch, assuming she probably packed one. She replied, "Truthfully, I usually just get so hungry on campus that I break down and eat regular food." I was deeply troubled by her desperation and how much she was hurting herself. Avoid letting yourself get too hungry while away from home by putting safe snacks in your purse or backpack like nuts or dried fruit, just in case.

Why Gluten Free Can Lead to Weight Gain

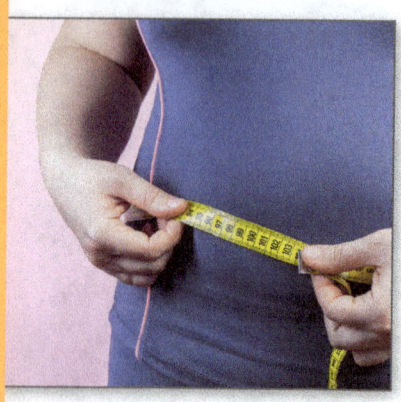

Damaged intestines are inefficient nutrient absorbers. Once your intestines start to heal on a gluten-free diet, you will absorb more of what you eat. You may be in the habit of eating a lot because you needed to previously. Another big factor is gluten-free baked goods are usually higher in carbs and fat to compensate for textural differences. Gluten-free diets are notoriously low in fiber as well. All these factors lead to weight gain. Here are a few hacks to help.

Eat a good breakfast. Your body burns more calories processing food in the morning so you net fewer. Breakfast is also the easiest meal to get a good dose of fiber with oatmeal, granola, cooked grain cereals, or whole grain gluten-free toast. You'll notice that you stay full longer and are more energetic throughout the day.

Make your biggest meal earlier in the day. Your body's ability to keep your blood sugar levels in proper balance, or glucose tolerance, decreases as the day goes on. Decreased glucose tolerance increases fat deposition. Dinner should be at least two and a half hours before you go to bed.

Increase your fiber/eat it first. Fiber has several powerful influences on appetite and calorie absorption. Fiber increases hormones that signal your body is full faster than other food components. Eat fruits, vegetables, beans, or whole grains and other fiber-rich food early in your meal to eat less overall. Fiber also traps fat and carbs and allows them to be absorbed more slowly.

Eat dessert and treats as part of a meal. Eating high-fat and high-carb foods as dessert at the end of a meal rather than by themselves as a snack lowers the blood sugar impact.

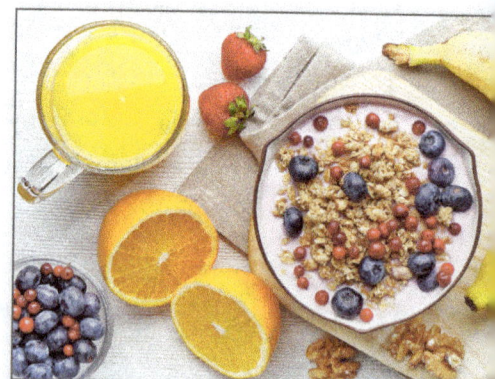

WHAT IS AN ESSENTIAL NUTRIENT?

An essential nutrient is one that is required for normal physiological functioning and growth, but cannot be produced by the body and must be consumed in the diet. These include nine amino acids, two fatty acids, thirteen vitamins, and fifteen minerals.

Essential Amino Acids

Our bodies produce all kinds of proteins to build, maintain, and run properly. They make our muscles, repair wounds, serve as messengers, store and transport nutrients, and function for immunity among other important functions. These amazing proteins are assembled from amino acids. The nine amino acids our bodies can't make in-house are histidine, isoleucine, leucine, lysine, methionine, phenylalanine, threonine, tryptophan, and valine. A complete protein is a single food source which contains all nine essential amino acids.

Essential Fatty Acids

Like proteins, fats or lipids in our bodies perform a host of necessary functions and fatty acids are the building blocks of these molecules. The two fatty acids our bodies can't manufacture are alpha-linolenic acid (an omega-3 fatty acid) and linoleic acid (an omega-6 fatty acid). The balance of omega-3 and omega-6 fatty acids strongly affects how well they function in our bodies. Standard diets usually contain too few omega-3s, so their presence is often called out on food and supplement packaging.

Vitamins

Vitamins are needed to make enzymes, regulate metabolism, and serve as antioxidants. The essential vitamins are: A, D, E, K, C, B. These are actually groups of related vitamins, but the only group we routinely see specified are vitamins in the B group: B1 (thiamine), B2 (riboflavin), B3 (niacin), B5 (pantothenic acid), B6 (pyridoxine), B7 (biotin), B9 (folate) and B12 (cobalamin).

Minerals

Different minerals are required to build structure, maintain acid base balance, regulate body systems, trigger nerve impulses and muscle contraction, and help release energy from food. The following are the essential minerals listed in order of decreasing recommended intake: potassium, chloride, sodium, calcium, phosphorus, magnesium, iron, zinc, manganese, copper, iodine, chromium, molybdenum, and selenium. Cobalt is part of vitamin B12 which is essential, so technically it belongs on the list of minerals too.

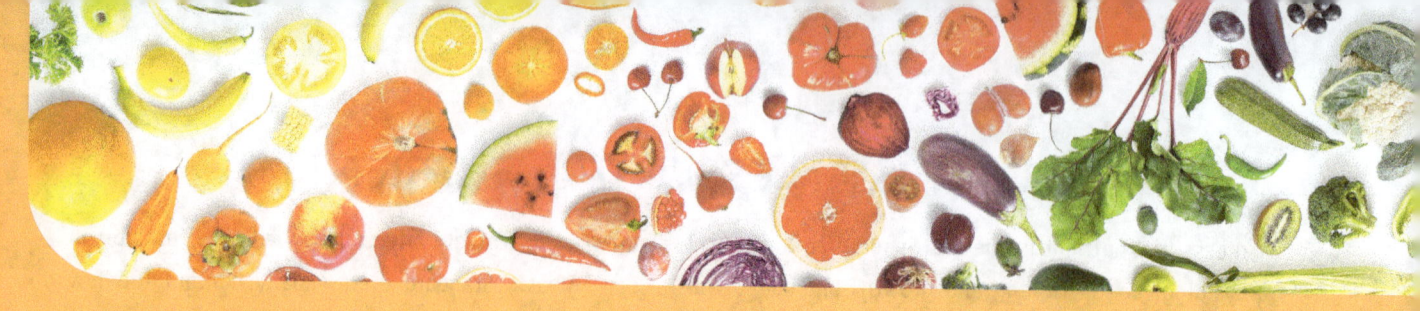

CHAPTER FIVE
GRAINS, NUTS and SEEDS

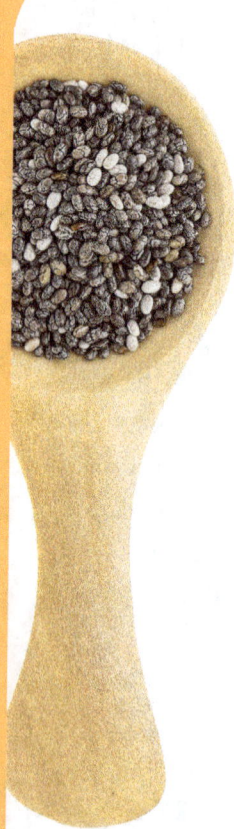

IF YOU ARE READING THIS BOOK to save money, eat better, or begin a gluten-free food storage program of your own, this chapter has the expanded information you need to dive deeper into adding power foods to your diet or home storage. The focus is on foods that are highly nutritious, inexpensive, and in most cases, storable. The emphasis on whole grains reflects my experimentation and study of food storage over the years. As you read this section, decide which of these great foods you want to experiment with. Then incorporate them into your life, diet, and storage.

Why Whole Grains?

A grain is considered "whole" if it contains all the parts of the grain (bran, endosperm, and germ). Grains that are not whole have one or more of these parts removed (usually the bran or germ), which removes fiber, healthy oils, and vitamins. Bran (the fibrous outer layer of the kernel), is the main difference in white flour and whole grain flour, and is removed because white flour makes lighter baked goods. The germ (the little bud in seeds that grows into a new plant) is often removed because it is high in oil which decreases the shelf life of flour. The removal of these elements benefits the seller or miller of the grain more than your nutrition.

There are two basic ways to use grains: cooked or ground into flour. Every grain can be cooked by boiling in water like rice. Once cooked it can be used in casseroles, soups, salads, and stir fries. Coarsely-ground grains can be cooked into porridge. You can grind your own grains to make flour or buy commercially ground gluten free grain flours for baking. Some grains can even be eaten raw like oatmeal in granola.

An easy way to start using whole grains is to buy one grain that sounds interesting and experiment. No special training or recipes are necessary. Simply add cooked grain to everything you already make, or in place of rice in recipes. Cook grains ahead and keep on hand in the fridge or freezer so they are easy to add to what you normally eat.

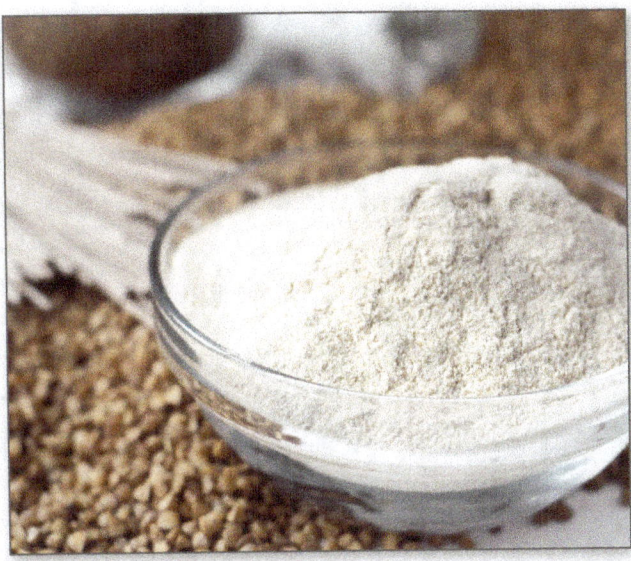

RICE GRAIN

Husk
Bran
White rice (Endosperm)
Germ (Embryo)

Gluten-Free Grains

Each grain contains a unique nutrient profile so eating a variety of grains is great for getting multiple nutrients your body requires. The following section is an introduction to gluten-free grains. Pick a few that sound interesting or are readily available and start experimenting.

Amaranth

The name Amaranth comes from the Greek word amarantos, or "one that does not wither," and is native to Peru. It is in the same family as pigweed and both seeds and leaves are edible. Though small, this grain is highly nutritious. Amaranth is very high in protein and is considered a complete protein. Uniquely, it is high in the amino acid lysine which is absent in most grains. It is also high in calcium, iron, magnesium, phosphorus and potassium.

Amaranth contains thickening properties, especially as a flour, and can be used to thicken soups, sauces and gravies. It can also be popped and used in salads as a crouton substitute, and in breads, cookies or snack bars. When boiled, it does not remain as single grains like rice, but rather forms a sweet, creamy, porridge-like consistency.

Amaranth's distinct and strong flavor is often described as sweet, earthy, grassy, or nutty, and should be combined with other grains for best flavor and performance in baked goods.

If you are milling amaranth into flour in a home mill, pour the grain in slowly while grinding so as not to plug the mill or blend it with other grains and mill the blend. Some mills are available with small grain hopper cups that slow the grain intake and automatically prevents plugging.

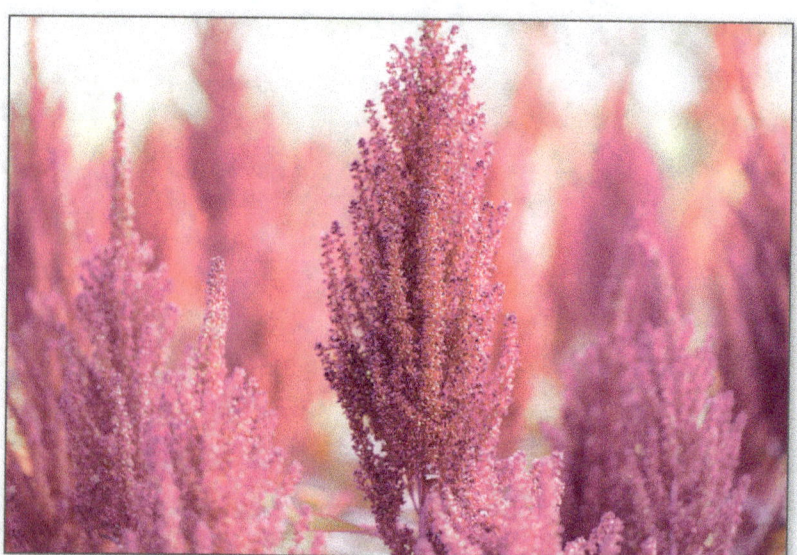

Amaranth flour is best used for baking at a 1:4 ratio with other flours because it performs better and imparts a milder flavor with other grains. Baked goods using 100% amaranth flour tend to be dense and gummy. Even the addition of 1 tbsp. of amaranth flour per cup of other grain flour yields better texture in gluten-free baked goods because the high protein content improves structure in baked goods.

Amaranth has a strong and distinct flavor which some love and others hate. I like it as porridge with butter and honey or sugar. It is slightly sweet on its own, but I prefer it a little sweeter. Its draw for me is it's a complete protein, and contains the amino acid lysine, which is an uncommon nutrient among grains. It is also good to add in low levels in baked goods to increase the structure. I keep some of this in food storage because it is so nutritious and good for flour, but I only keep small amounts I can rotate through because I don't like the flavor as it ages.

Amaranth leaves are also edible and the seeds can be sprouted and eaten as microgreens. Amaranth is in the pigweed family so some people who have seasonal allergies to pigweed will be allergic to amaranth grain. This also means that the leaves and seeds of the pigweed growing as a weed in your garden are edible and nutritious. When I heard this, I started chopping the leaves and adding them to main dishes instead of the spinach I usually sneak into food to nourish my family. No one noticed.

Storage: 2 years. Amaranth has a higher oil content than most grains so its shelf life is shorter.

Buckwheat

Native to Europe, buckwheat is not related to wheat in any way and is in the same plant family as rhubarb. The name is derived from the triangular shape of the seed, which resembles the larger seed of the beech tree, and therefore became "beech-wheat" or "buckwheat." It is a nutritional powerhouse because it is high in protein, zinc, copper, and manganese. Its high fiber content makes it a good choice for heart and bowel health. It contains all the essential amino acids, making it a complete protein. Buckwheat is also a low glycemic food (a measure of how much a food increases blood sugar levels).

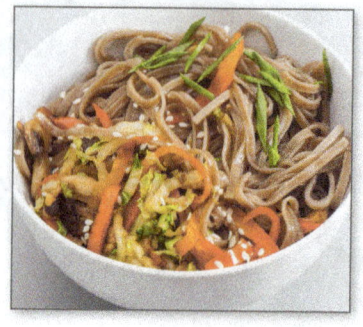

Buckwheat is familiar to many in pancakes, crepes, and Japanese soba noodles, but can also be used in breakfast cereals, stir-fries, risotto, breads, and muffins. Like oatmeal, it does not need to be cooked if soaked overnight, and makes a nutritious porridge the next day. Kasha is roasted buckwheat and is often served in breakfast cereals. Buckwheat can also be sprouted or ground into flour.

When used as flour, its high fiber content requires additional water or the dough will become gelatinous. Buckwheat flour performs well in quick breads and can replace up to 40% of the cornstarch in traditional gluten-free flours. It is often combined with other gluten-free flours for a milder flavor and improved texture of the final baked good.

When boiling buckwheat groats (whole kernel grain), care must be taken to keep them from breaking down into a mushy paste. This can be done by adding the appropriate amount of water, bringing it to a boil, then covering the pan and reducing the heat to a simmer. For salads, cook for 10 minutes. For fluffy grains, cook for 15 minutes. Remove from heat and drain any remaining water.

I have only recently begun to pay much attention to buckwheat. I definitely recommend playing around with it because it is nutritious and very versatile. My new way to eat buckwheat is to cook it like rice and add it to a stir fry. It is also a good addition to granola. Our recipe section features a very good buckwheat

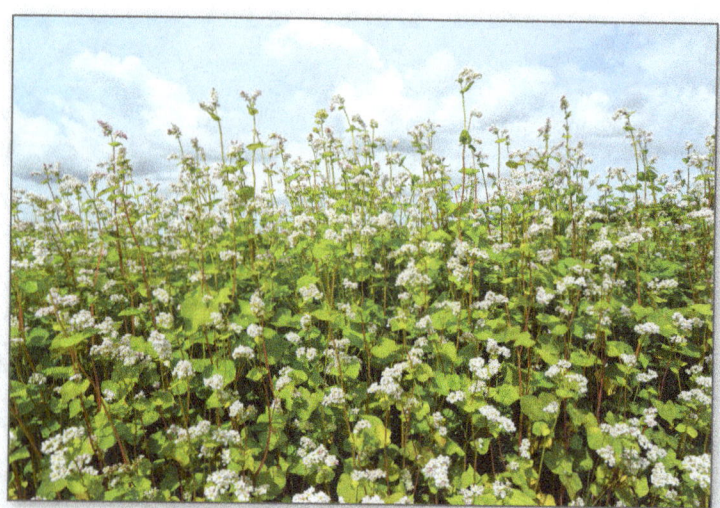

granola recipe (page 172-173). In low levels it adds a nice flavor and improves performance of gluten-free flour. The high fiber and quality protein make this worth storing and eating.

Storage: 2 years. I have stored buckwheat for up to six years under optimal storage conditions. I was surprised it was still good when I opened it. However, once opened, it began to age more quickly than I expected. This phenomenon is common in food that is stored well. Good storage slows the process, but the seeds are still old.

Millet

Although mostly used in birdseed in the U.S., millet is the 6th most important grain in the world, sustaining lives on one-third of the planet. This grain is drought tolerant, matures quickly, and will grow in many climates which explains why it is one of the oldest grains cultivated for human consumption. It is easy to digest and is one of the least allergenic grains.

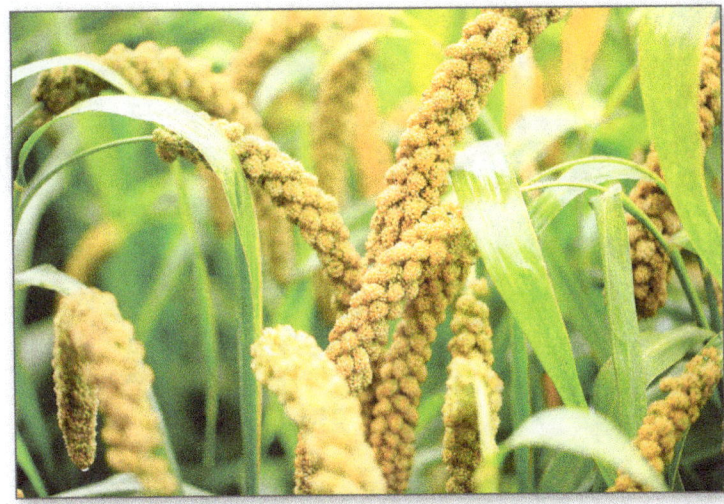

Millet has a mild corn-like flavor and can be cooked using varied amounts of water or ground for the following textures:

1. Crunchy for texture appeal in salads or other recipes when cooked with less water

2. Soft and fluffy like rice when cooked with more water

3. Ground then cooked as creamy porridge

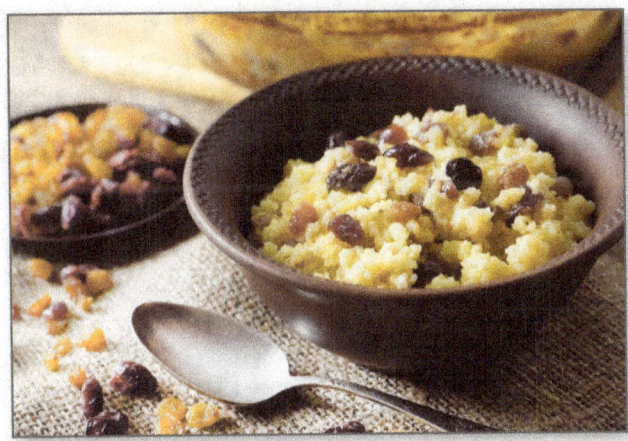

Cooked millet makes a delicious breakfast cereal in either whole or ground forms. For baked goods, millet flour is most often mixed with other grains, but can be used alone for quick breads like muffins and pancakes. Millet is recommended to be used in gluten-free flour blends at 30% or less of the total flour.

Toasting before grinding or cooking releases and deepens the flavor of the grain and eliminates the hint of bitterness sometimes found in millet. It is a good source of fiber, protein, and manganese, and is even more nutritious when sprouted.

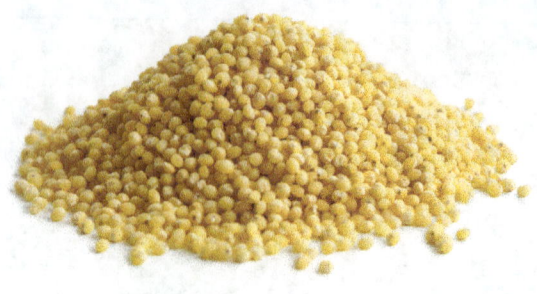

My favorite way to eat this is in place of rice or with butter and salt for breakfast. It's also a nice addition to flour blends, especially for cakes. It produces a lighter crumb.

Millet is a small grain, so if you are milling your own flour, pour it in a little at a time to avoid mill plugging or mix it with other grains.

Storage: 2-5 years.

Rice

Rice cultivation began 4,000 years ago in China. It has since spread throughout the world and is cultivated on every continent except Antarctica. Although white and brown rice are most familiar, many other colors are available. Each color possesses a slightly different nutritional profile.

When rice is harvested, the indigestible outer hull is removed and the whole grain rice is ready to cook and eat. Further milling removes the bran and germ layers and yields white rice. Since the oils and vitamins of the rice kernel are found in the bran layer, white rice has significantly lower nutritional value than brown or whole grain rice. Most white rice in the U.S. is fortified because so many of the B vitamins are lost in the additional milling. Brown and other colored rice become rancid more quickly and have a much shorter shelf life (only 6 to 12 months) than white rice and other grains. Fortified white rice does not become rancid as quickly, but loses most of its added vitamin potency after a year. It is also possible to wash off the fortifying vitamins if white rice is rinsed prior to cooking.

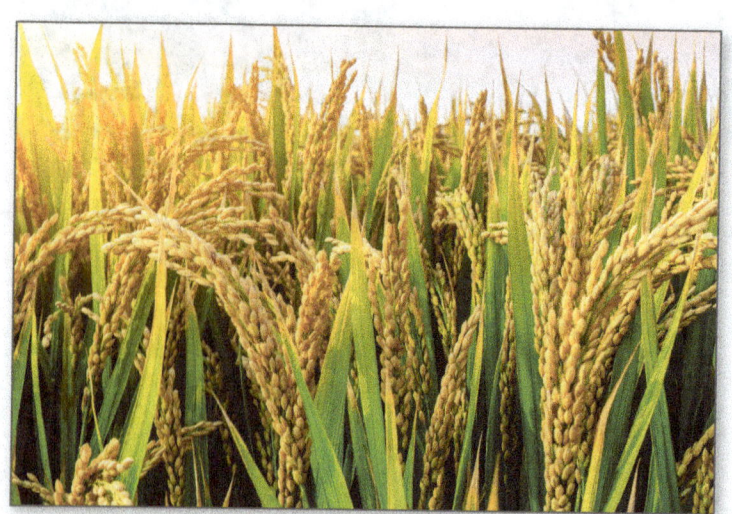

Brown rice has a much lower glycemic index than white rice which means it gives a slower insulin and blood sugar level spike than white rice. Brown rice is high in magnesium and B vitamins.

Rice is described by the length of its kernel: short, medium, or long grain. As the length of the kernel decreases, the starch increases. Short grain rice sticks together when cooked and is sometimes referred to as "sticky rice." If you are milling your own rice flour, it is best to use long and medium grain rice. Some gluten-free flours call for a small percentage of sweet rice flour which is made from very short grain rice like arborio. Sweet rice flour increases the starch content of the flour and improves texture, but will not perform well if used as the only grain in the flour. Short grain rice can be a good inclusion in long term storage if you plan to mill your own flour. It can be used in place of or in addition to refined starches to improve texture of baked goods.

Rice has the ability to take up arsenic while growing depending on the location and conditions during growth. The amount of arsenic most people ingest is not harmful. However, populations whose diets include a high proportion of rice, like people who eat gluten free, may be affected. The arsenic level in rice can be reduced by soaking and rinsing prior to cooking, or cooking like pasta with extra water, then draining prior to serving. Increasing the variety of grains you eat regularly will also lessen your exposure.

Storage: Colored rice 6-12 months. With excellent storage conditions you can stretch this time up to 18-24 months. If stored rice becomes rancid, and you still want or need to eat it, soak and rinse well before cooking and it will not taste rancid. Another hack is to add vinegar to the cooking water. When my neighbor first told me I could rescue my rancid brown rice, I was skeptical. Being the experimenter I am, I decided to put her folk wisdom to the test on some very old, very rancid brown rice from my storage room. I didn't tell my family about the experiment, and none of us could taste rancidity at all.

White rice, stored very well, can last 30 years. This shelf life was tested after being stored in #10 cans with low oxygen for 30 years in cool conditions. Though it had lost some of its nutritional value and did not taste as good as fresh, test subjects thought it was acceptable. This means that as a preparedness food, it is very good. Fortified white rice in consumer packaging maintains its added vitamin level for 1 year and loses most of the added vitamin potency by 3 years. White rice gets a bad name sometimes because it has a lot of calories, but in starvation conditions, that is critical. It is also cheap and easy to acquire.

Wild Rice

Wild rice is not rice at all, but rather a water grass that grows in small lakes or slow moving rivers. Rice is of the genus Oryza and wild rice is of the genus Zizania. Wild Rice is native to Connecticut waterways, with one variety from Texas. Wild rice is one of two grains native to North America and was called manoomin, or harvest berry, by Native Americans. Harvesting was done in a canoe with one person steering and another bending the grass over the canoe and beating it to knock the

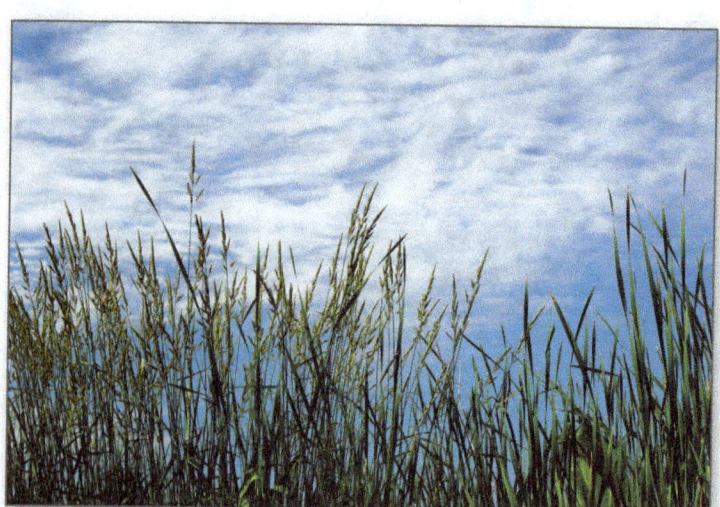

heads into the canoe. You can still purchase wild rice harvested this way but most is grown commercially in paddy fields.

Wild rice kernels are longer and thinner than rice and are a deep brown roasted color. It has a strong, rich, earthy flavor and is usually paired with meats or used in blends of different rices. This is an extremely fun grain to experiment adding to dishes. It retains more texture than rice and can change the flavor and texture of dishes in fun, delicious ways. It is cooked like rice but needs more water: 3 cups of water for every 1 cup of grain.

Wild rice is low in calories, high in fiber and has the 2nd highest grain protein content (oats are 1st) per 100 calories of all the grains. Like amaranth, it is high in lysine which is often the protein building limiting amino acid in vegan diets. It is also high in manganese, phosphorus, potassium and the B vitamins B6, niacin and folate.

Storage: Indefinite, or so says the Canoe® brand wild rice company because it contains almost no oil and is very dry. It is safe to assume that it can store a very long time. I have stored it with no noticeable changes for three years and counting. Also because of its low oil content it is less sensitive to higher storage temperatures than grains with higher oil contents. High nutrition and good storability are practical reasons to begin cooking and storing wild rice.

Sorghum

Sorghum, also called milo, is one of the top five cereal grains in the world because it is resistant to heat, drought, and insects. The most common varieties are red and white. In the U.S. it is primarily used in bird seed and animal feed, but is growing in popularity for human consumption. It can be cooked and used like rice or in salads, ground into flour for baked goods or thickening agents, popped, or served as a breakfast porridge. Though I don't pop sorghum regularly, I like it this way. It has good flavor, and is a crunchy, fun alternative to popcorn.

Sorghum is rich in complex carbohydrates, which gives it a lower glycemic index and keeps you feeling full longer. This grain is high in fiber and protein and contains both omega 3 and 6 oils. Though not a complete protein, the only missing

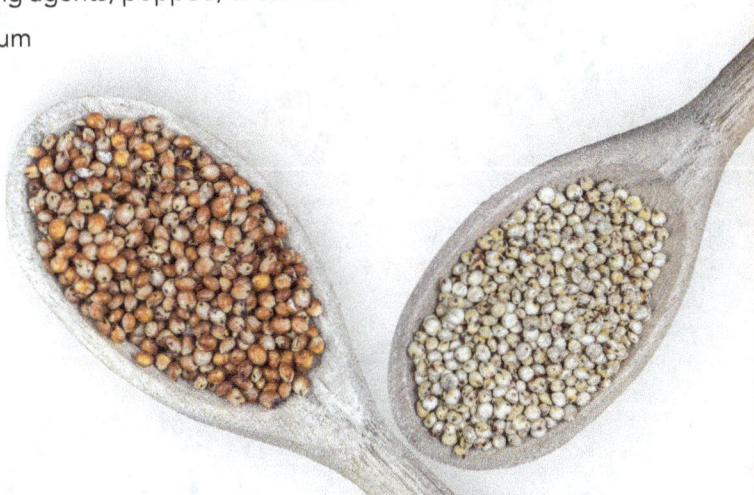

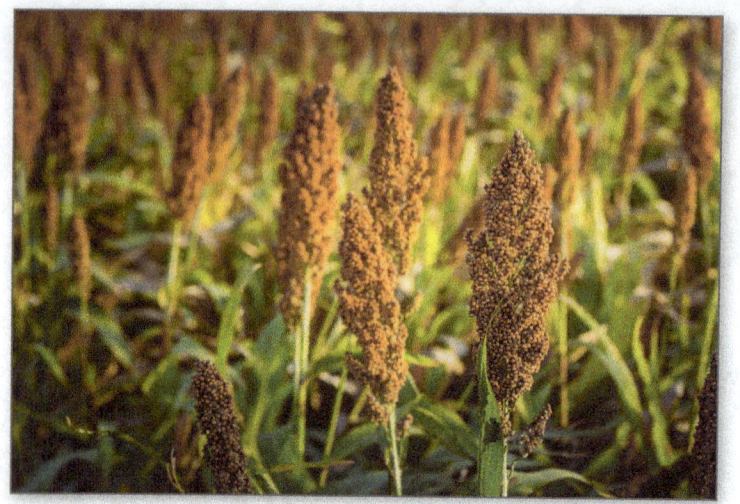

amino acid is lysine so it is good to pair with foods high in lysine like amaranth, mushrooms, cheese, eggs, and legumes. It also contains B vitamins and calcium, phosphorus, and potassium.

The boiling time and water to cook sorghum is longer than other grains and it retains a pleasant chewy texture that complements salads and stir fries especially well. It can be used alone for baking, but like other gluten-free flours, it is best when combined with other grain flours.

Sorghum and teff are tied for my favorite gluten-free grain. Sorghum's flavor is the most wheat-like of all the gluten-free grains. Yummy! It tastes even more wheat-like in flour when paired with teff flour. It makes a good replacement for pasta in salads. Toss cooked sorghum with fresh vegetables and add your favorite salad dressing for an easy delicious salad.

It is hard to get a smooth, fine flour when milling sorghum in a home grain mill. If you are planning to mill sorghum, experiment with it to see if you like the texture before you buy a lot of it. Some love the hardiness of a coarser flour, and some don't. I reached out to my sorghum supplier, Nu Life Market, for hints for the home sorghum miller. They explained that it is hard even with commercial mills to get a fine grind, and they must use multiple mill settings to produce their flour.

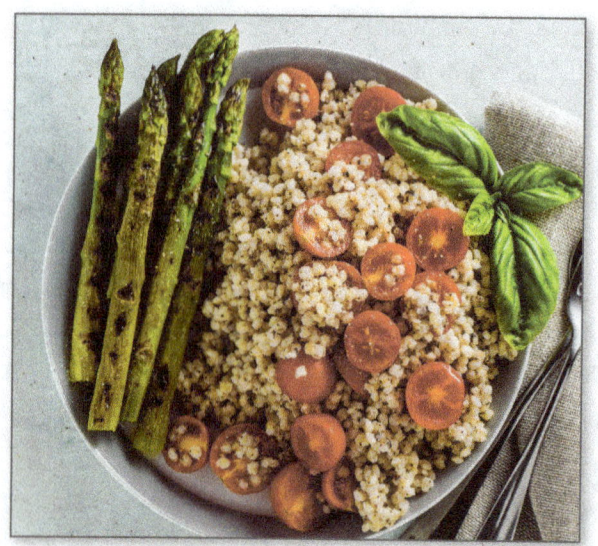

Storage: 2 years stored at room temperature in consumer packaging. In low oxygen, cool, dry conditions you can expect up to 10 years. I have stored sorghum for up to 10 years with very little change in taste or performance. If you like this grain, it fits well in long-term food storage programs.

Quinoa

Quinoa is an amazingly nutritious grain which can be added to your diet with very little effort. Native to the Andes, quinoa grows well in adverse conditions such as drought and poor soil quality. The plant produces a saponin (a soap-like compound) which functions as a natural insecticide making it pest resistant. It also has a long shelf life.

White quinoa is widely available, but red and black varieties can also be purchased. The colored varieties have a stronger flavor and have more texture when cooked. Quinoa contains all nine essential amino acids; as well as being high in the minerals iron, phosphorus, magnesium, calcium, and potassium; and vitamins E, riboflavin, and folate. Unlike wheat flour, gluten-free flours are not fortified with folate. Therefore, it is important to include folate-rich foods like quinoa in any gluten-free diet. Folate is essential for normal cell development, and deficiencies during pregnancy can cause spina bifida and other neural tube defects.

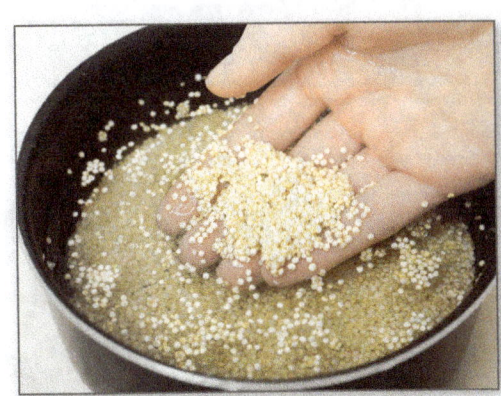

If you are new to whole grains, quinoa is one of the easiest to start adding into your diet. It is cooked just like rice with the same methods and proportions of water. It is also readily available in grocery stores. Though more expensive than rice, it is much more nutritious. Like all whole grains, it keeps you full and satisfied much longer than refined forms of grains.

Some quinoa comes pre-rinsed to remove the bitter saponin. If it is not labeled as pre-rinsed you need to rinse it prior to cooking. The rinse water will look slightly soapy. I like to either soak quinoa in water with 1 tablespoon of vinegar for a few minutes before rinsing or add 1-2 teaspoons of vinegar to cooking water. I stumbled upon this trick because quinoa can have a hint of bitterness. My thought was that since basic (opposite of acidic) flavors are bitter, I could counteract this effect with an acid, in this case, vinegar. It worked! In this same phase of experimenting I tried an 1/8 to 1/4 teaspoon of instant coffee in the cooking water. Another fun flavor

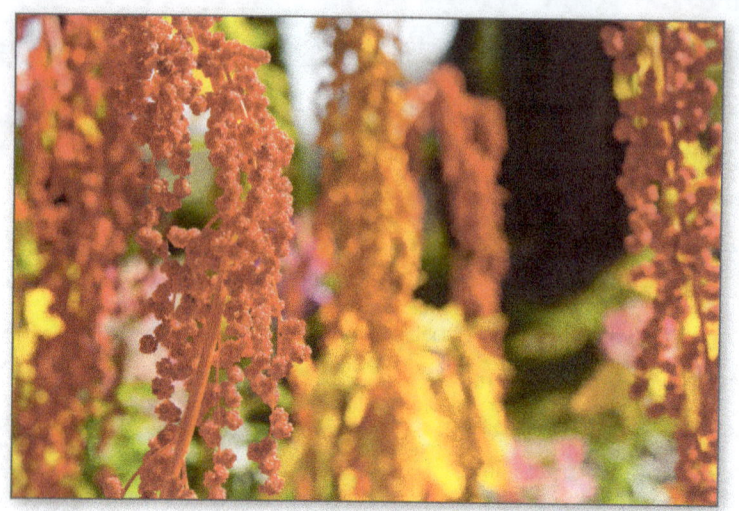

hack is to add a pleasant bitter flavor, for instance coffee, to something with an unpleasant bitter flavor. You don't notice the unwanted bitterness as much. The result of this experiment was to make the bitterness go away and make the quinoa taste roasted. Some of the people I tested this on really loved it.

My family eats quinoa primarily in place of rice. I also keep cooked quinoa in the fridge or freezer to sneak into other dishes to add nutrition and boost protein. One of my sons adds cooked quinoa to his quesadillas to make them more filling. Quinoa flour performs well, but tastes terrible. It enhances texture but should only be used in small percentages in flour blends if you want your creation to taste good.

Storage: 2 years in room temperatures or 5 in better conditions. With very good storage it will last 10.

Oats

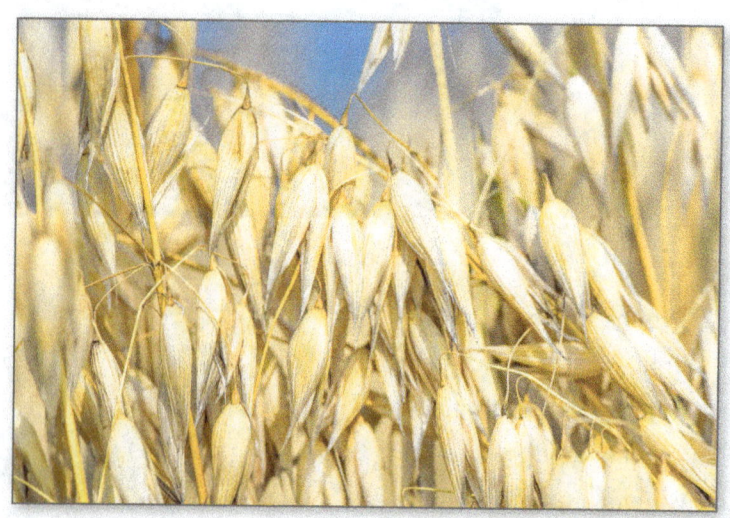

Oats are a very familiar whole grain. Oats are known for heart healthy beta-glucan fiber, complex carbohydrates, and protein. Beta glucans reduce cholesterol levels and are believed to reduce blood sugar after a carb-rich meal. Oats have been shown to help with weight loss because they digest slowly and increase satiety. They can be purchased as groats, steel cut, flour, and quick and regular rolled oats.

Oat bran, the most fiber-rich part of the kernel, can also be purchased and added to recipes, cereals, and smoothies to increase fiber content, although this is not a whole grain.

Oat Groats

A groat is any grain that has only the outer hull removed. Whole kernel oats are available, but less common than the other forms. Oats contain more fat than other grains, which is distributed throughout the groat rather than being concentrated in the germ. Most oats destined for human consumption are steam processed to reduce the enzymes which oxidize fat and turn it rancid. Groats are not steam treated, so they are especially prone to this oxidation and do not store well for long periods unlike oatmeal which has been steam treated and can last decades with proper storage.

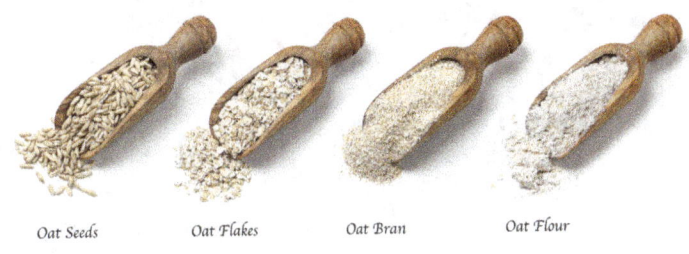

Oat Seeds   Oat Flakes   Oat Bran   Oat Flour

Steel Cut Oats

These are groats that have been cut into several pieces and are generally cooked and eaten as porridge. It should be noted that the more coarsely chopped they are, the longer they take to cook.

Flour

Oat flour improves the flavor, texture, and moisture of baked goods. In fact, I consider adding it to gluten-free flour as a baking hack, but it must be blended with other flours. It should make up no more than 25% of the total flour content. It is also prone to rancidity.

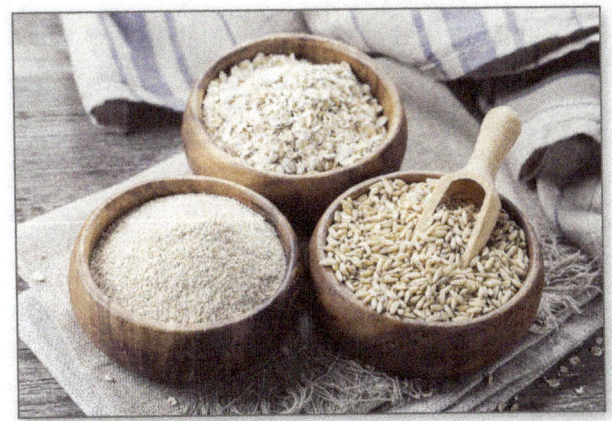

Regular Rolled Oatmeal

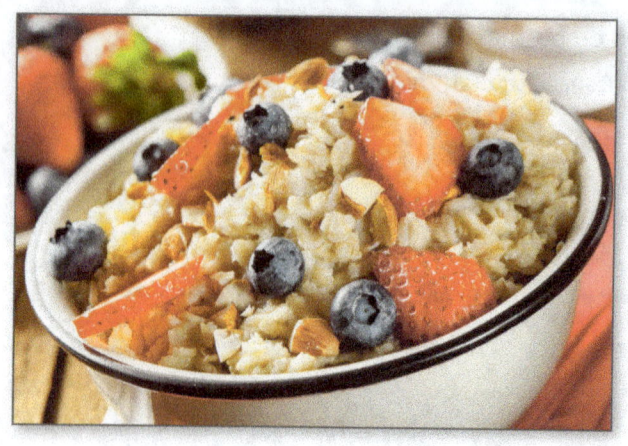

Oatmeal has been hulled, steam processed, then rolled flat and dried. This process increases the shelf life. Shelf life is highly variable depending on storage conditions and is longest when packaged in low oxygen conditions and kept cool.

Quick Oatmeal

Processed like regular rolled oats but is steamed longer and rolled flatter than non-instant oatmeal. This decreases the cooking time for consumers, but also increases the glycemic index, meaning that it is quickly digested and will increase blood sugar more rapidly. Quick oats also do not feel as filling as regular rolled oats.

Storage time: Groats and steel cut, 1-2 years. Oatmeal, 10-30 years. However, to get this kind of storage length for oatmeal it needs to be sealed in low oxygen environments and kept cool because of its high oil content. Number 10 cans with an O2 absorber work well.

Teff

Teff, the smallest of the true grains, is native to Ethiopia and Eritrea in the horn of Africa and is grown in a wide range of conditions. It is most commonly milled into flour and used to make injera, an Ethiopian sourdough flatbread. It can range in color from deep red-brown to almost white and has a wheat-like taste. Darker varieties have a stronger, more molasses-like flavor than lighter varieties.

Teff is a rich source of protein, fiber, and manganese, and has the highest calcium content of any grain. Because the grain is so small, it is impossible to separate its bran and germ, so all forms of teff are 100% whole grain. Teff costs more than other grains because it has a lower yield, is difficult to harvest, and is grown in a limited number of places. However, the excellent flavor, good baking performance, nutrition, and length of storage make it well worth the price.

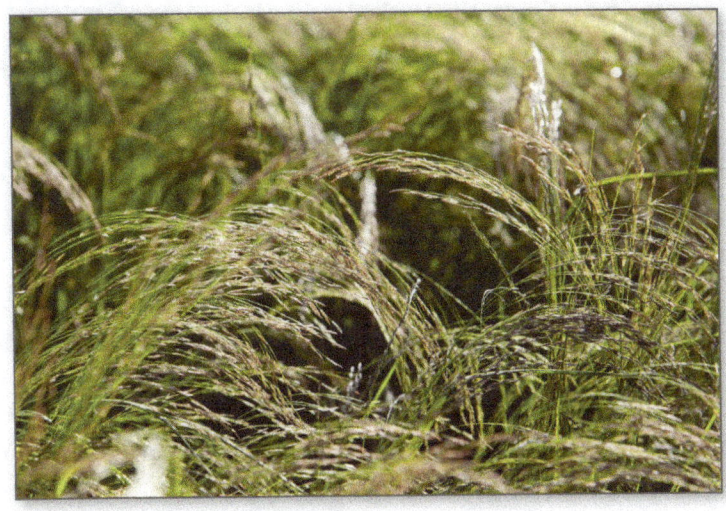

My favorite way to use teff is in gluten-free flour blends along with sorghum. It tastes great. I also like to keep cooked teff around to slip into other dishes to boost nutrition or as a meat extender in recipes. Many grains can replace rice in recipes, but not teff because of its size and texture. If you want to eat it like rice it is best to mix with other small grains with similar cooking times like quinoa, millet, and buckwheat (see recipe on page 184). The Teff Company has a lot of good recipes on their website: www.teffco.com.

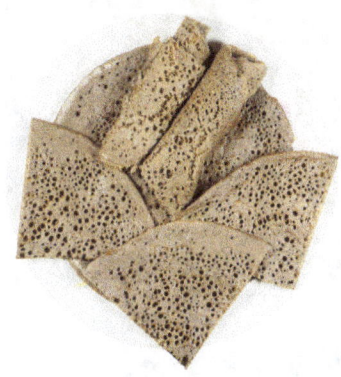

Storage: 2 years in consumer packaging at room temperature. I have had success storing teff with no detectable changes for 6 years. Based on my discussions with growers, teff may store well for much longer like 20 years. If you are interested in adopting a long-term food storage program, I strongly recommend you experiment with, eat, and store teff.

Corn

Corn is considered a vegetable when it is eaten fresh, or a grain when it is dried. Most corn grown in the U.S. is fed to animals and turned into vegetable oil, although it's excellent human food, too. It is readily available, easy to grow in backyard gardens, can be eaten in many forms, and is liked by most children. Sweet corn and popcorn are the most common varieties consumed in whole form by

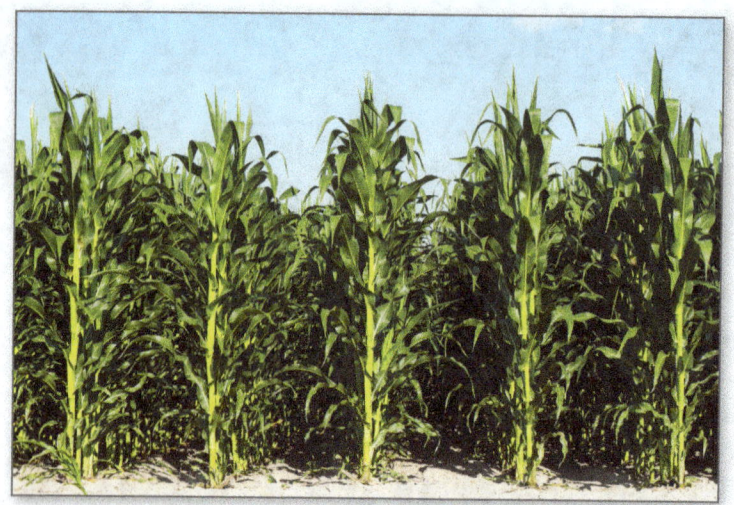

people. Field or dent corn has a high starch content and is used mainly for animal feed and industrial uses other than consumption.

Native to the Americas, corn's origin was unknown for many years since it does not grow wild anywhere on Earth. In recent years, genetic tests have revealed a very close genetic makeup to a plant called Teosite from Mexico, which is now believed to be corn's early ancestor.

Nutritionally, corn boasts the highest vitamin A content of any grain, 10 times higher than other grains. It is also high in other antioxidants

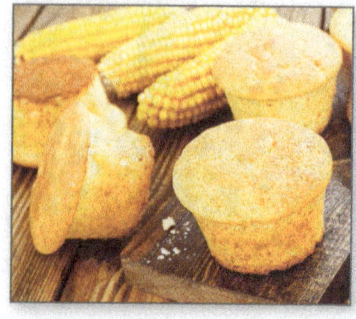

and carotenoids like lutein and zeaxanthin which are associated with eye health. Blue and purple corn boast the same antioxidants (anthocyanins) as blueberries.

Corn can also be coarsely ground to be used in hot breakfast cereal or in baked goods such as cornmeal muffins. It can also be ground into a finer flour and used in a wider variety of baked goods. Coarser grinds yield a slightly gritty texture which is denser and more crumbly than finer cornmeal and flour. Most commercially available meals and flour have the germ removed prior to milling since the high oil content causes it to become rancid quickly. Since the germ is not removed in home-ground flour it contains all the natural corn oils.

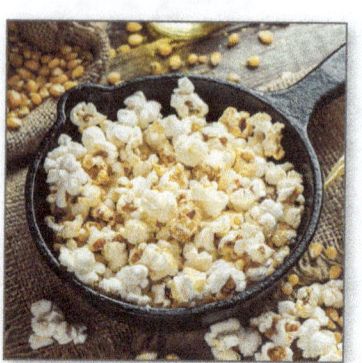

Popcorn is one of the easiest forms of corn to buy in bulk and store. It is also easy to rotate since it is long lasting and makes an extremely cheap and tasty snack. It's low water content also makes it ideal for storage. Popcorn kernels can also be milled into cornmeal and flour, although it is harder to mill into a fine flour.

Storage: 1-2 years at room temperature and 5+ in good storage conditions.

Ways to Cook Grains

Grain is usually rinsed prior to cooking. All grains are cooked by simmering but there are three different methods: pasta, absorption and pilaf. The pasta method uses excess water, boiling until soft, followed by draining extra water, and is best suited to larger grains like sorghum, oats and rice. Like pasta, salted water is brought to a boil then the grain is added and cooked until tender. Drain in a colander and let sit for 5 minutes. Rice cooked this way has a lower arsenic content because arsenic released in cooking is drained away. The rule of thumb ratio for cooking grains with the pasta method is 1 cup grain to 6 cups water with ½ tsp salt.

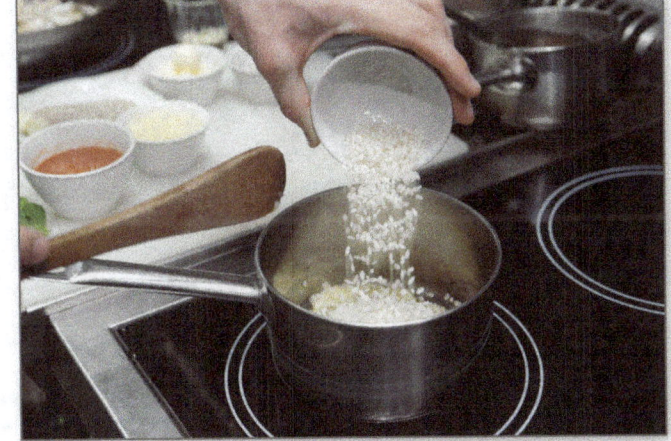

The absorption and pilaf methods are similar and use a grain-specific prescribed amount of water, just enough to hydrate the grains. These two methods, absorption and pilaf, use the same volume of water to grain ratio. For the absorption method add grain and appropriate water volume to a saucepan, stir to distribute grains and water evenly then bring to a boil. Once it reaches a full boil, place a tight fitting lid on the pan and reduce the heat to low and simmer until tender. Since this method is designed to absorb all available water, opening the lid frequently can cause too much water to be lost leaving grain crunchy or burning on the bottom. When water is fully absorbed remove the pan from heat and let sit for 5-10 minutes to finish cooking. This is similar to the warm cycle in rice cookers. Have you ever noticed that if you open a rice cooker immediately after the cook light turns off the rice is slightly crunchy? Finally fluff grain with a fork and serve. If you prefer a fluffy to a sticky grain, place a towel between the pot and the lid for the resting period to absorb excess water.

In the pilaf method, grains are first cooked slightly in butter or oil. This gives a slightly richer, roasted flavor and improved texture. Heat oil in a large saucepan over medium heat. Use 2 Tbsp oil per cup of grain. Next add grains to the pan and stir as grains are cooking. Grains may stick at first until all grains are coated. After several minutes the grains will start to turn a little opaque. Next add liquid and increase heat and bring to a boil then reduce and simmer as you would with the absorption method. America's Test Kitchen has a short video demonstrating the absorption and pilaf method at https://www.youtube.com/watch?v=68PPJuF-gnUw

Why Eat Beans?

Beans are an amazing food! But let's start with bean terminology. Beans are the plants or fruit of the Fabaceae or Leguminosae families, commonly called the bean, pea, or legume family. When used as dry grains they are sometimes called pulses. This group also includes peas, peanuts, and lentils. This section is about beans cooked without their pods rather than in pods like green or string beans. Legumes come in a host of varieties like chickpea, kidney, black, navy, pinto, red, and lentils – all of which are in most grocery stores. There are many more varieties available online and in specialty stores like Asian markets. You can buy them dry (cheapest), canned (easiest), or sprouted (different nutrients). Beans are such a powerhouse, you should probably consider eating them every day, or at least more often than you do now. Each bean has its own unique nutrients so it is good to enjoy a variety of different beans as well.

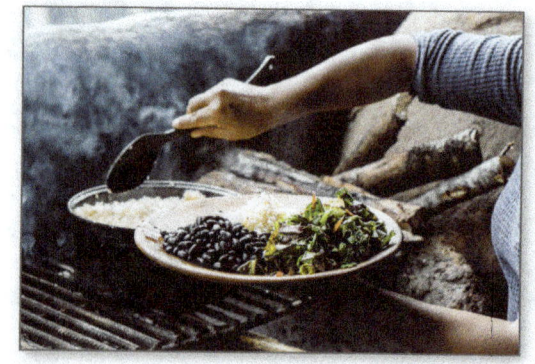

Big Deal Nutrients in Beans/Legumes

Protein is one of the key nutrients found in beans. Meat and dairy are also high in protein, but they come with a lot of calories and saturated fats. Beans are a very storable source of protein.

Folate is a nutrient people with celiac disease need to pay attention to. It is a critical nutrient typically low in gluten-free diets and is poorly absorbed in cases of intestinal damage. Folate is essential for DNA creation and repair, brain and nerve function, liver and heart health, and red blood cell formation. It is also critical to get adequate levels before and during pregnancy to prevent neural tube birth defects like spina bifida. The black eyed pea has the highest level of folate of all the beans, with kidney beans coming in second.

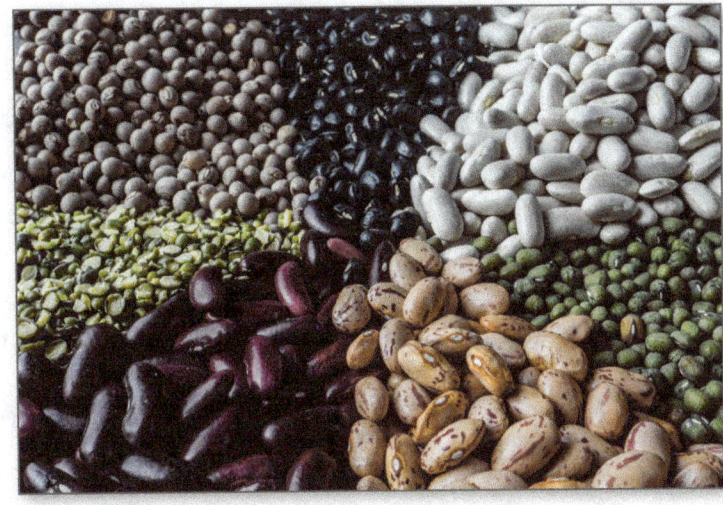

Note: Folate is naturally occurring vitamin B9 and folic acid is the synthetic version. These two forms are usually referred to synonymously.

Minerals vary by type of bean but include iron, manganese, magnesium, and potassium.

Fiber is an often underappreciated nutrient. The daily recommended intake is 25 grams for females and 38 grams for males. How much does the average American eat every day? 10-15 grams.

One of the benefits of eating the recommended dose of fiber daily is weight loss. Fiber makes you feel full faster than any other food component. If you are not usually a bean consumer, try this experiment. Eat a bean-based main dish like rice and beans first. Then notice whether you eat or feel like eating smaller servings of the side dishes and dessert. You will probably be surprised.

Fibrous foods like beans contain complex carbohydrates that are slower to digest so eating beans is a great way to reduce spikes in blood glucose levels. Frequent bean meals are perfect for diabetics and pre-diabetics.

Fiber also reduces cholesterol by trapping it which allows your body to excrete rather than absorb it. Eating more beans tends to naturally decrease meat consumption, so they are a double whammy for lowering cholesterol—less consumed and less absorbed. Fibrous foods also help normalize blood pressure. If you are worried about heart disease, eating beans regularly is a smart move.

Common Bean Varieties

This section describes the nutrient profiles of several of the most common bean/legume varieties. Choose some you find interesting to experiment with.

Chickpeas/Garbanzo Beans

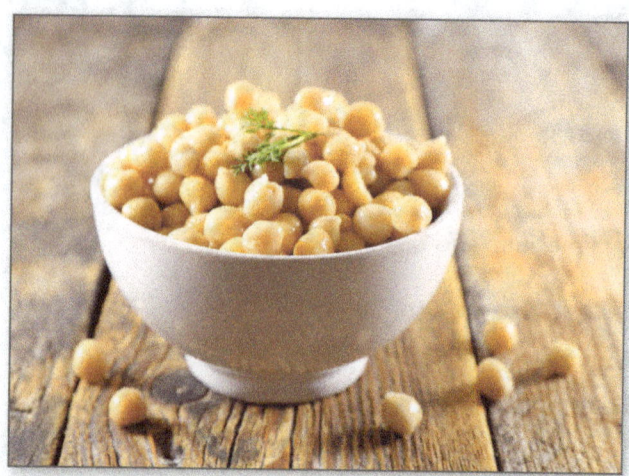

Chickpeas are native to the Mediterranean and are common in Mediterranean, Indian, and Middle Eastern cuisines. They are main ingredients in falafel and hummus and are common salad toppings. The two types of chickpeas are: Kabuli, which are large, white, and mild flavored (also called garbanzo beans), and Desi, a smaller darker bean with a yellow center. India has the highest production and consumption rate, but in the U.S. the largest producing states are Montana, Washington, and Idaho.

Chickpeas can be used in soups and curries, roasted for delightful crispy snacks, or used for flour. For the gluten-free baker, chickpea flour is an amazing addition especially in breads. I was first introduced to chickpea flour in gluten-free bread by a food science intern working for me. She started with my No Fail Bread recipe (page 251) and substituted chickpea flour in different proportions. The flavor was mild and the texture was good. I really got excited about it when a chickpea flour company sent me samples of their flour and some recipes. They were phenomenal! Chickpea has the mildest flavor of the bean flours with high protein content (great to improve

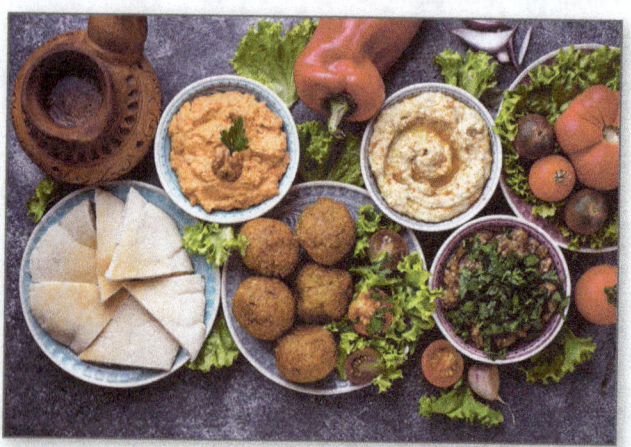

structure of baked goods) and naturally high folate. It was the perfect ingredient in my quest to make the gluten-free diet more nutritious.

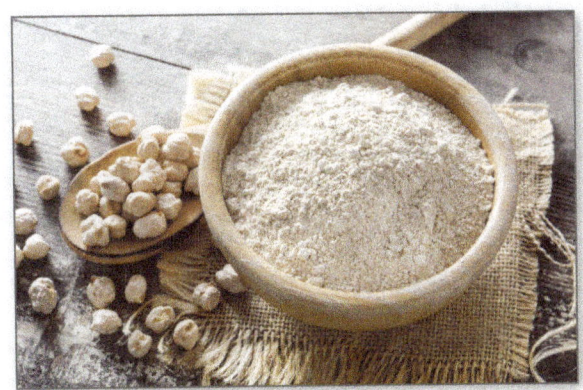

One cup of cooked chickpeas delivers: Calories 269, Protein 14.5 grams, Fiber 12.5 g, Folate 71% of RDI, Manganese 84% of RDI, Copper 29% RDI, Iron 26% RDI.

Storage: 2-3 years at room temperature. Well stored (i.e low oxygen, light, and temperature), 5-10 years.

Lentils

Lentils are native to the Middle East but spread rapidly through Europe, Asia, and North Africa. They are a main ingredient in curries and are used as thickeners. In Ethiopia, lentils are often the first solid food given to infants. One of the most convenient things about lentils is the short, no-soak cooking time. They are completely cooked in 40 minutes which makes them an easy nutrition booster for soups and stews. They can also be used as a meat substitute in vegan versions of burger patties, sloppy joes, and taco filling (pages 215-218). Toasting makes them a crunchy topping for salad.

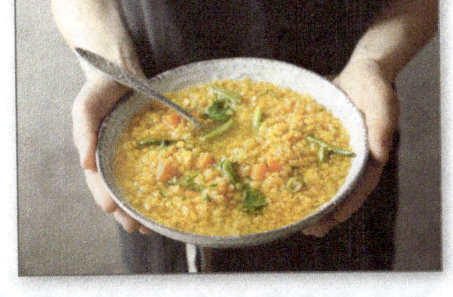

There are several types of lentils: Brown, green, red or yellow, and specialty.

Brown is the most common type of lentil and ranges in color from khaki to almost black and has a mild earthy flavor. These hold their shape well and are a good addition to soups, salads, and meat replacements like meat loaf or patties.

Green lentils are very similar to brown lentils but have a stronger, slightly peppery taste.

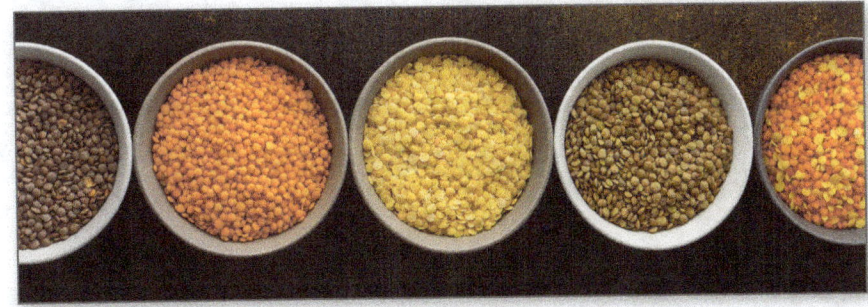

Red and yellow lentils range in color from golden yellow to orange to red. These varieties often come split which shortens the cooking time and yields a softer texture, making them good for soups or stews, or pureed and used as a thickener in recipes. They have a slight sweet and nutty flavor and give characteristic flavor to some Indian or Middle Eastern dishes like dhal, a thick curry stew.

The most common specialty lentils are black, beluga, and puy. These seeds are smaller than common varieties and have a rich earthy flavor.

One cup of cooked lentils contains: Calories 230, Protein 17.9 grams, Fiber 15.6 grams, Folate 90% RDI, Manganese: 49% RDI, Copper 29% RDI, Thiamin (Vit B1) 22% RDI.

Storage: 1-2 years at room temperature. 5+ years with good conditions.

Dried Peas

Though recipes abound for delicious fresh or frozen peas, this section is about dried peas which lend themselves to recipes that call for dry beans and lentils. Different varieties are grown for fresh and frozen peas versus dried peas. Peas destined for drying are left on the vine in the pod and harvested later than for vegetable peas. The mature seeds have a higher starch content and are more suited for drying and storing.

Split pea soup is the most common way these peas are used, but are easily exchanged for lentils in most recipes and give different flavor and nutrition. In addition to soups and stews they can be transformed into crispy snacks and croutons similar to roasted chickpeas, or turned into easy nutritious wraps similar to lentils.

One cup of cooked dried peas contains: Calories 125, Protein 8.2 grams, Fiber 8.8 grams, Folate 24% RDI, Manganese 22%, Vitamin K 48% RDI, Thiamine (Vit B1) 30% RDI.

Storage: 2-3 years at room temperature, and up to 5 in ideal conditions.

Kidney Beans

These beans are very recognizable by their large size, red color, and distinctive kidney shape. All the beans have low glycemic indices, but kidney beans are among the lowest. They are commonly used in chili and are a delicious powerhouse of nutrition. Kidney beans should always be fully cooked, as raw beans contain a toxin destroyed by cooking.

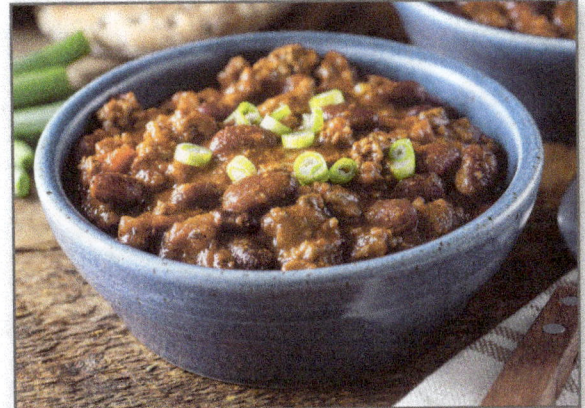

One cup of cooked kidney beans contains: Calories 215, Protein 13.4 grams, Fiber 13.6 grams, Folate 23% RDI, Manganese 22% RDI, Thiamin (Vit B1) 20% RDI, Copper 17% RDI, Iron 17% RDI.

Storage: 5-10 years.

Black Beans

If you search the internet for the healthiest bean, you will find lists with various rankings. Some rank for protein, others antioxidants or other traits, but black beans are always one of the top beans. They are delicious, easy to find, and boast a high antioxidant and protein content. Black beans are familiar in Central and South American cuisines. This is definitely a winner for regular eating and adding to home storage.

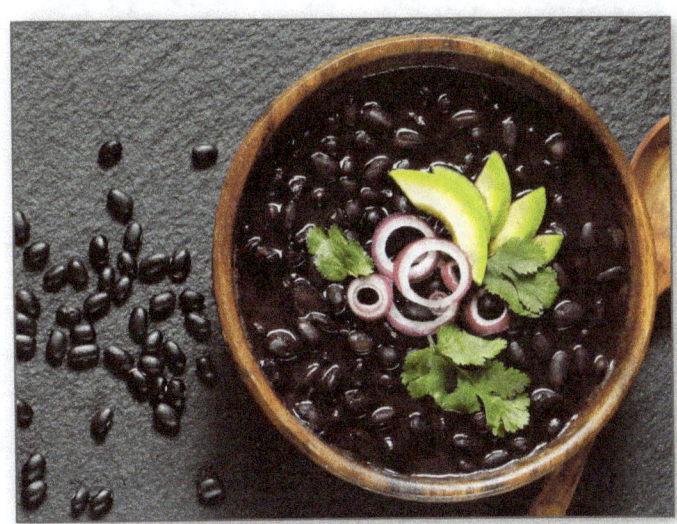

One cup of cooked black beans contains: Calories 227, Protein 15.2 grams, Fiber 15 grams, Folate 64% RDI, Manganese 38% RDI, Thiamine (Vit B1) 28% RDI, Iron 20% RDI.

Storage: 5-30 years

Soybeans

Soybeans are a legume native to Asia. They were introduced to the United States in the 1800s and now 50% of all soybeans are grown here. Soybeans can be purchased dry, canned, or frozen. Edamame are fresh soybeans harvested while still immature. This is analogous to green beans that are eaten in the pod. Though

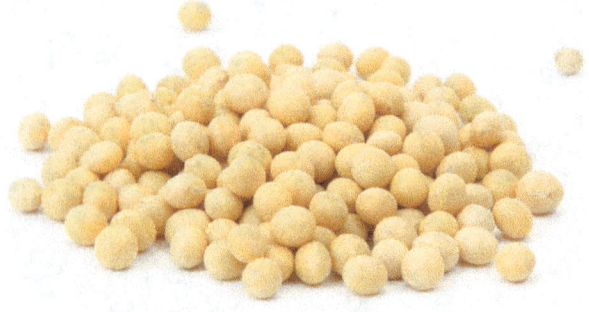

there are many different varieties and colors of soybeans, the most common variety is light yellow and round with a tiny dark spot.

Because soy has the highest and best protein content of any bean, a mild flavor and high oil content, it is used to make a myriad of products like tofu, soymilk, soy sauce, protein drinks, tempeh, cooking oil, edamame, and soy flour. If you are not allergic, there is a lot to like about soy.

Dried soybeans are not available in all grocery stores but are common in Asian markets. If you have never tried them, they are definitely worth buying at least once to try. They are soaked and cooked like other dry beans but take longer and become tender rather than soft. They should be soaked in the refrigerator to prevent fermentation.

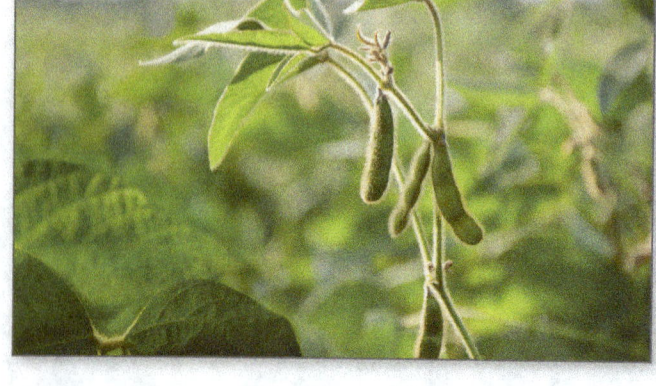

Each cup of cooked soybeans contains: Calories 298, Protein 28 grams, Fiber 10 grams, Manganese 71% RDI, Iron 49% RDI, Phosphorus 42% RDI, Vitamin K 41% RDI, Riboflavin (Vit B2) 29% RDI, Folate 23% RDI. For more information on soy and health benefits visit https://pubmed.ncbi.nlm.nih.gov/28838083/.

Storage: 3 years at room temperature, longer with optimal storage.

Pinto Beans

The pinto bean is the most popular bean in America and is most commonly known for its starring role in chili con carne and refried beans. In Mexico and the Southwest United States, they are the most commonly grown bean. They are cheap, easy to find, and nutritious. They figure heavily in cuisines of Spain, Mexico, and Brazil, and it's easy to find delicious recipes which include them.

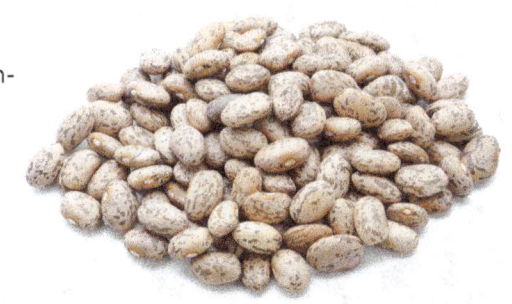

One cup of cooked pinto beans contains: Calories 245, Protein 15.4 grams, Fiber 15.4 grams, Folate 74% RDI, Manganese 39% RDI, Copper 29% RDI, Thiamine (Vit B1) 22% RDI.

Storage: 1-2 years at room temperature, and 5-30 with optimal storage.

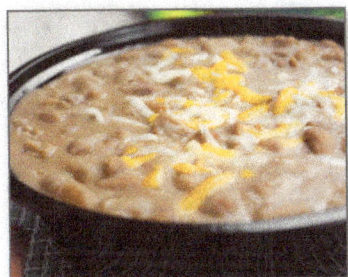

Nuts & Seeds

Nuts and seeds have been part of human diets as long as we can determine. It makes perfect sense; they are packed with heart healthy fats, fiber, plant proteins, minerals and vitamins, and antioxidants. Choose whichever kind you like best and start eating them regularly. Then branch out and try others to expand the nutrients you eat. Almonds are popular, but try some hazelnuts, pecans, walnuts or pistachios for a change. Snack on peanuts (a legume we call a nut) or seeds like pumpkin, sunflower, pine nuts, or pomegranate. Toss in some flax, chia, hemp, or sesame with your smoothie, granola, salads, or stir fry. Nut flours can also be a healthful and texture improving element of gluten-free flours.

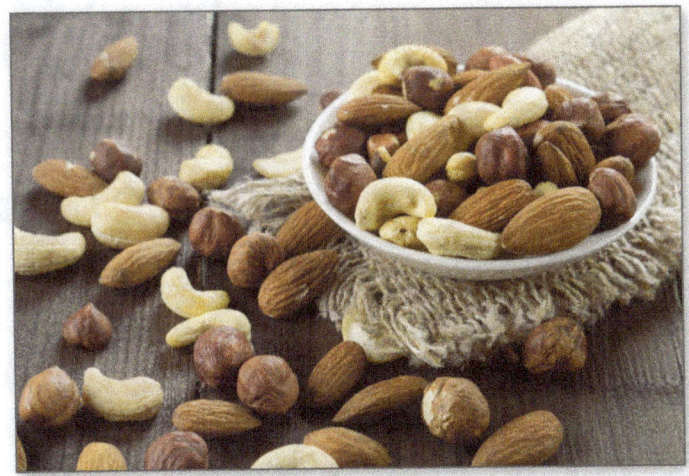

There is enough evidence of the health benefits of nuts that they are included in the government dietary recommendations of the U.S. and Canada.

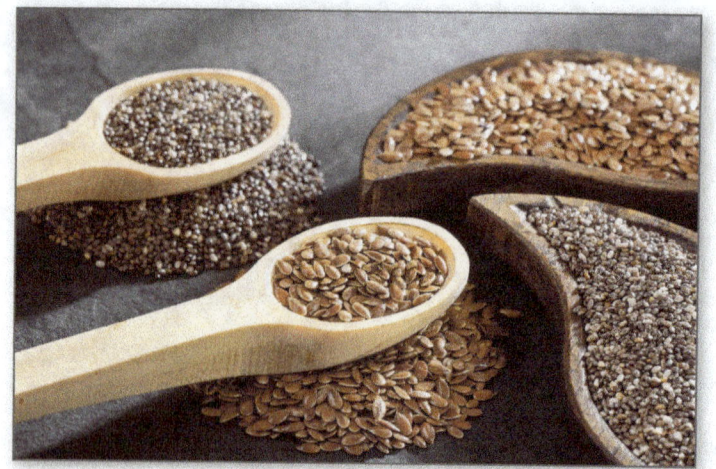

The FDA allows the statement that a 1.5 oz serving per day of most nuts as part of a healthy diet low in saturated fat and cholesterol may reduce the risk of heart disease.

Since this book is written for the gluten free who may also be allergic to other foods, I want to call out two specific seeds: flax and chia. These two seeds are very nutritious with high fiber and omega 3 fatty acids which make them exceptionally heart healthy, and can also be used as an egg substitute. They won't work for all egg replacement needs but generally work well in baking. Flax also increases shelf life of baked goods, which is a plus since most gluten-free foods stale quickly.

To make one flax or chia egg: Stir 1 tablespoon of *ground* flax or chia seed into 3 tablespoons of hot water. Stir well and let sit for 3-5 minutes until they have a gelatinous consistency. Add to your recipe as you would an egg. Hint: the more finely the seeds are ground, the better result you will get.

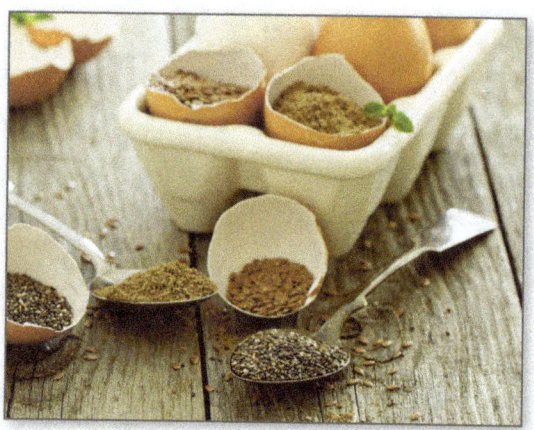

Storing Nuts and Seeds

Because nuts and seeds contain a lot of natural fats, they don't store well for long periods of time. Nutritionally, these would be ideal foods to store but not in freshness and longevity. Most nuts are only good for about a year. The high unsaturated fat levels makes them very sensitive to heat and oxygen, so for longer term storage pack them in airtight, opaque, containers and keep them in the freezer. This extends the shelf life to up to two years.

If you use flax or chia and want to keep a larger supply on hand for storage, choose chia. It lasts longer and there is less variability in quality. Chia is usually packaged for consumers with a two-year shelf life which can be extended to four with good packaging in a fridge or freezer. Unlike flax, chia seeds do not need to be ground for your body to absorb the nutrients and have a mild flavor.

Flax has some advantages over chia; it improves baked good texture more than chia, and contains slightly more ALA or alpha-linolenic acid, an omega 3 fatty acid. The main disadvantage of flax is storage length, but there are some keys to getting it to last longer. Use the universal shelf life rules of storing without light, heat and oxygen and store high quality whole seeds. Whole seeds store twice as long as ground seeds with freezer storage being 2 years for ground and 4 years for whole seeds. Keep in mind that your body cannot extract the nutrients from unground flax well, so you will require a coffee grinder to mill your own whole seeds before consuming.

HOW CAN I JUDGE FLAX QUALITY?

Since flax storage length, nutritional quality, and flavor is greatly affected by the quality of the seed, it is important to know what good flax looks like. The seeds should all look plump and glossy. Shrunken or thin seeds are immature seeds which develop rancidity more quickly.

High-quality flax should contain no weed seeds. If you see different seeds, commonly little round black seeds, it was not grown in a low-weed field or was not sorted well post-harvest. Organically grown flax is typically of lower quality than non-organic flax because of weeds in the field. Flax does not compete strongly with other plants and has decreased levels of omega 3 fatty acids and other nutrients as a result. Increased weed competition also causes some areas in fields to mature more slowly and can cause immature seeds to be harvested along with the mature seeds thereby reducing shelf life.

GRAIN & BEAN COOKING CHART

	METHOD	RATIO OF STAPLE TO WATER	SETTING AND COOK TIME	YIELD (FOR 1 CUP DRY STAPLE)
Brown Rice	Stovetop	1:2	Bring to boil, then simmer, covered, for 30 minutes	2 cups
	Pressure cooker	1:1 1/4	Manual for 15 minutes	
	Slow cooker	1: 1 1/2	High for 2 1/2 hours Low for 5 hours	
Quinoa	Stovetop	1:1 1/2	Bring to boil, then simmer, covered, for 20 minutes	3 cups
	Pressure cooker	1:1	Manual for 1 minute	
	Slow cooker	1:1 1/2	High for 2 1/2 hours Low for 5 hours	
Beans	Stovetop	1:3	Soak overnight, then bring to boil and simmer for 45 to 60 mintues	2 1/4 cups
	Pressure cooker	1:3	Dry: Manual for 25 to 30 minutes Soaked: Manual for 8 to 10 minutes	
	Slow cooker	1:3	Soak overnight, then cook on high for 3 to 4 hours or low for 6 to 8 hours	
Lentils	Stovetop	1:3	Bring to boil, reduce heat, and simmer for 25 minutes	2 1/2 cups
	Pressure cooker	1:3	Dry: Manual for 10 mintues Soaking uneccessary.	
	Slow cooker	1:3	High for 3 to 4 hours Low for 6 to 8 hours	
Chickpeas	Stovetop	1:3	Soak overnight, bring to a boil, and simmer for 35 to 40 minutes	2 1/2 to 3 cups
	Pressure cooker	1:3	Dry: Manual for 35 to 40 minutes	
	Slow cooker	1:3	Soak overnight, then cook on high for 3 to 4 hours or low for 6 to 8 hours	

	METHOD	RATIO OF STAPLE TO WATER	SETTING AND COOK TIME	YIELD (FOR 1 CUP DRY STAPLE)
Amaranth	Stovetop	1:3	Boil and then let simmer for 20 mintues stiring occasionally. Can be toasted before cooking by browning in the pan before adding water.	2
	Pressure cooker	1:2	Pressure cook on high for 5 minutes.	
Buckwheat	Stovetop	1:2	Bring water to a boil. Add buckwheat and simmer for 10-15 minutes. Drain excess water	
	Pressure cooker	1:1 1/3	Pressure on high for 5 minutes then let sit for 8 minutes before releasing pressure	
	Slow cooker	1:2	Cook for 2 hrs on high or 4 hrs on low	
Millet	Stovetop	1:2	Bring to a boil. Reduce heat and simmer for about 20 mins.	1:3.5
	Pressure cooker	1:1 3/4	Pressure cook on high for 10 minutes.	
	Slow cooker	1: 3 1/2	Cook on low for 4-5 hours or on high 1 1/2 - 2 1/2 hours.	
Oats Steel Cut	Stovetop	1: 3 1/2 - 4	Bring to a boil. Reduce heat and simmer for about 20 mins stiring occasionally.	1:3
	Pressure cooker	1: 1 1/2	Cook on high for 4 minutes	
	Slow cooker	1:4	Cook on low for 7-8 hours or on high for 4-5 hours.	

GRAIN & BEAN COOKING CHART (CONTINUED)

	METHOD	RATIO OF STAPLE TO WATER	SETTING AND COOK TIME	YIELD (FOR 1 CUP DRY STAPLE)
White Rice	Stovetop	1:2	Bring to a boil. Reduce heat to low and simmer for about 20 minutes.	1:3
	Oven		Use glass baking dish covered with foil 45-60 mins	
	Slow cooker		Spray crock w/ cooking spray. Cook on high 1 1/2 - 2 hours. Stir occasionally	
Sorghum	Stovetop	1:3	Bring to a boil. Reduce heat and simmer for about 45 mins.	
	Pressure cooker	1: 2.5	Pressure on high for 22 mins	
	Slow cooker	1: 2.5	Turn on high and cook until desired firmness is achieved approx. 2 hrs	
Teff	Stovetop	1:3	Bring to a boil. Simmer for 20 minutes. Can be toasted prior to boiling.	2 Cups
	Pressure cooker	1:2	Pressure on high for 3 minutes	
	Slow cooker	1: 1 1/2	Cook on high for 2 - 2 1/2 hours	

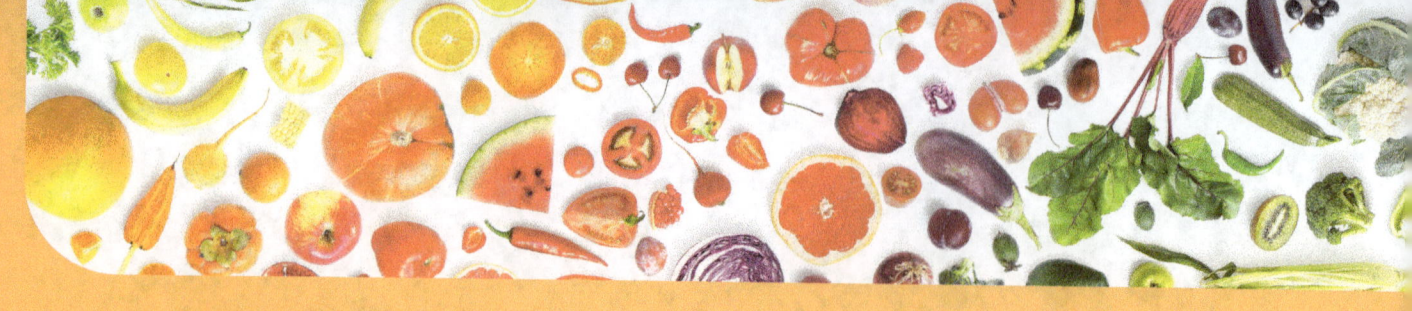

CHAPTER SIX
How to **CONVERT RECIPES** to Gluten Free

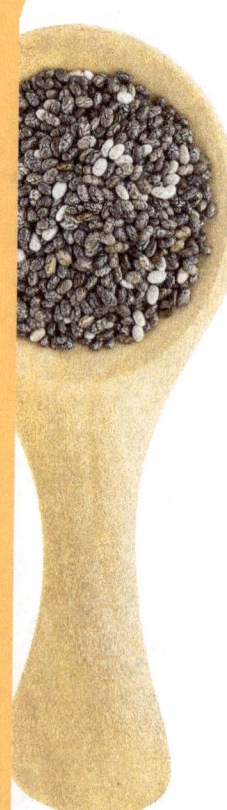

EVERY PERSON AND FAMILY HAS FAVORITE RECIPES and holiday food traditions. It can be painful to give these up, but fortunately many can be converted to a gluten-free version.

In fact, many already are. Before you convert your own recipe, check to see if someone else has done the work for you. Search the internet by the name of your recipe and see what you find. There are a lot of great resources among bloggers and on Pinterest.

Converting Your Own Favorites

The first step in conversion is to examine your recipe critically. Look at each ingredient and figure out what it does. Recipes include ingredients that build structure, serve as filler or flavor carriers, provide texture, add flavor and, in baked goods, leaven. Some elements have a dual function. Once you figure out what your ingredients do, you can better understand what they can be replaced with to transform the dish to gluten free.

For practice let's analyze a recipe that contains gluten.

MACARONI SALAD

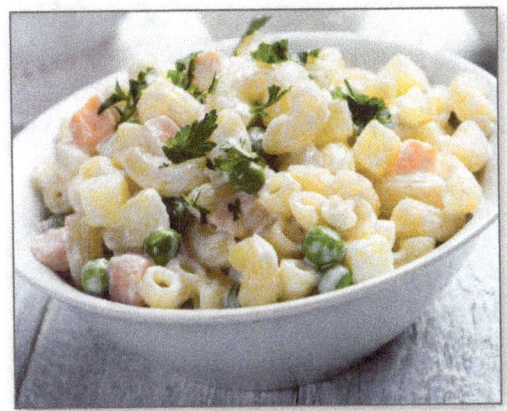

Ingredient	Function
4 C uncooked macaroni	filler/flavor carrier
1 C mayonnaise	texture and flavor
¼ C vinegar	flavor
2/3 C sugar	flavor
1 ½ tbsp yellow mustard	flavor
1 ½ tsp salt	flavor
½ tsp black pepper	flavor
1 chopped onion	flavor and texture, possibly color
1 chopped bell pepper	flavor, texture and color
¼ C grated carrot	flavor, texture and color
2 tbsp chopped pimento	flavor, texture and color

Now, look at your own favorite recipes. What are your ingredients doing? What is the most satisfying thing for you about this dish? Is it the flavor, texture, or your memories of the food? These questions can help you pick the best strategy for converting each recipe.

Strategy #1: Swap Ingredients with Gluten-Free Versions

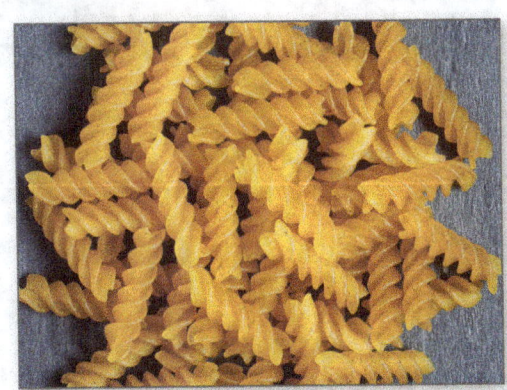

Most of the ingredients in macaroni salad are already gluten free, except for macaroni. In this case, you can use gluten-free macaroni in place of the traditional macaroni and leave the rest of the recipe alone.

Strategy #2: Keep Flavor and Texture Ingredients but Change Fillers or Flavor Carriers

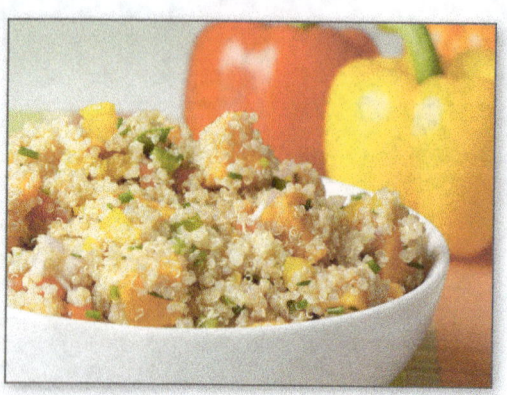

If there were no gluten-free macaroni available, or you didn't like the performance or taste of gluten-free macaroni, you could create the sauce as usual and add another filler such as quinoa, rice, sorghum, or potatoes.

The strategy of pulling the flavor and texture ingredients out of the recipe then placing them on another filler food works well for casseroles, too. Fillers you might consider for your next meal are cooked gluten-free grains like rice, quinoa, sorghum, potatoes (chunks, shreds, tater tots), or corn tortillas.

Strategy #3: Create Your Own Recipes

Below is a list of the essential seasonings of common ethnic foods. You can use these seasonings to create your own recipes and sauces. Commercial seasoning blends can also be used, just make sure they are gluten free. Copy the flavors you love and put them in different dishes that are gluten or dairy free.

I often use this strategy when making stir fry dishes. I recently asked my son if he got tired of stir fry since we usually eat this dish once every 10 days. His

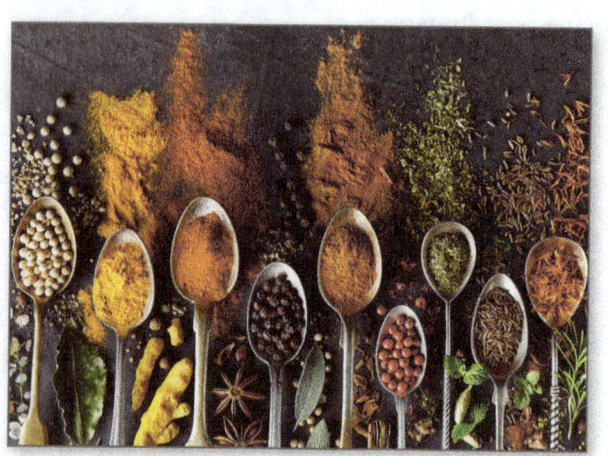

answer was, "No, it always tastes different." My stir fry starts with sauteing onions, celery, shredded carrots, and bell peppers (and sometimes meat). Then I add garlic, followed by a cooked grain. Beans and nuts are a good addition at this point as well. Finally, I ask my children what type of ethnic dish they are in the mood for, (e.g. Greek, Mexican, Italian), and use the seasonings from their selected flavor profile.

Another way to use the ethnic seasoning lists below is to create your own replacement ingredients. Suppose you discover the enchilada sauce you have used for years contains gluten. You can use the seasonings below added to tomato sauce as a replacement. You may want to eventually switch to a gluten-free brand, but this works fine in a pinch.

Mexican	Italian	French	Greek	Indian	Middle Eastern
Garlic	Garlic	Garlic	Parsley	Curry	Cumin
Onion	Onion	Bay leaves	Oregano	Cardamom	Ginger
Cumin	Oregano	Basil	Marjoram	Chiles	Basil
Chili powder	Basil	Thyme	Dill	Nutmeg	Dill
Peppers	Fennel	Tarragon	Mint	Masala	Marjoram
Oregano	Olive oil	Parsley	Lemon	Cinnamon	Parsley
	Sage	Chives	Cumin	Ginger	
	Marjoram		Olive Oil	Mustard Seed	
	Chervil		Rosemary		

Converting Baked Goods Recipes

Converting your favorite baked treats to gluten free is not as straightforward as converting other types of food. The easiest way to convert baked recipes like cookies, cakes, muffins, biscuits, and so forth, is to find a good commercial, all-purpose, gluten-free flour and swap it out in your recipe. This is especially helpful when you first start a gluten-free diet. However, converting baked goods in general is harder than other recipes and requires more experimentation because each flour behaves very differently from traditional flour, and even other gluten-free flours. The chemistry of gluten-free baking is different than with wheat flour.

Exchanging wheat flour with a good gluten-free flour does not work to convert traditional yeast breads from a gluten-full recipe—a specific gluten-free recipe must be used. Principles and hacks for gluten-free baking are explored in depth in Section 4: Cooking and Baking. If you really want to dive into making your own gluten-free bread I suggest the books *Gluten-Free Artisan Bread in Five Minutes a Day*[1] by Jeff Hertzberg and Zoe Francois, and *Gluten Free on a Shoestring Bakes Bread*[2] by Nicole Hunn.

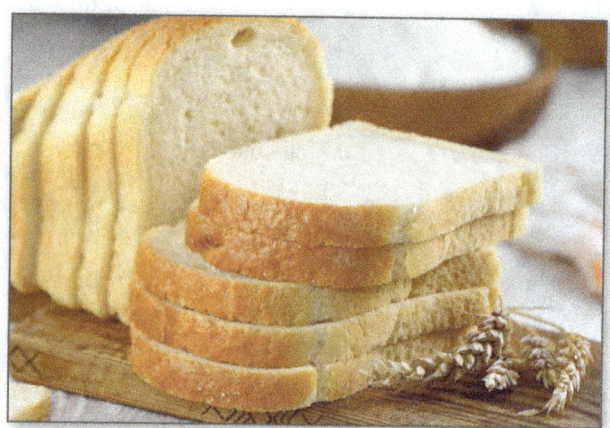

Regular Wheat Flour Bread

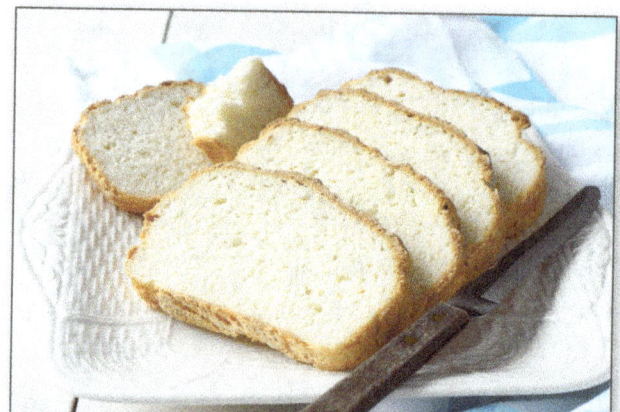

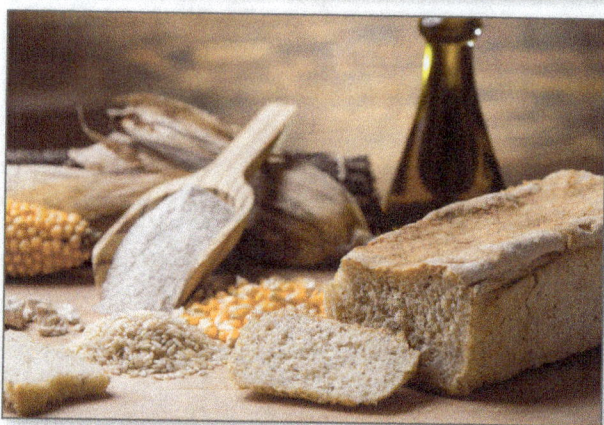

Gluten Free Bread

[1]Hertzberg, J., & François, Z. (2014). Gluten-Free Artisan Bread in Five Minutes a Day. St. Martin's Press.

[2]Hunn, N. (2013). Gluten-Free on a Shoestring Bakes Bread: Biscuits, Bagels, Buns, and More. Da Capo Lifelong Books.

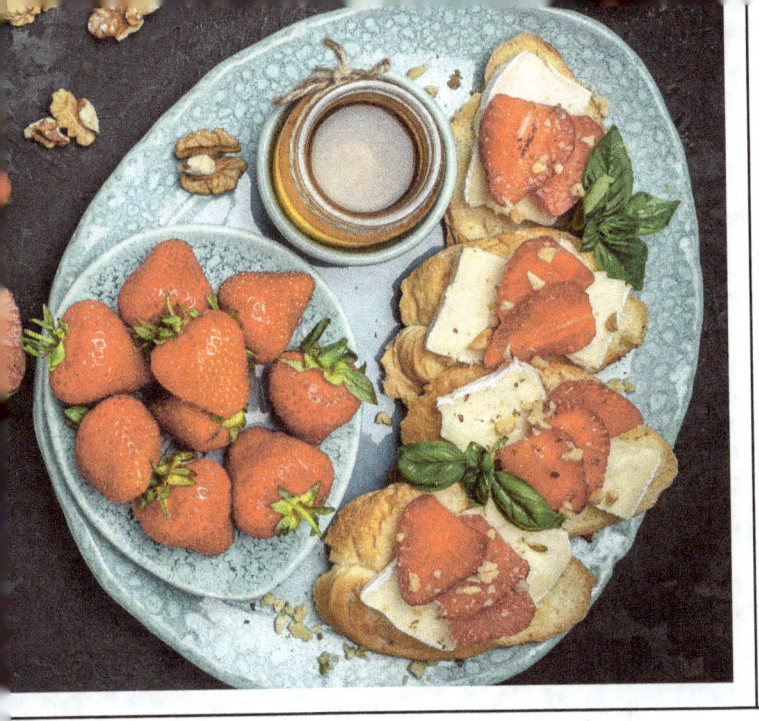

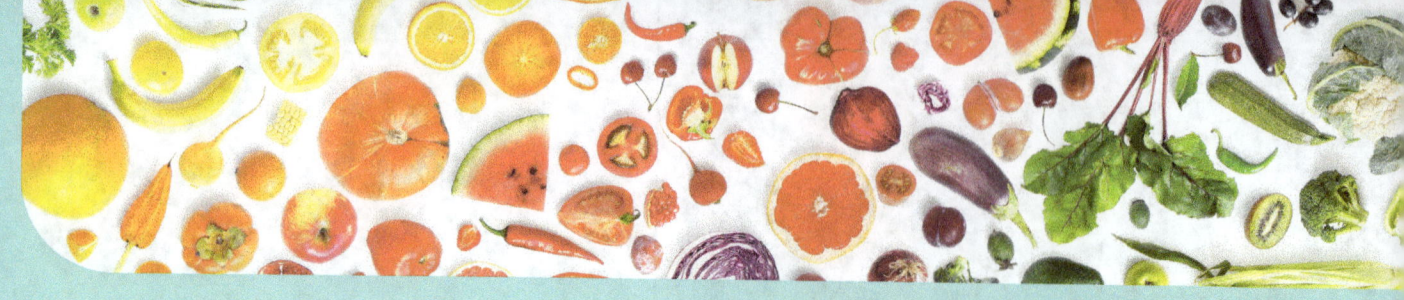

CHAPTER SEVEN

Five Strategies to MAKE COOKING CONVENIENT

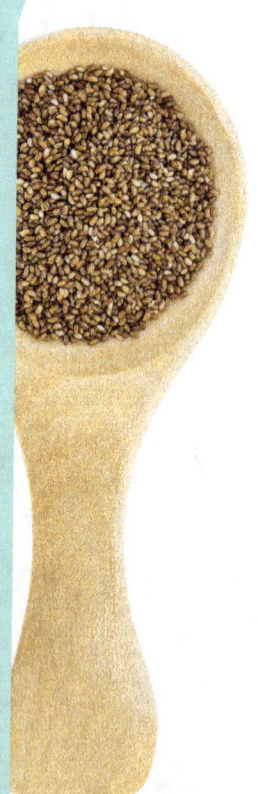

LET'S FACE IT: GOING GLUTEN FREE MEANS COOKING MORE YOURSELF.
Fortunately, there are great benefits. A study by the University of Washington School of Public Health[1] found that cooking more meals at home improved diet while lowering cost per meal. Throw in knowing your food is safe, and it sounds like a great option. Unfortunately, it isn't always. Sometimes there is no time or energy to cook. This chapter outlines four strategies I learned as a busy mother of five to "bank" time associated with cooking. Cooking still takes time, but these ideas make cooking happen when time is available.

Strategy 1: Keep a Well-Stocked Pantry

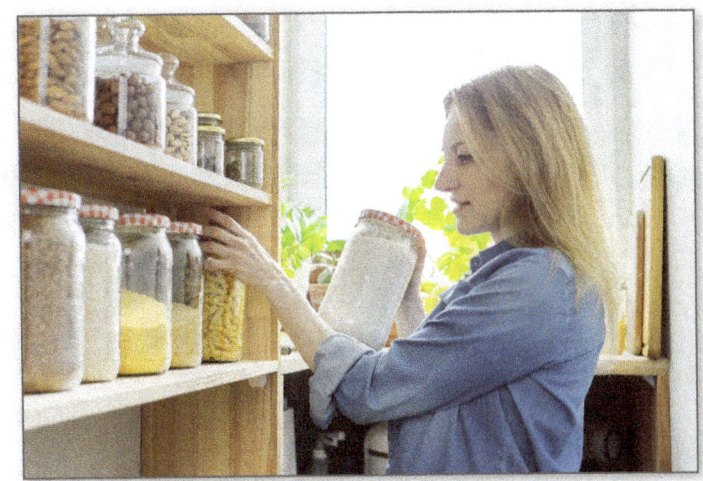

Nothing is more inconvenient than starting to cook something and not having all the ingredients. Keep the ingredients for your go-to recipes on-hand at all times. In fact, keep a few extras so you don't run out. Running to the store in the middle of a recipe is frustrating and inefficient.

Strategy 2: Plan Ahead—Cook Ahead

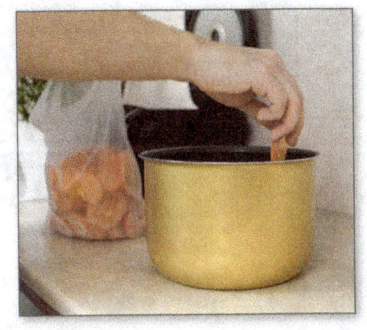

Think about what you will eat tomorrow after dinner tonight. Then you can make preparations before it's a rush. Get the meat out of the freezer tonight so it's ready to cook tomorrow. Start your oatmeal or other hot cereal in the slow cooker before bed tonight. Pack part of your lunch. Put all the ingredients for a slow cooker recipe in the crock and refrigerate so you can pull it out and start it before dashing out to work in the morning. You get the idea —start sooner!

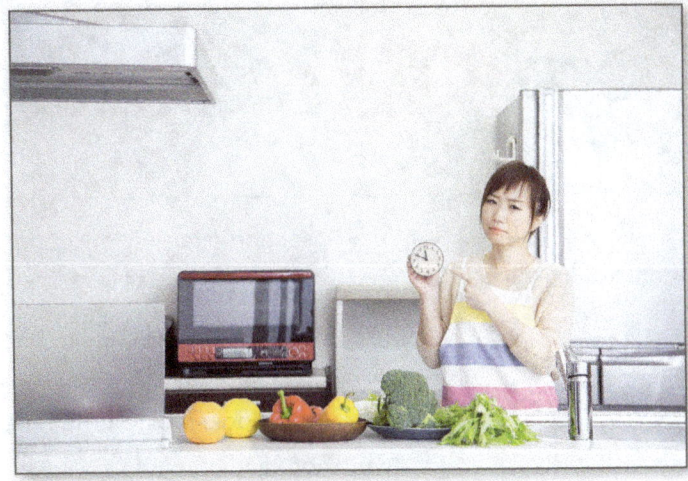

Planning ahead pairs perfectly with cooking ahead. Make big batches of your favorite foods by doubling recipes. This adds a few minutes to prep time but results in twice the amount of food with one setup and cleanup. You cut the time to make the second batch almost in half. The additional food can be frozen until needed. I use this strategy often for chili and other bean dishes, broth, sloppy joe filling, and casseroles.

Another cook ahead trick is to cook gluten-free whole grains and keep a container of pre-cooked grains in the fridge or freezer. It makes incorporating this power food into your diet easy when they are cooked and ready to go. They are conveniently available to eat as a breakfast cereal, add to stir fry, or create other dishes.

Strategy 3: Make your own mixes

This is especially helpful for making baked goods. To try this, make a favorite recipe like cookies and prepare additional mixes at the same time. Place one or more zippered storage bags open on your counter. Measure each dry ingredient

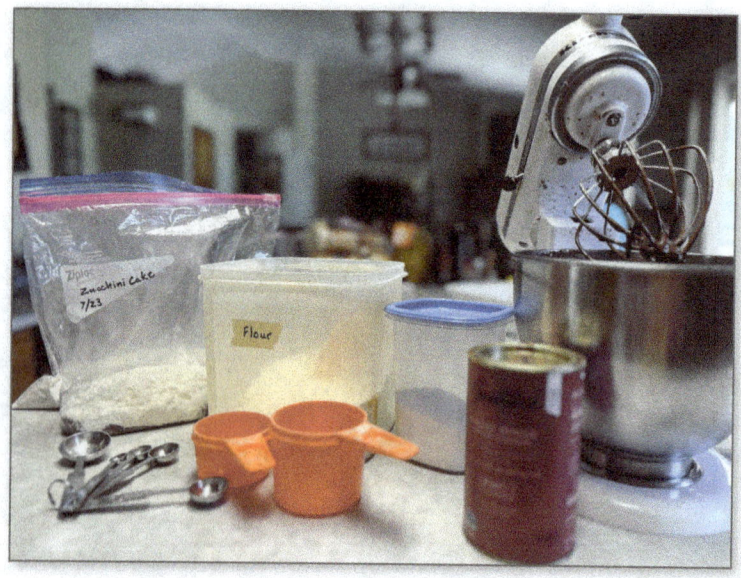

into each bag. Put one in the mixing bowl for your current batch, and one in each open bag for future batches. When all the dry ingredients are in the bags, simply zip them up and put them in an airtight container, and store in a cool place. Finish the batch in the mixer and bake. Next time you want cookies, you only need to cream your butter and sugar, add eggs, and add your premeasured mix.

You can also make mixes following a recipe specifically designed as a mix. We have included recipes for cream soup, cake, brownies, pancakes, and muffins in our "mixes" recipe

Make an additional mix while making a batch

section (starting on page 256). Many of these recipes were adapted from the book Make-A-Mix: 306 recipes to save time and money by Eliason, Harvard and Westover (ISBN1-55561-073-0). This is an older book but is still available online and in many libraries in several editions. Though I have not tried every recipe in this book, most of the baked goods need only the addition of the proper amount of xanthan gum.

Strategy 4: Pre-Prep Recipe Steps and Freeze

Prepping frequently-used ingredients and freezing ahead can also save time and dirty dishes. Think of a recipe you make often, and the ingredients and steps you take to prepare it. Do you brown meat and onions for main dishes routinely? If so, cook a large batch of meat and onions and freeze them in portions for one recipe. Vegetables like onion, celery, and peppers can be chopped ahead and frozen.

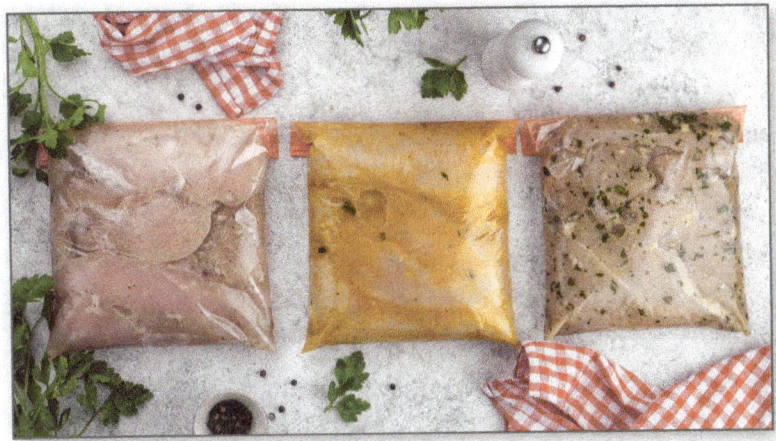

Freeze food at different points in the recipe to maximize convenience. Consider which point in the recipe is best to freeze for your preferences: before or after it is cooked? If you prefer freshly-baked, you should freeze the batter or dough before baking your food. If you want quicker access to the food, or want to run your oven less, freeze after it is baked.

Let's consider cookies as an example. Suppose you double a recipe of cookie dough. You can either bake the whole batch, then freeze finished cookies; or make dough balls and freeze those. The advantage of baking first is that cookies are ready to eat as soon as they are thawed. Energy is saved because the oven is used once. The

TIP

Freeze chopped veggies on a cookie sheet. Once frozen, remove and place in glass mason jars and return them to the freezer. Tray freezing first allows pieces to be individually frozen so individual portions can be removed without thawing. You don't have to use glass jars, but they will keep strong-smelling vegetables like onions and peppers from flavoring other food in the freezer—unlike plastic containers.

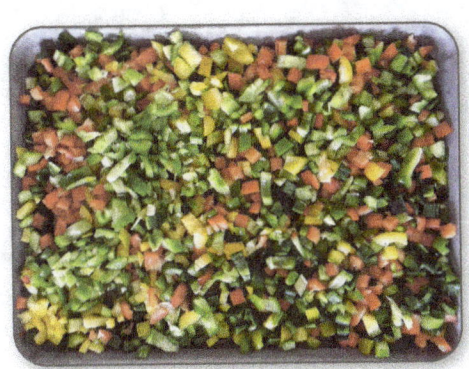

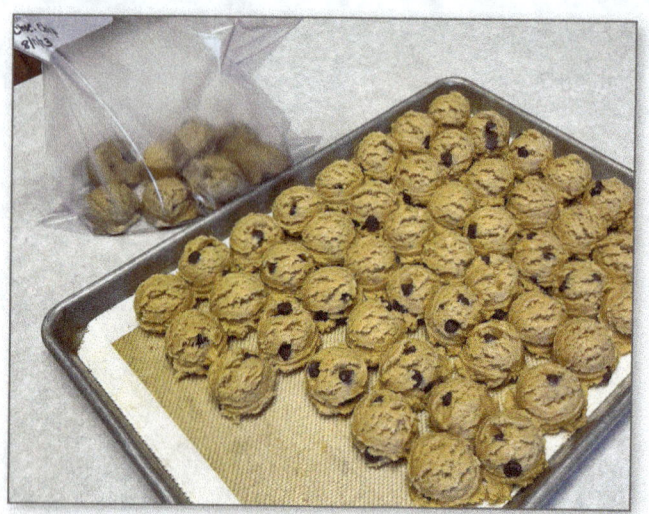
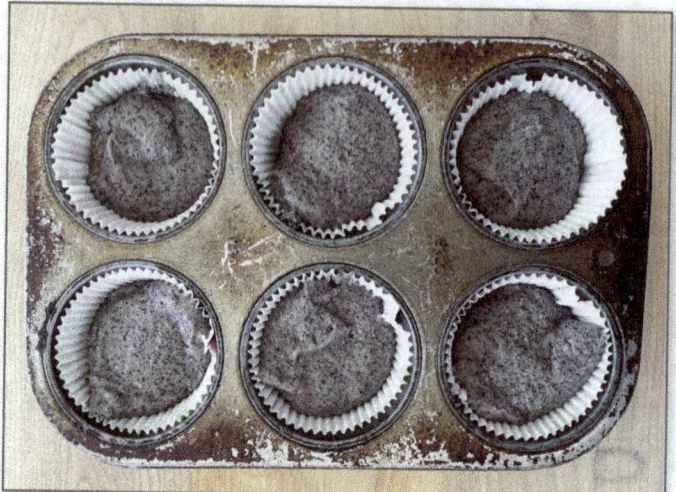

advantage of freezing dough balls is that you can enjoy fresh baked cookies any time you want or eat raw cookie dough to your heart's content. Cakes and muffins can also be frozen as a batter in cupcake papers. Once frozen, it is best to move to an airtight freezer container. You can also bake cakes or muffins first then freeze.

Strategy 5: Adapt a Few Key Recipes

Making variations of favorite recipes saves time and failures. You probably won't have to consult a recipe since you know it already and most likely have the necessary ingredients on-hand. For instance, I have two cake recipes, two cookie recipes, and a stir fry recipe (described in Chapter 6: Converting Recipes) used for 95% of all the foods I make in those categories, but they are not always the same flavor. These recipes are easy to change with additions, flavorings, and seasonings.

For example, one of my cake recipes is a quick chocolate zucchini cake. I use it often and don't need to glance back and forth at the recipe. When making a non-chocolate flavor, I omit the cocoa and add the equivalent amount of flour. I have also added extracts or spices to change the flavor, and other fruits and vegetables to replace zucchini, including squash, apples, pears and carrots. We have included the recipe in our recipe section (page 240-241).

---

[1]James, S. (2017, June 1). Cooking at home tonight? It's most likely cheaper and healthier, UW study finds. Retrieved May 4, 2023, from https://sph.washington.edu/news-events/news/cooking-home-tonight-its-most-likely-cheaper-and-healthier-uw-study-finds

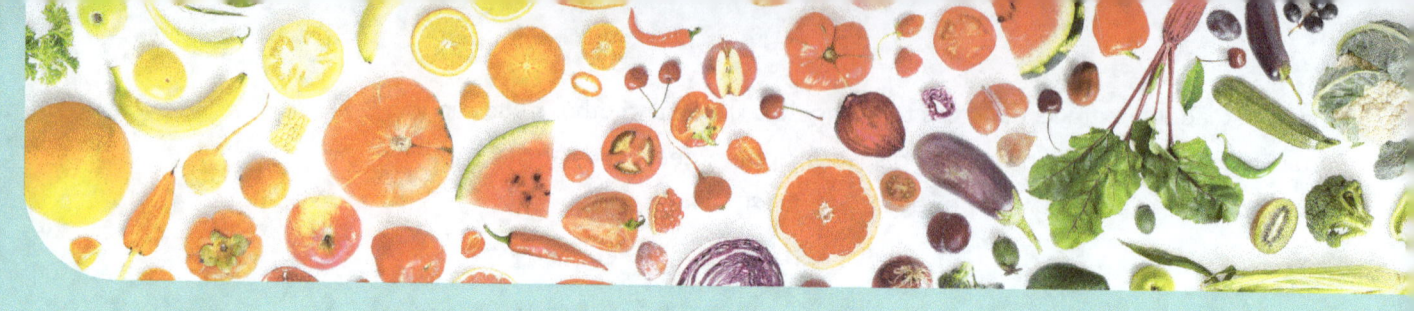

CHAPTER EIGHT
Gluten Free BAKING

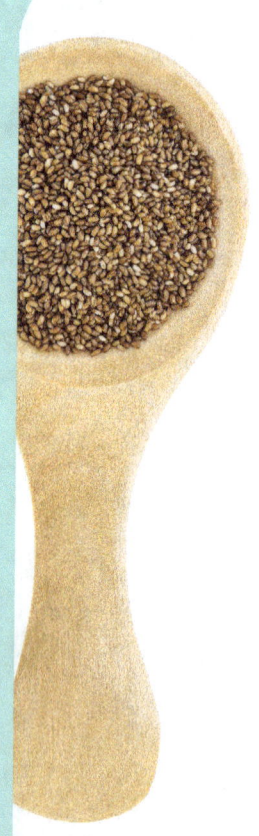

Charting Your Course in Gluten-Free Baking

Everyone likes some kind of baked goods but before you jump into the world of gluten-free home baking, be sure to honestly acknowledge your values and habits. This will greatly decrease your frustration throughout the process of mastering gluten-free baking. Answer the questions below to determine your approach in the kitchen.

- What drives my diet choices most: time, money, or nutrition?

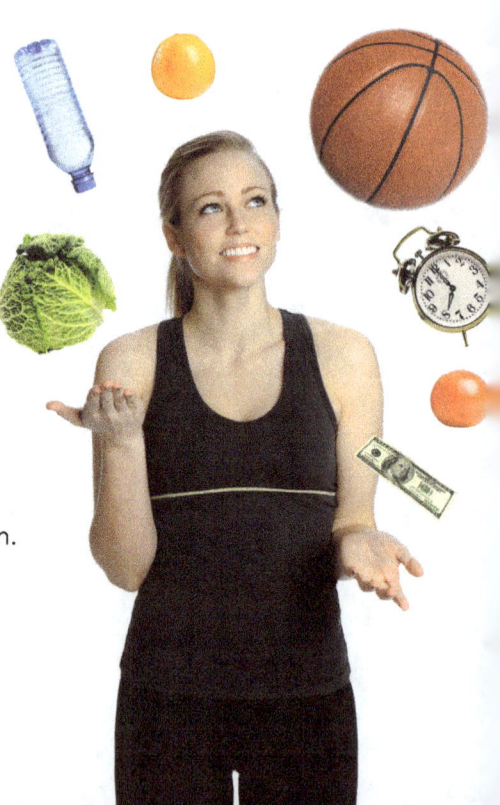

- Do I like to cook or bake?

- How much time am I willing to spend in the kitchen?

- Am I patient with kitchen experimentation and failure?

- Does my budget allow me to purchase pre-made gluten-free baked goods?

- Do I want to implement a more healthful diet?

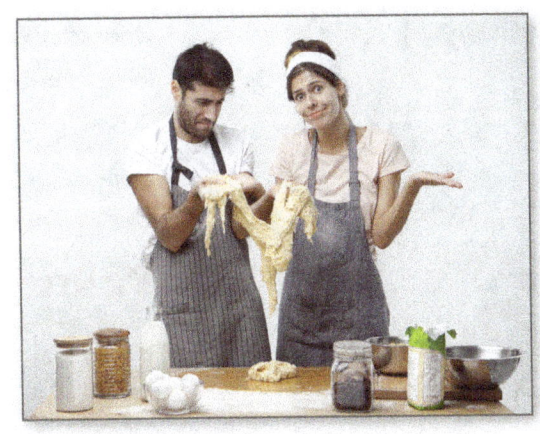

Don't like to cook or bake? You can purchase ready-made gluten-free foods. They are quick, easy, and widely available at many different food markets. On the downside, they are quite expensive, have high amounts of sugar, and are often calorie-dense and nutrient low. Convenient but expensive.

Don't like to bake and have a tight budget of time, money, or patience? Using pre-packaged gluten-free baking mixes can save time and overcome lack of experience. Walmart's gluten-free aisle is a good place to start if you are on a tight budget. Take advantage of sales and coupons as well. Find a good all-purpose commercially produced flour blend for the times you need to use flour (see Chapter 9: All About Flour). You can also find a few easy-to-make treat recipes and bake ahead and freeze (see Chapter 7: Five Strategies to Make Cooking Convenient).

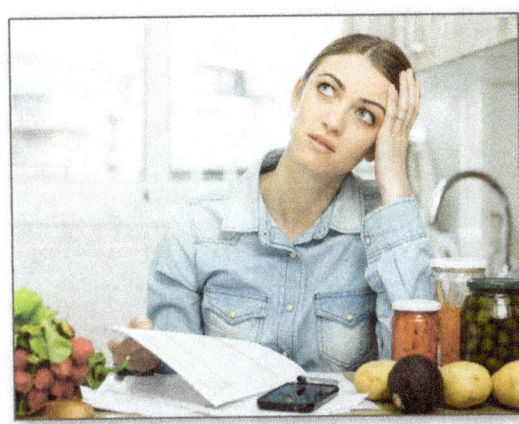

To select for budget and nutrition, buy some prepared foods and treats but change your diet focus to naturally gluten-free foods. Fruits and vegetables are delicious and take little prep time. Think outside the box for dessert options, like yogurt with gluten-free granola and fresh fruit. You can also look for whole grain flours for baking. There are several commercially available gluten-free options. King Arthur® is a good partly whole grain option, and Tree Street® Grains make excellent 100% whole grain flours or make your own (see recipes on pages 245-248).

If you like baking but have a low failure tolerance or are new to gluten-free baking, start with a good commercial flour blend and substitute into your previous wheat flour recipes. Start with quick breads, muffins and brownies before branching out to cookies and breads. This is a good place to start even if you were an experienced baker before going gluten free. From there, you can expand to other recipes.

Failures in the Kitchen

One of the frustrating things about being diagnosed with celiac, gluten intolerance, or allergy is losing cooking knowledge overnight. How you cook and bake, and what and where you can eat, are changed instantly. Baking is a special challenge to master until you learn a few principles related to gluten-free baking success. In the meantime, you will have cooking failures. Don't despair—failures are opportunities to learn. No one started cooking gluten free knowing what to do!

A wise kindergarten teacher once told me that children naturally believe, "If it's worth doing, it's worth doing badly." The price of learning is failure. Children are not afraid of failure. They fail many times every day. As an adult, you may not be as comfortable with failure but it's the price of improvement. People I've taught in gluten-free cooking classes often express an unwillingness to experiment due to high ingredient cost. Eating gluten free is expensive, but keep

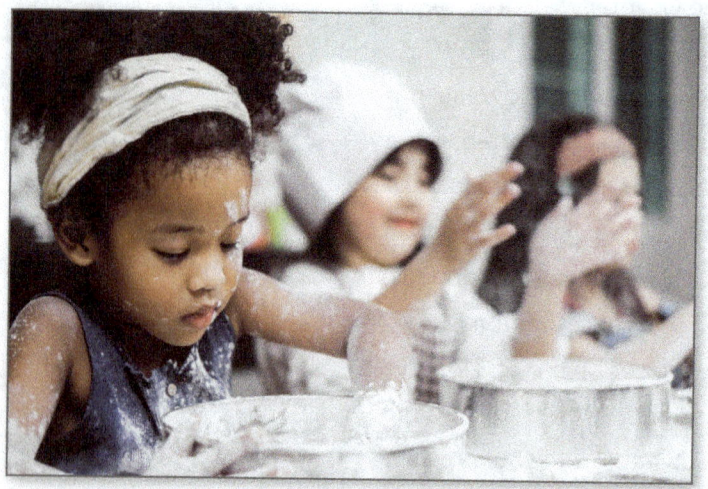

it in perspective. Gluten-free flour costs roughly five times more than white all-purpose flour from wheat. *But even so,* your whole recipe is going to cost only a few dollars. Compare that to the time and cost of attending a cooking class. Experimenting is a cheap education.

Still, failure is painful. One tactic to reduce failures is to concentrate on learning one or two foods at a time. Another key to quicker success is understanding principles to enable you to figure out what went wrong in the recipe. I recommend cookbooks like Nicole Hunn's *Gluten-Free on a Shoestring* series, and America's Test Kitchen *How Can It Be Gluten-Free* books as a great place to start learning gluten-free cooking principles. It is helpful to read the non-recipe pages of cookbooks for information as well as recipes.

Beginning Baking Tips

Follow the Recipe

Gluten-free flour is not as forgiving as wheat flour. Follow the recipe exactly the first time. If it succeeds, you will know the recipe is sound. Then if you vary ingredients later and the outcome changes, you will know why.

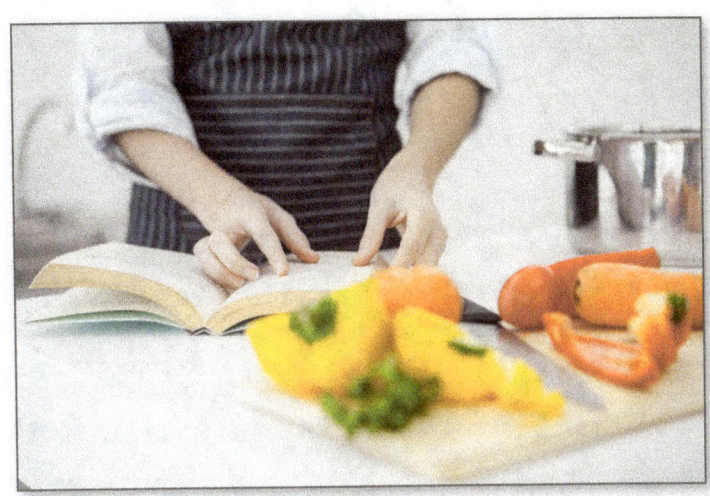

How to Measure Flour

It is a good idea to stir flour blends before measuring since heavier ingredients in the blend can settle out. Unless the recipe indicates the method of measuring flour, measure by lightly spooning flour into your measuring cup then leveling. Gluten-free flours are not standardized and contain highly packable ingredients, so scooping directly from the package will add too much to your recipe. **The absolute best way to measure gluten-free flour is to weigh it** because measuring by volume is highly variable between cooks. Look for recipes that include weights and you will achieve more consistent results.

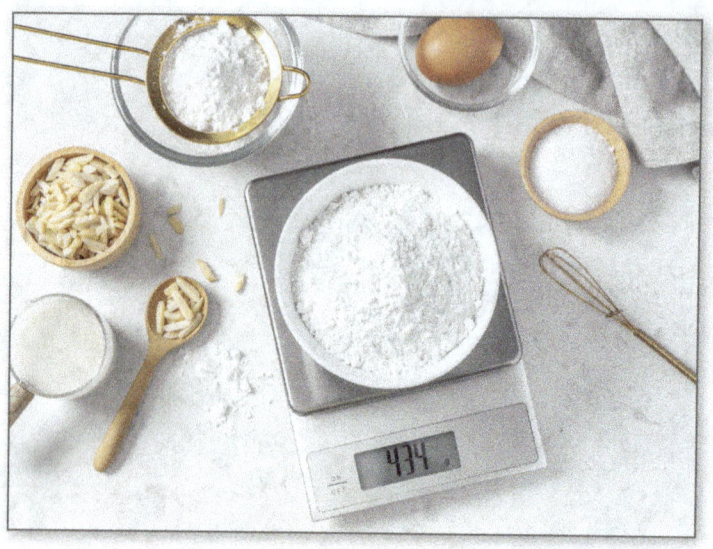

Measuring flour is faster than weighing, and if you measure consistently you can progress from weighing to measuring with recipes you use often. To master precision, measure your ingredients before putting them on a scale. Measure using the same cups and methods each time. Whenever I create a new baking mix for my company, I have multiple employees make it up following package directions. The variability in the final products is huge because of the ingredients they measure and add. However, my results are very uniform because I use the same measuring procedure every time.

Pay Attention to the Before and After Appearance

Each gluten-free flour performs differently, mostly because of different hydration rates among components. Notice the consistency of the batter or dough before you bake, then note your final result. Did it fall? Is it dry? What is the consistency? Liquid volume almost always needs to be adjusted between flour blends, so if you learn what a type of dough or batter (e.g. cookie, bread, muffin) is supposed to look like, you can adjust better on future recipes.

One way to hedge your bets when making a recipe with a new flour blend is to add ½ cup less flour than the recipe calls for then bake one cookie or muffin. If the cookie spreads too much or the muffin doesn't have enough structure to support itself, add the rest of the flour then bake the whole batch.

Don't Forget the Gums

Most recipes, except for some pancake and crepe recipes, require a gum like xanthan or guar to replace the structure-building elements of gluten. Check your flour's ingredient list. If your flour blend does not include a gum, you must add it.

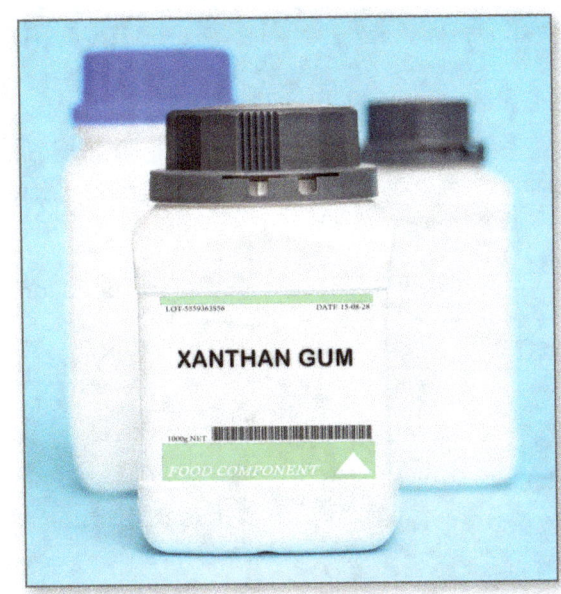

Most commercial blends add xanthan from 1 to 2% of the flour weight. In home cooking, the rule of thumb is ¼ tsp – 1 tsp per cup of flour. A quarter tsp is usually used for pancakes, ½ tsp is a good all-purpose flour starting point, and 1 tsp is usually best for high-structure recipes like bread or recipes made with coarser home milled flour. If your recipe is crumbly and falls apart, increase your gums. If it is gummy and rubbery, decrease the amount of gum.

Recipes with weights of ingredients often give a measured amount for gums since the weight of a teaspoon of gum is below the accuracy threshold of most kitchen scales. Use 4 grams as the weight of a teaspoon of xanthan gum. We experimented in our test kitchen with different people and different measuring spoon sets and the weight was pretty consistent at 4 grams.

Add Flavor with Different Gluten-Free Flours

Many people don't realize how flavorful wheat flour is until they try gluten-free flour. Gluten-free flours with high percentages of rice flour and starch are bland — experiment with adding other grain flours besides rice. Our favorites are sorghum and teff based on flavor and texture effects.

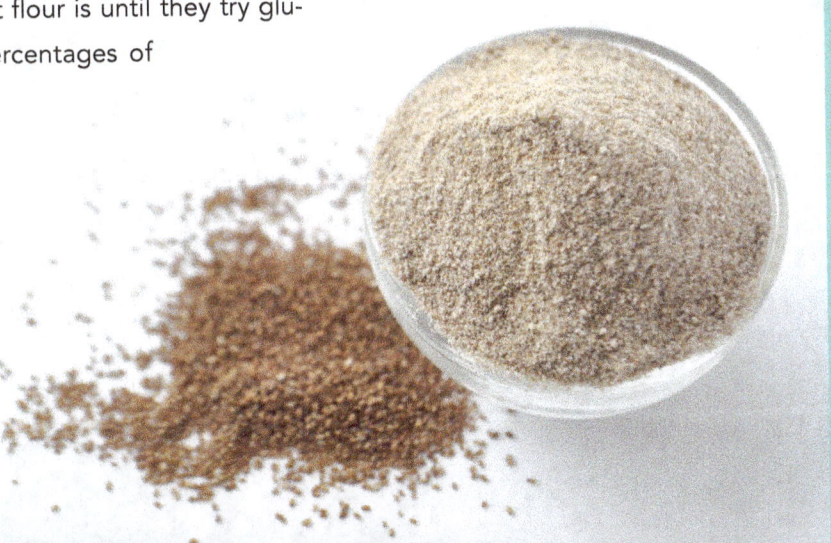

Adjust Gluten-Free Baking Time

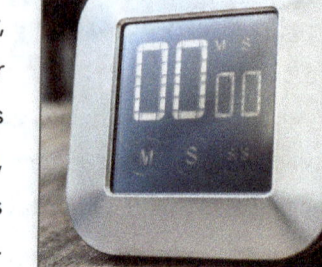

To adequately hydrate the starches in the flour, gluten-free batters contain more water than their analogous wheat flour batters, which increases baking time. Some recipes, most notably bread, look done long before they really are. If recipes need more baking time but are getting too brown, they can be covered

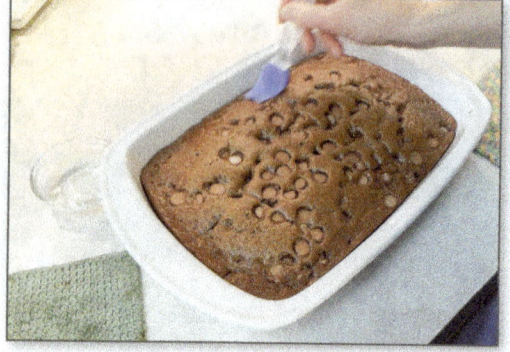

lightly with foil part way through baking. Sometimes the edges of baked goods like cake get too dry in the time it takes to adequately bake the center. When this happens, brush the edges with a little water using a pastry brush while the cake is still warm. For breads, brush with oil, butter, or butter substitute to keep the crust soft after baking.

Decrease Grittiness

Allowing batters to sit up to 30 minutes before baking allows time for starches to become fully hydrated. This will decrease the grittiness sometimes associated with gluten-free baked goods. Some flours, especially rice, are more prone to grittiness. When creating your own flour blend, buy ultra-fine flours, especially rice flour.

Start with Small Batches

Use small batches to test recipes first. Once you know a strategy or recipe works, you can make more. Gluten-free baked goods also stale much faster than foods made with wheat, so smaller batches can reduce waste due to freshness problems. If you make large batches, freeze to preserve.

Mix Generously

With the exception of bread, wheat flour recipes instruct minimal stirring because mixing makes gluten toughen. Gluten-free recipes can't get tough this way and extra beating of batter often improves texture by facilitating air incorporation and more time to hydrate starches and gums, so go ahead and whip it up.

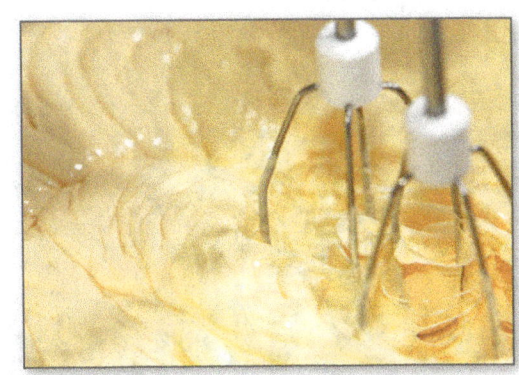

Limiting Greasiness

Sometimes baked recipes that have been converted to gluten free have a greasy mouthfeel or changed texture. This effect can be very pronounced in cookie recipes. Possible solutions are to reduce the oil or butter a bit, or swap some of the butter for oil. If you want to experiment, try a batch of cookies made with shortening and one made with oil. You will probably be surprised.

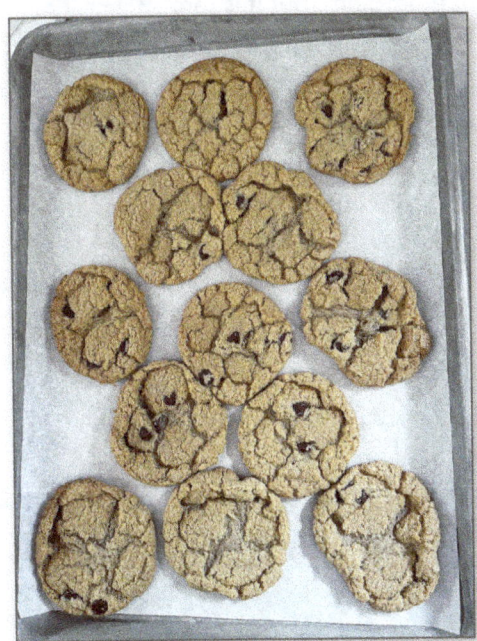

Gluten free cookies made with oil

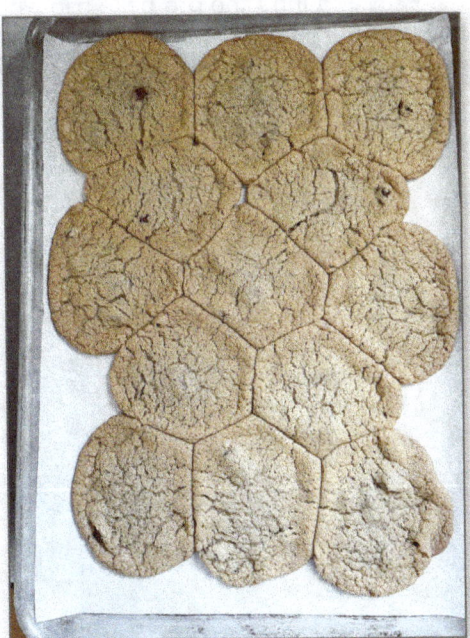

Gluten free cookies made with shortening

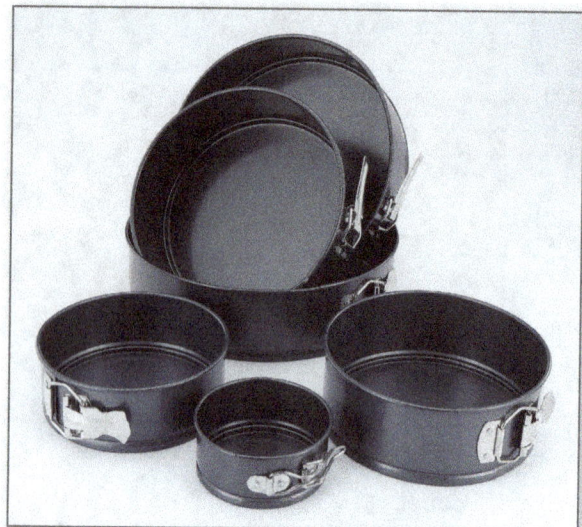

Pan Size Matters

You probably already know this and just didn't realize it. The walls of pans support the structure of baked goods as they set up during baking. This is why certain cakes like angel food are traditionally baked in tube or loaf pans. A regular cake pan has too much distance from the sides to support angel food batter during baking. This applies to even more gluten-free batters, especially breads.

If a recipe instructs a certain pan size, use that size. If you don't have the right pan size, use the closest size you have. Be aware that the recipe might turn out with a lower than expected rise in your larger pan. Because of this, I don't use wide bread pans or let batter rise above the edge of the pan before baking. Some high-protein breads can rise higher than the top during the pre-bake rise without a problem, but it is rare.

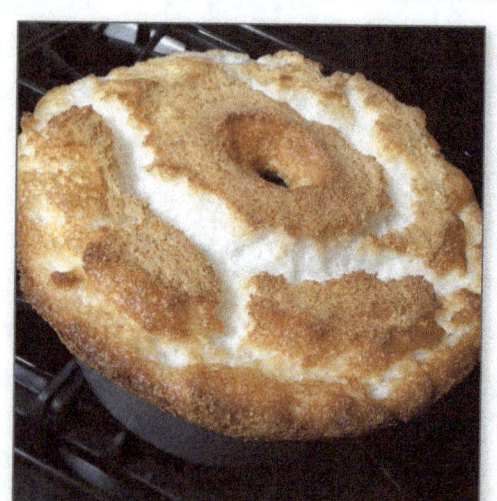

TROUBLESHOOTING IN BAKING

BAKED GOOD	PROBLEM	POSSIBLE SOLUTIONS
Cakes	Greasy	Substitute oil for all or part of butter
	Dense	Decrease fat or use fat containing dairy or chocolate instead
	Gummy Center/Falls	Increase baking time
		Decrease oven temperature (rises in oven then falls before baking is finished)
		Add structure builders like eggs, gums, or starch
	Gritty	Allow batter to rest for 15-30 minutes, use blend with less rice flour
Muffins/ Quick Breads	Crumbly	Add eggs or gums
	Dry	Decrease flour, bake less
	Dense	Add a little extra leavening
	Gritty	Let batter rest 15-30 minutes before baking
Cookies	Spread too much	Add more flour in small increment
		Add/increase gums
		Chill dough prior to baking
	Gritty	Replace some of the shortening in the recipe with liquid oil or melted butter
	Hard texture	Replace white sugar with brown sugar
Yeast Breads	Flat loaves	Use more liquid in recipe
		Add high protein flour to the blend
		Use smaller pan to allow more support of dough
		Don't allow loaf to rise to the top of the pan or add a foil collar to support the loaf
	Dense or cake like texture	Add psyllium
	Gummy center	Bake longer. Internal temperature should be 205 - 210° F
		Note: Temperature should not be checked until the recipe baking time is up. Checking too soon can cause bread to fall.

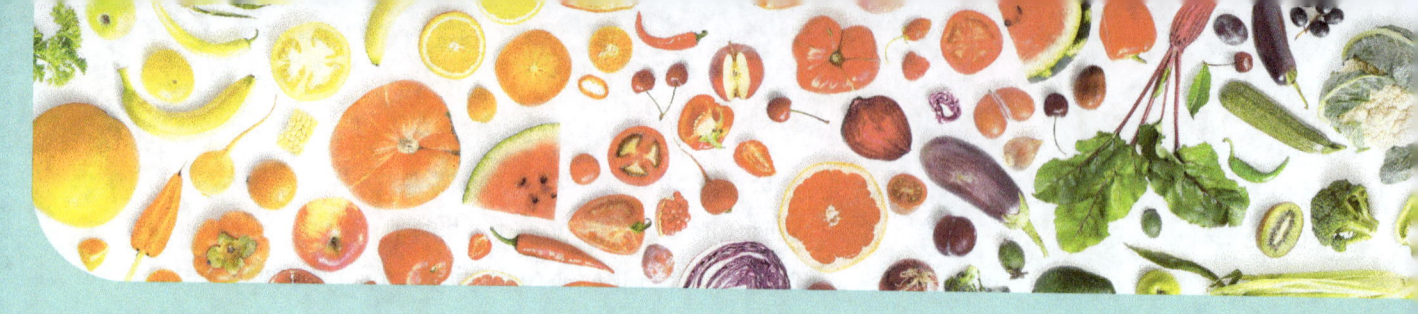

CHAPTER NINE
REPLACING Wheat Flour

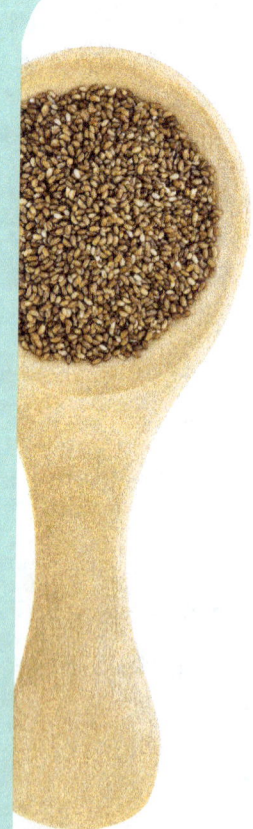

WHEN IT COMES TO GLUTEN-FREE FLOUR, not much of what you know about wheat flour applies. This chapter is all about finding or making flour that works for you. Understanding the functions of flour will also help you troubleshoot problems as they arise.

Finding Your First Flour

We recommend starting your gluten-free baking journey with a commercially-available, gluten-free flour blend. This will make your transition more natural, especially if you are new to cooking or baking at home. Many brands of gluten-free flour perform well in non-yeast bread recipes. Keep in mind that there is no truly "all purpose" flour in the world of gluten free, and you will need a different flour for bread than other baked items.

Try one flour blend at a time when baking. Do not be discouraged if you try multiple brands before you find one that performs to your satisfaction in your recipes. Read reviews of flours or look for advice on social media groups to find flour blends that sound promising.

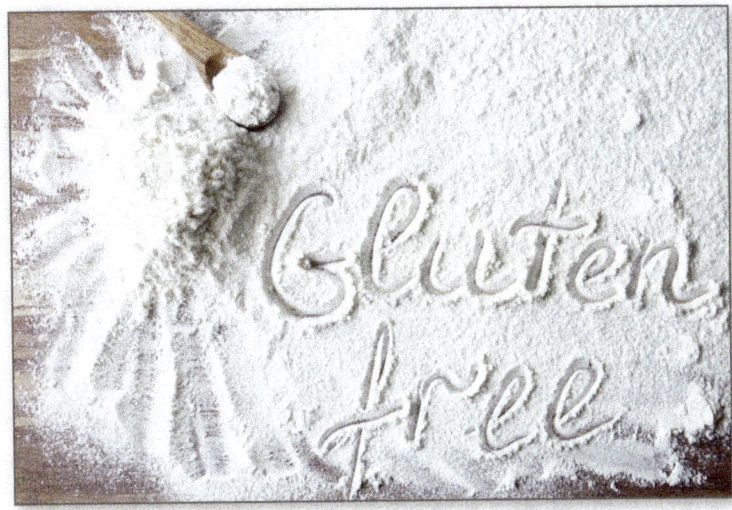

Flours that can best replace white flour cup for cup in recipes have several common characteristics: they are a blend of different flours, have a high starch content, and contain xanthan or guar gum. These fluffy white-type flours often use white and brown rice as the main ingredients. If you like the texture that a flour blend provides but find it bland tasting, add 1 tsp-1 tbsp teff flour per cup of flour to improve flavor. To do this, I add the teff to the measuring cup first then fill with the flour blend.

Understanding the Functions of Flour

Knowing what regular wheat flour does in recipes is tremendously helpful in troubleshooting problems and converting recipes. This section explains the main functional properties of flour and how to correct for weaknesses in gluten-free systems.

Function 1: Thickening

Wheat flour is often used to thicken sauces and gravies. It contains protein and fats which act as binders and stabilizers in the sauce as well as starch, which thickens. The cheapest and easiest replacement is cornstarch and it works in most applications.

Cornstarch has a few limitations, however. It is pure starch, which does not bind some ingredients in sauce as well as flour. In the case of sauces that use a rue, like white sauce, use a gluten-free flour blend. The flours and xanthan gum in the blend can bind and stabilize these ingredients. Corn starch can also break down if heated too high. Its maximum thickening happens just below boiling temperature.

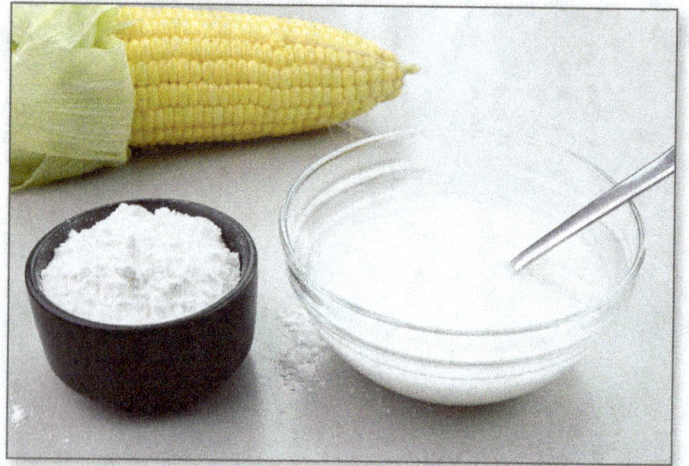

Thickening for Cooking: To use cornstarch as a sauce thickener, first mix thoroughly with cold water until it forms a smooth slurry. Add the slurry near the end of cooking to avoid overcooking. Generally, less cornstarch is needed to thicken than traditional flour.

Thickening for Baking: Another less obvious need for thickening is in batters. A batter must be thick enough to support the gas bubbles being formed by leaveners like baking powder or yeast until the batter has baked enough to set the structure. If the batter lacks sufficient thickening, bubbles collapse and the finished product will be dense and flat. Knowing this gives you possible solutions. For instance, starches and gums can be added. Gluten-free batters also thicken as they sit. This gives starches and gums time to hydrate and thicken, which also decreases falling and grittiness common in gluten-free baked goods.

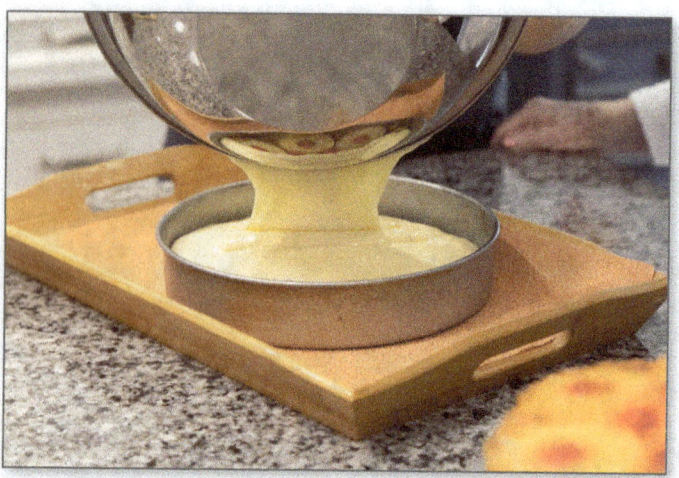

Function 2: Building Structure

Wheat flour's most important function in baking is forming the structure of the food. Gluten is a wheat protein that forms a stretchy network in the presence of water and heat. This network surrounds and stabilizes the starch granules that swell in the batter and holds them while the structure solidifies through baking. Lack of structure can cause batters to collapse, and finished products to be dense and undercooked in the middle. This is visually evident in gluten-free breads that lack sufficient structure. The top of the loaf may be fluffy with lots of baked-in air pockets, while the bottom is more dense and has visibly smaller air pockets. Or, your baked good may look perfect in the oven, but later on when you pull it out, it totally collapses. In such cases, the leavening worked but the structure capacity of the batter was insufficient.

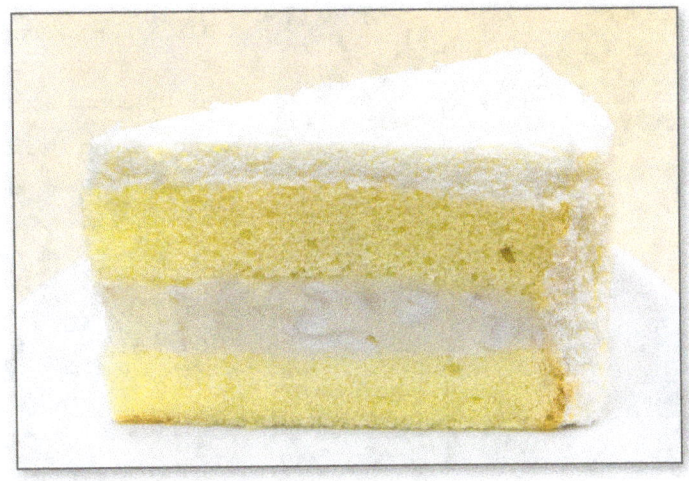

Note the texture of this cake. The batter had sufficient thickening and structure elements to hold and retain the air pockets that make it light.

Most gluten-free flour blends are high in starch but lack sufficient binding and structure building ability without structure builders included. Common structure building additives are **xanthan**, **guar**, or **psyllium (fiber)**. These also help retain moisture, and improve shelf life and texture. Gums are usually included in commercially-available flour blends, but if not, you can add them yourself.

Flour structure problems can also be improved by increasing the protein content of the flour blend with additions of powdered milk, bean flours, eggs, or soy. Eggs can be extremely important in building structure and binding ingredients in gluten-free recipes as well. Don't be surprised to see eggs in gluten-free recipes which don't usually contain eggs, like biscuits. They can make an amazing difference in the lightness of baked goods.

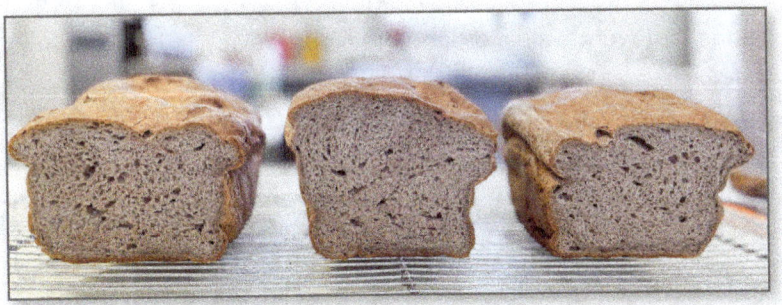

These loaves were made with bean flours of different protein levels. The middle loaf has the highest protein content. Note that it has the highest rise and fewer collapsed air cells at the bottom of the loaf.

Function 3: Coating

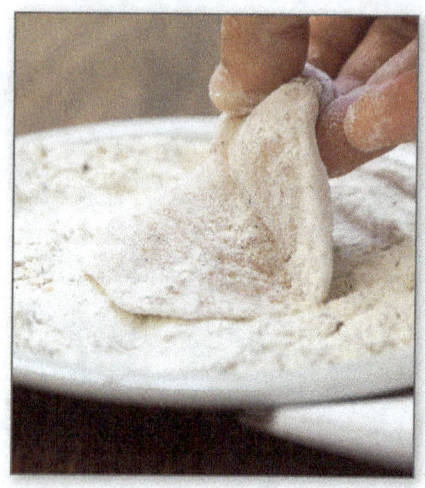

Flour functions as a coating in breaded recipes. The starch in wheat flour aids browning and crisping, and the protein helps bind breading to food. A

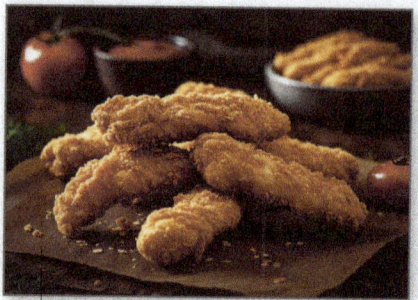

cornstarch dusting followed by an egg dip can work well for breading foods. Try gluten-free versions of cereals like cornflakes and crispy rice, crushed potato or corn chips, or make your own gluten-free bread crumbs for final breading.

Creating Your Own Flour

If you like baking, blending your own flour opens up the world of gluten-free baking and can save money. No single gluten-free grain has the composition of wheat, so combinations of grains, starches, and gums must be used to achieve the same properties as traditional flour. Each ingredient has a different effect on the recipe, and blending your own allows you to select for your own preferences in flavor, nutrition, and performance. Many commercial blends lean heavily on rice and starch because it is cheap and provides good texture, but comes at the price of flavor and nutrition.

Recipes for flour blends abound on the internet and in cookbooks, and can serve as your starting point. After experimentation, most cooks settle into one or two blends that work well in their own favorite recipes. Understanding a little more about what's in a blend and why it's there will make it easier to evaluate and adapt flour recipes to suit yourself.

Finding the Balance

Good flour blends find the right balance of starch and protein by using a mix of high-protein flours and starch, either from refined starches or starchy grain flours. Too much protein can leave a recipe heavy, under-leavened, and pasty. Too little protein and recipes take on a starchy taste and tex-

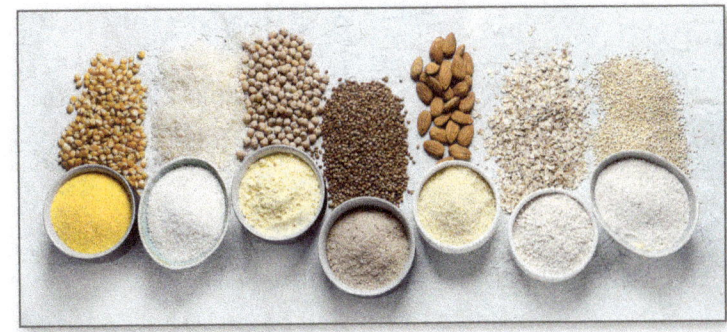

ture. Protein and starch provide structure in different ways and times throughout the baking process, and both are needed.

Choose which protein-containing flours you want to add based on what you want the texture and flavor of the finished product to be. For instance, **bean flour** is wonderfully nutritious and has high protein but tastes like beans and is best suited for stronger-flavored recipes. Chickpea is the mildest of the bean flours.

Oat flour can add creaminess and improve texture. **Nut flours** like almond add flavor and moist-
ness but give a denser crumb. The table of flours
on pages 94-97 gives more information about the
specifics of different flours to help you choose.

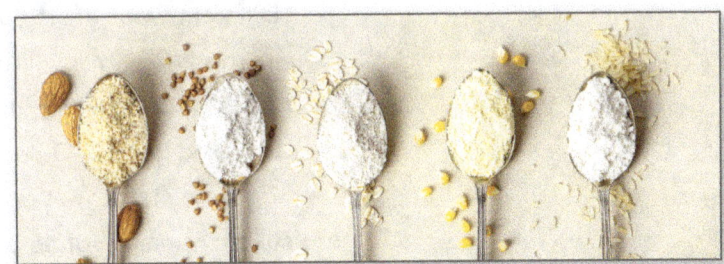

Select for Flavor and Color

The flavor and color of flour should complement the overall appeal of the finished product. For instance, brown teff tastes like wheat with a hint of molasses, and has a flat brown color rather than golden brown. If the flat brown color looks un-appetizing in the recipe, use a lighter-colored ivory teff instead. Some flours like bean, quinoa, and buckwheat have flavors that can detract from the desired flavor of your recipe.

Adding Starch

With the right blend of grains you can do without refined starches like corn or tapioca in a flour blend because grains naturally contain starch—see the recipe for Jaylee's 100% whole-grain flour in the recipe section (page 246). Hundred percent whole-grain, gluten-free flours boast high nutrition and flavor but give slightly denser, coarser texture (think of whole wheat vs. white bread). One hundred percent whole grain flours are well suited for bread, pancakes, muffins, and graham crackers.

You can also choose a happy medium result with whole grain flours plus added starch. With this blend you get a more thickened batter and a lighter texture from the starch, while rounding out the flavor and boosting nutrition with whole grains. My whole grain all-purpose flour recipes contain 25% starch (see Jaylee's Whole Grain All Purpose Flour recipe on pages 248-249).

Different types of starches may also be mixed to make subtle differences in texture. This is why many flour-blend recipes call for different starches. **Tapioca starch** (also called tapioca flour) is the most all-purpose and gives a nice, springy chew to baked goods. Other starches commonly used in combinations are **cornstarch**, **potato starch** (not potato flour), and **arrowroot**. A small addition of **potato starch** increases softness and mellows flavor and is often included in flour for rolls and cookies.

Adding Gums

Chapter 8 described the need for gums like guar and xanthan to build structure. Almost all recipes will require one to succeed. Xanthan is considered the best for almost everything. If xanthan bothers you, see our flours table on p. 94-97 for replacement equivalents. Yeast breads and pizza crusts are greatly improved with either psyllium or a mix of xanthan and psyllium. Psyllium powder can be found in health food stores and is the main ingredient in Metamucil®.

Some bakers prefer to use flour that comes with a percentage of xanthan added already rather than having to add it for each recipe. Some prefer to use flour without xanthan included and add their own to each recipe for more control of the final texture. I found this to be an issue while trying to make a good pancake from commercial flours which included xanthan gum. No matter what recipe I tried, the pancakes felt like a sponge in my mouth. When I used flour without xanthan and added my own at a lower level the pancakes were much better.

There are general rules about how much xanthan or guar to use per cup of flour (see pg 81), but in our tests the needed level changed with the fineness of the flour. I discovered this phenomenon by testing home-milled flour and commercially-milled flour in duplicate recipes. A coarser flour needs slightly increased gum levels.

Choosing Starch to Grain Flour Ratios

The proportion of grain flour to starch in your blend makes a big difference in performance and texture. Are you a fluffy white lover? A hearty whole grain type? My own preference is fluffy white for cookies and biscuits, but a partially whole grain for most other things, and 100% whole grain for certain breads, muffins and pancakes. Considering what you want your texture, flavor, and nutritional outcome to be can help you choose where to start in your experimenting. If aiming for a more "white" flour effect, start with 60% starch and 40% grain flour. If you want a whole grain flour, start with 30% starch and 70% grain flour ratio.

FLOURS

STARCHY FLOURS/ STARCH	FLAVOR	CHARACTERISTICS	TIPS
White Rice	Neutral	Makes crusts crisp, builds structure, gritty and dry in high percentages	Buy the finest grind and blend w/ other flours to decrease grittiness
Brown Rice	Nutty, earthy, can magnify off flavors in other ingredients	Gritty in high concentrations	Buy finest grind possible
Sweet Rice/Gluti-nous Rice	Neutral	Best in blends, binds moisture	
Potato Starch (not flour)	Neutral- slight starchy taste	Adds softness to baked goods. Can be heavy in high concentrations.	Best used sparingly w/ other starches. Requires more water and longer baking times.
Tapioca Starch/ Flour	Neutral	Very versatile, light, elastic texture	
Corn Starch	Neutral	Makes crusts crispy, "starchy" effect in high concentrations	Use half as much if replacing tapioca
WHOLE GRAIN & PROTEIN FLOURS			
Sorghum	Most wheat-like flavor	Slight grainy texture	Graininess improved by eggs and oil and combination with starch
Teff	Earthy, wheaty, hint of molasses	Heavy if used alone	Available in brown or ivory varieties. Ivory is milder and has a more white flour look.
Millet	Mild corn like flavor	Can be used alone but gives better rise, especially in yeast breads with other flours	Absorbs less water than other flours- decrease water in recipe
Corn	Sweet mild flavor	May give coarse texture, flavor blends and enhances other flours	Varied coarseness changes texture
Oat	Sweet, mild, nutty	Adds softness, sweetness	Adding to flour blends adds moisture and shelf life

USAGE	NUTRITION	OTHER
Most applications	Minimal due to high starch content	
	Contains oils, fiber, and vitamins absent in white rice	Short shelf life- store in cool place
Good thickener for soups and sauces. Binds and holds moisture to decrease grit. Helps bind water in whole grain flour blends. Good in breads, pastries and cakes	Minimal due to high starch content	Made from short grain or sticky rice. Easy to find in Asian markets. Can be considered as pure starch in flour blends.
Excellent addition to breads, cookies and cakes	Minimal due to high starch content	Can be substitued with sweet rice or arrowroot
Good thickener and binder, replaces flour coating in breaded recipes.	Minimal- mostly starch	Can be overly chewy in excess concentration
Exellent thickener for soups and sauces. Good coating for breaded recipes.	Minimal	
Excellent in combination with other flours, good in muffins, pancakes, crackers and cookies	High in complex carbohydrates, protein and fiber	Good replacement for oat flour in recipes
Works well in all applications. Best blended with other flours.	High in protein, fiber and minerals	Adding a Tbsp per cup of commercial blend all-purpose flour improves flavor
Good in crackers, quick breads and as a blend in other flours	Most easily digested grain, least allergenic	Flour stores for 4-6 months
Best in quick breads or in combinations with other flours	Highest concentration of antioxidants in grains	
Can be used alone in pancakes and muffins. Best used at 25% or less in other flour blends	Good source of fiber	Grind oatmeal in blender of food processor to make your own oat flour

(continued on next page)

FLOURS (CONTINUED)

WHOLE GRAIN & PROTEIN FLOURS	FLAVOR	CHARACTERISTICS	TIPS
Amaranth	Slightly sweet, earthy, strong	Best in blends, binds moisture	Use at 10-15% or less to increase structure in baked goods
Buckwheat	Nutty, earthy, strong	Absorbs water well, builds structure	Increase water in recipe
Quinoa	Earthy, grassy, slightly bitter	Light fluffy flour- can taste grassy in high concentrations	Use in blends for breads to add structure/protein
Almond	Nutty	High oil content adds richness, crisps crusts.	Sold as almond flour or meal
Chickpea	Slightly sweet, distinct	Adds softness, richness	As little as 1 Tbs/cup of flour improves texture, nutrition
Other Beans	Beany	Performs like chickpea with stronger flavor	
BINDERS			
Xanthan Gum	Neutral	Adds structure and dough stretch abscent in GF flour	
Guar Gum	Neutral	Adds structure and dough stretch abscent in GF flour	
Psyllium Husk	Wheat like	Builds structure and makes lighter texture especially in yeast breads.	
OTHER			
Ground Flax	Nutty	Serves as a binder and egg replacer	Finer grinds improve texture and replace eggs best
Chia	Neutral	Functions and nutrition similar to flax	

USAGE	NUTRITION	OTHER
Most applications if used in blends	Considered a superfood because of high protein and nutrient content	
Crepes, muffins, pancakes, quick breads	A complete protein, high in fiber and antioxidants	Can allow a decrease in starch percentage in flour blends
Good in most baked goods especially bread, cookies, savory pastry	Complete protein, high in minerals	
Especially good in cookies and cakes, adds structure	High in protein and healthy fats	Improves shelf life of baked goods
Serves as a thickener and structure builder	High in protein and B vitamins	Most wheat based flours are fortified with B vitamins and folate. Chickpea adds these naturally.
Similar to chickpea		The darker the bean the stronger the flavor
Best texture control when level is changed for specific recipes		Most commercial all-purpose flours contain 2% xanthan. Weight of flour x .02=xanthan weight to add.
Replaces xanthan 1:1 except in cookies which require 1:3		
Replaces xanthan 1:2 except in cookies which require 1:5		
Good in any baked good, especially breads and whole grain applications. Increases shelf life. If grinding from whole seeds use a coffee grinder-not a grain mill.	High in fiber and omega 3 fatty acids	Flax has a short shelf life and can develop off flavors quickly. Freezing preserves freshness.
		Has much longer shelf life than flax

Learning from an Experiment in Baking

This section walks you through one of my experiments to help you understand the practical applications of creating your own flour and recipes outlined in the section above. It also shows my thought process during experiments. I made one change at a time so the effect of each change would be obvious.

I chose this particular bread recipe because it is a no-fail type bread recipe. In other words, it's a muffin/quick bread recipe, plus yeast. The first round of the experiment was designed to show the properties of each flour. I replaced the entire volume of flour with one flour at a time. I used finely-ground commercial flours for this experiment.

Combine the following dry ingredients and mix well:

2 ¼ C Flour

2 tbsp Sugar

1 tbsp Yeast

2 tsp Baking Powder

¼ tsp Salt

1 tsp Xanthan Gum

1 tsp Psyllium Husk

Add:

1 ¼ C Water

2 tbsp oil

2 eggs

Stir to combine, then beat on high for 3 minutes. Place batter in a greased 8.5" x 4.5" loaf pan (the Pyrex size). Allow to rise about 1/2 inch from the top of the pan. Do not let batter rise to the top of the pan before baking. Bake at 350° F for 55 minutes or until internal temperature reaches 200-205° F. Place a sheet of foil lightly on top of the loaf halfway through baking to prevent over browning.

Remove from oven and allow to cool. Remove from pan and cut when completely cooled.

The Results

My first round of experimenting was to determine the properties of individual flours, so I used only one type of flour per batch with no added starches. Here is what I learned.

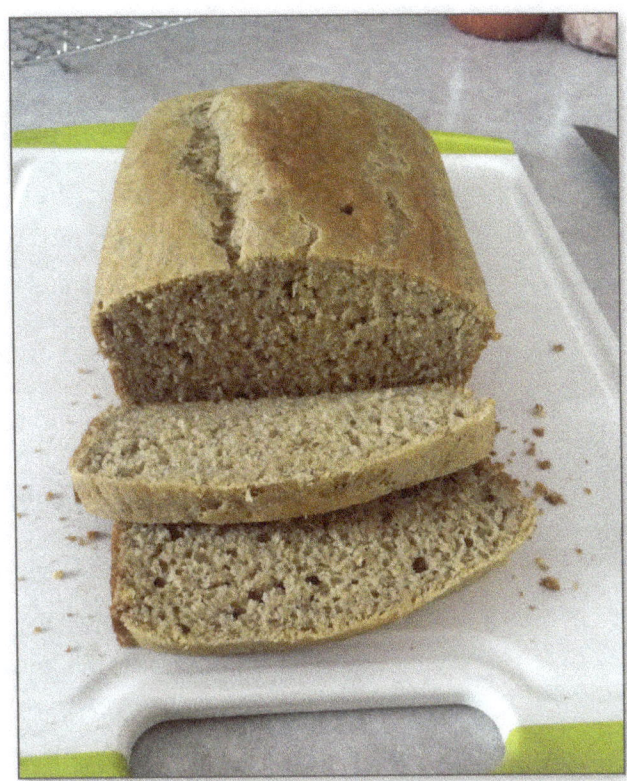

Rice flour: Brown, white, and parboiled. All varieties had decent texture and rise with slight graininess. No off tastes except the parboiled, which had a slight taste of evergreen. Parboiled rice is instant rice and has been partially cooked then dried to cook up faster. I theorized it would absorb water faster and give a better texture. That was wrong, and I didn't like the flavor.

Sorghum flour: Red or white worked equally well. Sorghum has a neutral wheat-like flavor and performed very well with rise and texture.

Teff flour: Brown or ivory both worked well. Teff has a high nutrient content, good flavor and performance. Brown teff has a stronger, molasses-like flavor, and ivory teff has a malt like flavor. Ivory teff made the loaf look more like white bread.

Corn flour: Unsurprisingly, produced a texture and flavor like cornbread but gave decent rise.

Buckwheat flour: Gave very nice texture because of its high protein and fiber content. It also required more water than the recipe called for because of the fiber. Flavor was not universally liked.

Millet flour: Had a distinct, but not unpleasant flavor. Produced a light, cake-like texture that did not absorb as much water as other flours. Water was decreased to prevent the loaf falling.

Quinoa flour: The texture was good, but the flavor was terrible. I threw that loaf in the garden and let the birds eat it. No one in the family would eat that one, not even me. Definitely a flour to add in small proportions.

Amaranth and oat flours both fell, and were gummy when used as the only flour in the recipe.

Lessons Learned from Initial Testing

Use any combination of the flours that will work alone, and the recipe will not fail. Knowing this gives you the power to change to your own tastes and specific allergies. I used this knowledge to help Kristi, a friend with multiple allergies, make a bread that she was not allergic to. We simply plugged in three flours totaling 2 ¼ C which she could eat: in her case teff, brown rice, and sweet rice. She had not eaten any form of bread for years and was overjoyed to have it back in her life.

Experiment Round Two

Next, I experimented adding in other flours and starches. I really love whole grain because of its wonderful nutrition and flavor, but still love the texture of white bread. Most of the things I bake are a compromise between these two ideals leaning more heavily towards whole grain, especially for breads and muffins. However, for cookies and cake I demand no nutrition, only decadent pleasure!

For these experiments I measured the flour and weighed it, too. I prefer weighing gluten-free flour (see chapter 8) to decrease failures, but since I develop products and recipes for consumers, I do both. My next addition was starch in the form of sweet rice flour since it has a very high starch content. When I measured,

I used 2 cups of grain flours and ¼ cup of starch. Weighed out, this calculates to 10% starch and 90% grain flour. Starch definitely improved the texture.

Next was the addition of minor flours, ones that cannot be used alone but can add important nutrients or textural properties. These went into the recipe at about ¼ cup. This is 10% but I found they can go into the blend at up to 25%.

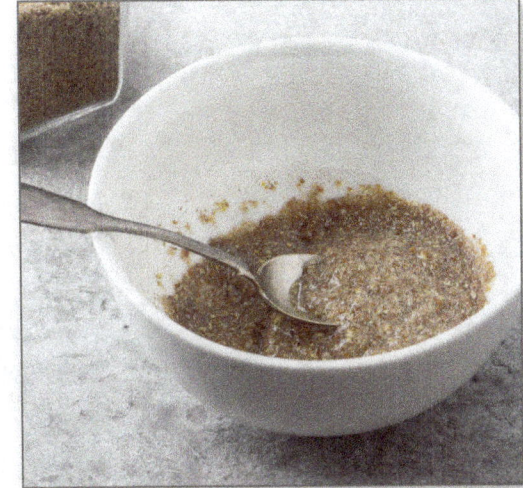

Amaranth, oats, and chickpea added more protein and improved the structure and rising ability. Amaranth and chickpea have nutrients that are often missing in gluten-free diets like lysine, and folate. Oats added smoothness to the final mouthfeel but also added a slight bitterness. Bitterness in oats surprised me because I think of oats as sweet and nutty, but I discovered that they have bitterness, too.

Experiment Round Three: Replacing Eggs

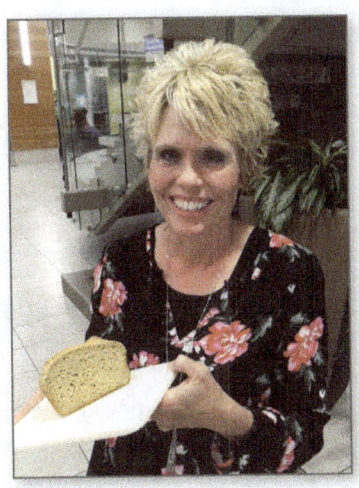

My friend Kristi is also allergic to eggs. From my experiments above, I knew which grains would work alone in no-fail bread. That was easy. I tried a "flax egg." Ground flax is my favorite egg replacement for baked goods because it extends shelf life and has a good flavor if you use fresh, quality flax.

For each egg in a recipe whisk 1 Tbsp ground flax into 3 Tbsp of warm water and allow to sit a few minutes until it develops a thick and egg-like consistency. The finer the flax is ground, the better this works. Ground chia seed will also work for egg replacement following the same instructions.

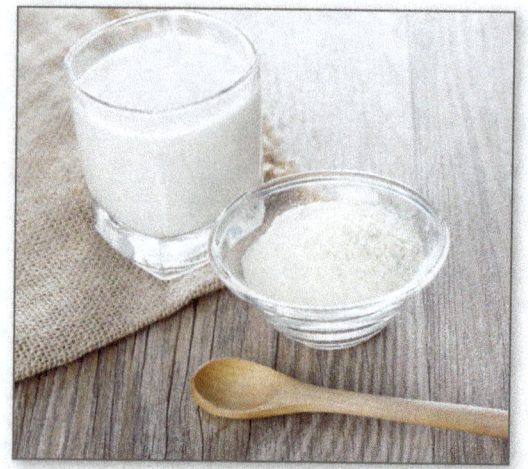

Adding Milk

I try to make gluten-free food without milk because so many people who can't eat gluten can't eat milk either. In fact, all my company's products are gluten AND dairy free. I did not even experiment with it for years, but gave in and tested it when I decided to write this book.

If you tolerate it, milk is a wonderful addition—almost a secret ingredient. A gluten-free baking hack. It is easy to add to a recipe in liquid form or by adding powdered milk to your flour blend. It improves texture and rounds out and enriches flavor. It can also mask some off flavors from gluten-free grains, and has the nutritional benefit of increasing protein and calcium. The *Gluten Free on a Shoestring* books and blog have several very good flour recipes that include milk you might try.

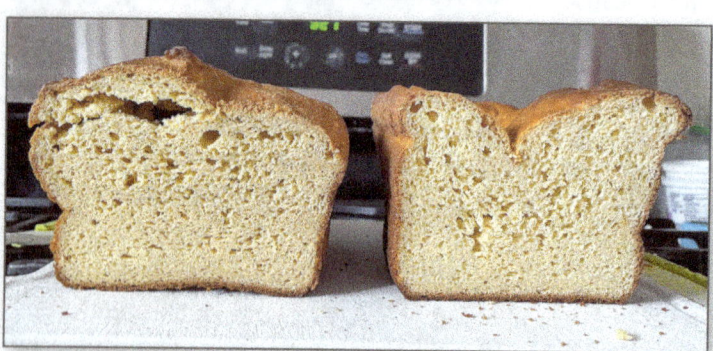

The recipe is the same for both loaves except that the liquid in the recipe on the left is milk. Note that the top did not collapse because of the increased structure the milk protein added.

Flour Texture Baking Experiment

When it came time to work on recipes for baking mixes for the book, I decided to test side by side three kinds of flour in a homemade white cake mix recipe (see page 262): home milled whole-grain, commercially milled whole grain, and a traditional high-starch, gluten free commercial white flour. For the whole grain milled and commercial whole grain blends we used the Jaylee's All-Purpose recipe on page 248-249. Our fluffy white commercial blend was my go to blend, Grandpa's Kitchen. The cakes came out with different textures and flavors but all were very good.

The Results

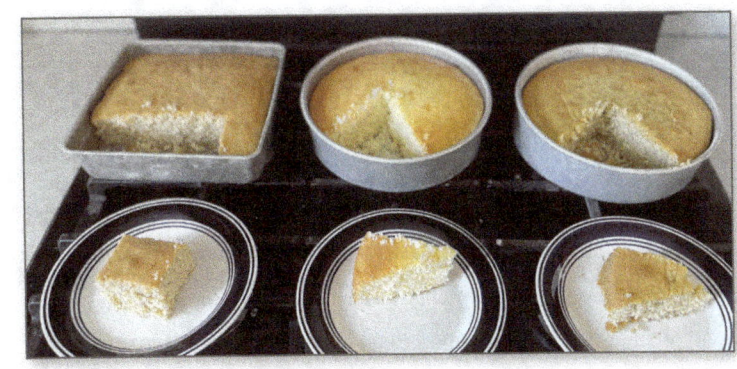

Commercially-produced, white gluten-free flour blend: The texture and flavor were just like a commercial cake mix. It had a similar light airy feel and tasted of vanilla. The second day it was still good but slightly dry, and the third day had significant drying. If you want a cake to taste like all the cakes you had before you were gluten free, this is the way to go.

Commercially-ground, whole grain flours blended at home: We used the same grain flours and proportions as the home ground flour in the trial below. This blend produced the best texture of all the flours. It was smoother and moister than the white flour and tasted like vanilla with a hint of whole grain flavor. It stayed moist longer than the high-starch flour but as it aged the bitterness of the flour intensified, though never becoming horrible.

Home-milled whole grain: This cake had the best flavor of all. It tasted like vanilla with a more prominent grain flavor without bitterness. The texture was cake-like except it had tiny grain pieces that could be felt when chewed, like you might expect in cornbread. This cake finished baking before the others because the flour absorbed more water. Remarkably, it was still moist and delicious at five days old, at which point my oldest son came to visit and ate all that was left.

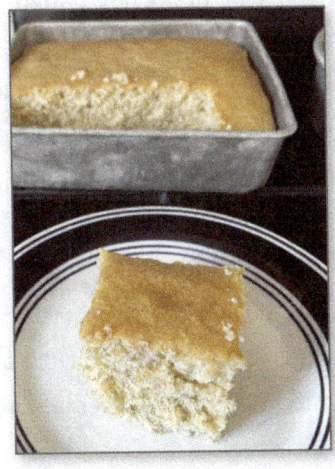
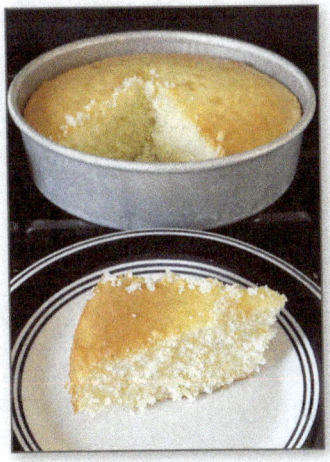
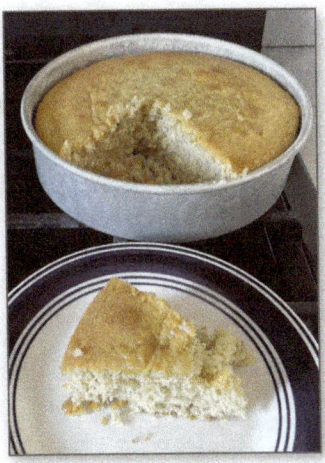

Commercial Milled Whole Grain

Commercial White Flour

Home Milled Whole Grain

MILLING YOUR OWN FLOUR

My gluten-free mix business did not begin with baked goods and flour, rather with a personal desire to have *everyone* eat together. I was looking for a dish which could be prepared without special recipes or training, had broad appeal, and would allow the people in my groups to eat together without even noticing a difference. The solution was gluten- and dairy-free cream soups which fit into every casserole recipe. As I spent more time in the gluten-free community, I realized how pathetic the nutrition in gluten-free food is. It bothered me that celiacs were cheated out of nourishing food!

About that time, I became friends with another local businessman: Dave Cobia, owner of Tree Street Grains, who had a mission to increase nutrition by using whole grains and milling them fresh. He created

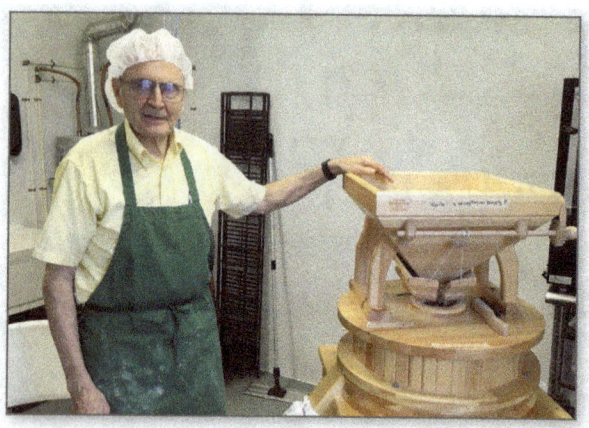

Dave Cobia milling grains

a 9-grain, 100% whole grain flour which was gluten free and actually performed well in recipes! I wanted his secret. I started buying his flour and making ancient grain muffin mixes to add a nutritious product to my line. Soon, I offered to buy the company. It took him several years, and turning 83, before I finally convinced him that he should sell to me. That was the beginning of my research and promotion of freshly-milled, gluten-free flours.

With the growing number of commercially available whole grain flours, why would anyone want to mill their own? It is definitely something not everyone can or wants to do, but there are some good reasons to consider it.

Reasons to Mill Your Own Flour

The flavor of freshly-milled flour is phenomenal. There is really no comparison between older flour and fresh flour. I knew that this was true from my days of milling wheat in my home kitchen, but I had no idea that in gluten-free flours it made an even bigger difference.

Another friend who owns a gluten-free flour company, Grandpa's Kitchen, said that she didn't put much sorghum flour in her blend because she didn't like the taste. I was puzzled because my experience with sorghum is a sweet, wheat-like flavor. The difference was she was buying her sorghum flour commercially, while I was milling my own. Later, I tried commercially milled sorghum flour and discovered that it had a little aftertaste not present in the freshly-ground version. If you are adventurous, home milling lends itself to all sorts of flavor experiments like roasting the grain first, combining different grains, or milling herbs into the flour.

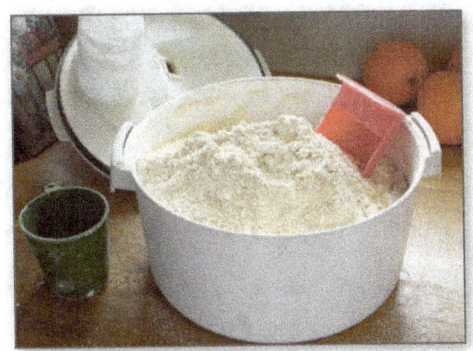

The nutrition of freshly-milled flour is unparalleled as well. Food exposed to air deteriorates—it's why we put plastic wrap on food. Flour particles are small and have more surface area exposed to oxidize and lose nutrients compared to an intact grain kernel. Nature also makes seeds resistant to degrading, preserving their ability to grow later. This doesn't mean you can't mill flour in advance of your needs, but it should be stored in the freezer for optimum nutrition and small batches are ideal. Many commercial flours also have the nutrient-rich bran layer and germ removed. Home-milled flour contains all the parts of the grain: bran, germ and endosperm.

Home milling gives you 100% control over what is in your flour. There are no added preservatives or bleaching agents. The flour is often less expensive than commercially milled, gluten-free flours when grains are purchased in bulk. However, this is not always the case since grain type and source pricing vary.

For long-term food storage and self-sufficiency, grains and a mill are indispensable. Flour maintains its peak nutrition for less than a year under ideal storage while intact grains store well for years. Home flour milling is popular among emergency preparedness groups and artisan bread bakers.

Considerations Before Embarking on Home Milling

Upfront cost of a grain mill. Grain mills range in price from $60 for an inexpensive hand mill to $500 for a top-line electric model. Mills also require countertop or cupboard space. A few things can be ground into flour in a blender, coffee grinder, or food processor like nuts, oatmeal, and potato flakes; but other grains are better suited to mills designed for grains. It is possible to grind grains in the blender but only in small batches and care must be taken not to overwork your blender.

A learning curve exists. Home-milled flour does not perform like commercial flours, so recipes must be tweaked. The flour tends to be slightly coarser and absorbs more water. Additionally, home ground usually requires more xanthan gum than the same recipe made with a commercial flour.

It takes extra time. Having to mill flour as part of each baking event adds time to the process and can be a hassle. Flour can be stored in the freezer for later use, but can pick up flavors or moisture from the freezer if not stored properly. If you know you don't like baking or are always in a hurry, home milling is probably not for you. Instead, eat your whole grains cooked and buy flour.

You might not like the texture. If you have food texture issues or like all things fluffy white, you probably won't like the texture of home milled flour.

Burr Mills vs. Impact Mills

There are two basic types of grain mills: burr and impact.

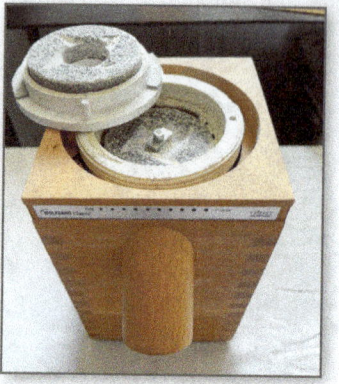

Burr Mill

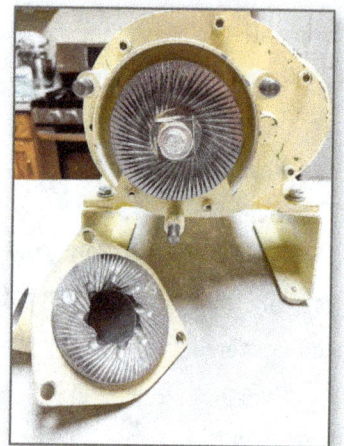

Impact Mill

Burr mills have two stone or steel plates, one stationary and one rotating. As grain is fed between the rotating stones it is ground into flour. These grind in varying coarseness from flour to meals, and will grind more types of seeds. Burr mills, and particularly stone mills, keep grain a little cooler than impact mills which can affect nutrient levels and shelf life. Oils in the grains are sensitive to heat and become rancid more quickly when they get hot in milling. Although, in the small batches milled for most home baking, the temperature rise is usually insignificant. Burr mills are available in electric and hand-crank versions.

Impact mills (also called micronizing mills) grind with two steel plates with concentric rings of teeth or fins. These spin at very high RPMs and grain is cut into smaller and smaller sizes as it is impacted. These mills generate more heat while milling than burr mills. Micronizing mills produce finer flour than burr mills but will not mill coarser than meal. In my own kitchen, I have a micronizing flour mill for baking needs and a small hand crank mill to make my cracked grain cereal.

Deciding on a Mill

Once you decide you want to buy a mill, use the questions below to determine which type of mill you will buy.

1. **What power source do you want? Electric, Manual, or Convertible?**

    An electric mill is faster and easier to use. If you plan to mill frequently, or more than two cups at a time, the electric is the way to go because cranking enough flour for several loaves of bread is tedious and tiring.

    If emergency preparedness for no electricity events is your goal, you should go with a manual or convertible model. Manual grinding is easier with a mill with a long handle and large flywheel. If you get a convertible model, make sure it will perform well in electric or manual mode. Those who want an off-the-grid backup that's easier may want to research the Wondermill Jr., which has an adapter for a power drill or a belt which can be motor or bicycle driven. It also has changeable stone or burr milling plates. In my own case, I chose

Wondermill Jr.
photo used with permission

a cheap hand grinder for non-electric backup and a nice electric for regular use.

2. **What kind of milling mechanism do you want? Burr or impact?**

    I own both types, and find that for most baking purposes either is fine. Impact mills produce a finer flour, but home milling won't produce the ultrafine flours you can purchase no matter which type of mill you have. When I want the best of both worlds (e.g. hearty flavor and nutrition of fresh and the texture of ultrafine), I mix home and commercial flours. Burr mills can also grind a coarser texture which is nice for hot cereal. Some burr mills can be taken apart and cleaned at home. Impact/micronizing mills cannot, but never need to be unless you grind something outside of the manufacturer's directions, like nuts or flax seeds. In that case, a factory repair is necessary.

3. **What will you be milling? Dry, wet, oily, or a combination?**

    Grains are dry, nuts are oily, and sprouted grains are wet. Some burr mills are a possibility with ingredients other than grains and beans that are dry, but not all burr mills will do wet or oily foods. Those that do may require adapter parts. An example of this type of mill is the Wondermill Jr. If you want to mill more than dry ingredients, check the manufacturer's instructions before purchasing. Oily and wet foods like nuts and flaxseeds can usually be ground in a coffee grinder or blender/food processor which is a cheap, good option for this type of milling.

4. How often will you mill?

If you love baking and anticipate using your mill often, get a good electric model. One deterrent to milling can be having to get the mill out everytime you want to make flour, so look for a mill that fits on your countertop, or in a convenient and accessible cupboard.

A note to those who have been home millers prior to going gluten free: you will never get a mill which has run wheat or other gluten-containing grain to be completely gluten free. If you have celiac disease, sell your old mill and buy a new one. If you are merely gluten intolerant, decide if you are willing to suffer the consequences of trace amounts of gluten. If your mill is a type that can be taken apart, brush it out. Otherwise or in addition to that, run large quantities of the cheapest gluten-free grain you can find, probably rice, through it. If you want to test for gluten after this procedure, there is a home test kit called EZ Gluten available online at https://ezgluten.com/.

If you are just beginning to mill flour, I recommend the book *The Essential Home-Ground Flour Book* by Sue Becker (ISBN 978-0-7788-0534-2). It includes information about the nutrition and performance of different grains, how to choose a mill plus lots of recipes, both glutenous and gluten free. Of note, I find her recipes need a little more xanthan gum than they call for in some cases, but this may be a difference in how fine our respective mills grind.

Some Thoughts on Mills From the Owner of Six Mills

You may be thinking, "Six mills? Really?" I currently own two small commercial mills, a Wolfgang (now branded as Mockmill), a Nutrimill, a Back to Basics hand crank mill (now branded as Victorio), and one made by a local machine shop. Each has its own good and bad features. There

Small Commercial Mill

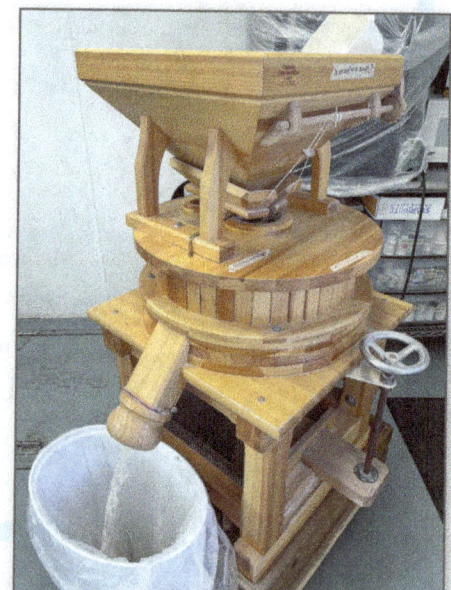

are many other mills available on the market, many of them very good as well. Look at reviews and visit a store that sells several types of mills to get an idea of what you want.

The Mockmill is a stone mill. It is pretty and has a small countertop footprint. It is easy to adjust and makes both flour and coarsely ground grains, a nice grind for breakfast porridge. Fineness of flour is determined by how close the mill stones are set together. If I plug it up, I can take it apart and clean it, and it is relatively quiet. It does not mill flour quite as finely as my Nutrimill, a burr mill. This coarseness is more noticeable with harder grains like sorghum.

The Nutrimill has a slightly bigger countertop presence than the Wolfgang, but not by much. It is loud, so I start it milling and step away. The sound of milling changes when it gets close to empty, so I return and tend it at that point. My K-Tec was also a loud mill and I ran that one outside for noise control. The flour fineness is controlled in two ways: by adjusting the fineness setting and by the grain flow rate. You can grind slower with a coarser setting, or faster with a finer setting, and get the same result. My Nutrimill's coarsest setting only grinds as fine as coarse cornmeal which is not a very good cracked grain porridge maker. This mill grinds sorghum a bit finer than my Wolfgang. This is overall my preferred mill.

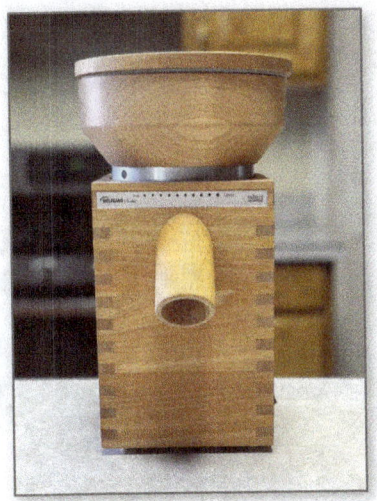

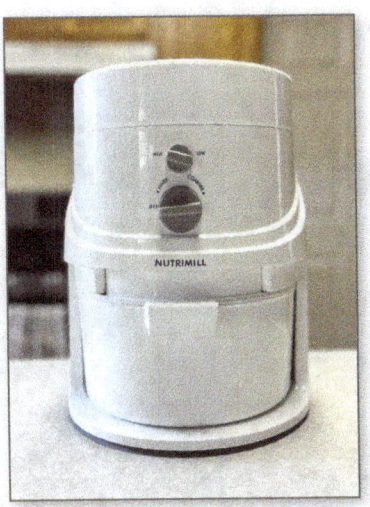

The hand crank Back to Basics mill was purchased as a preparedness backup for no electricity emergencies. I would hate to have it be my only means of making flour. It doesn't grind very finely and it takes a long time to mill a significant volume. I use this one for making breakfast cereal often. It is small and inexpensive.

Since I have all these mills, I use different ones for different purposes. Some are dedicated gluten free and others are not. If I just had one, I would go with the Mockmill, a stone mill, because it is the most versatile. If I only intended to mill flour, I would definitely choose the Nutrimill, a burr or micronizing mill, because I like finer flour. If I only planned on milling flour as a last resort in the event of disaster with no electricity, or if I only wanted cracked cereals, I would keep a small hand mill as my only mill.

Helpful Home-Milling Hints

- If milling a blend of grains, mix them together in the mill hopper. Place the predominant grain in first then add the others and mix with your hand.
- Blending grains together allows small grains like teff to mill more finely than if they are milled alone.

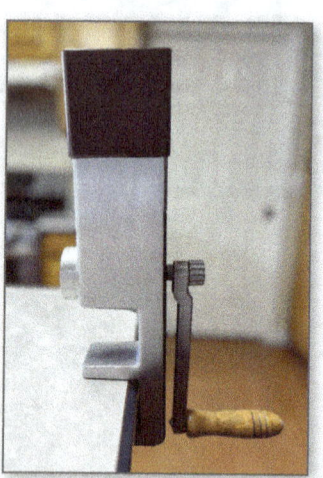
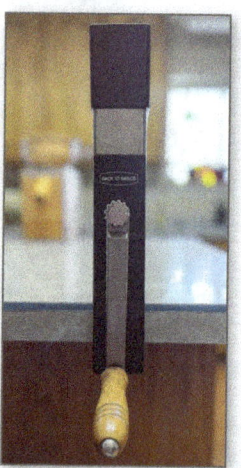

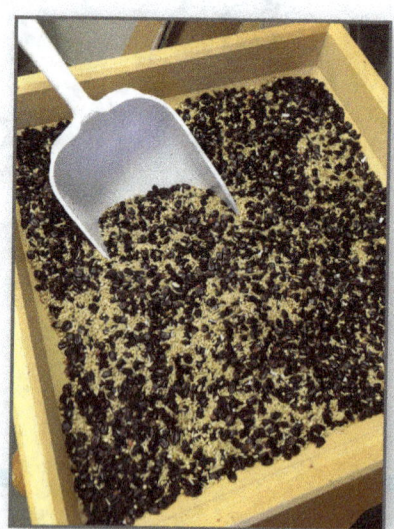

- Flour performs best and maintains optimum nutrition if it mills at a lower temperature and cools quickly. Some grains mill hotter than others naturally. Harder grains mill hotter than softer grains. This is another reason to mix grains to mill. You should not chill grains prior to milling however. This causes water to condense on the grains and milling suffers.

- Fineness is controlled by adjusting the speed of the grain flow and the closeness of the milling stones. Finer flours produce lighter baked goods with better rise.

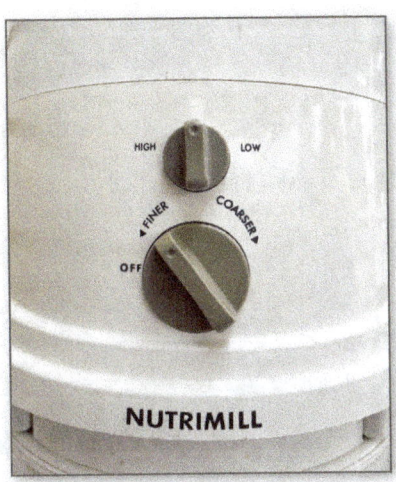

The top knob controls grain flow rate and the bottom knob controls space of stones or plates.

- Sometimes home milled bean flours can be slightly bitter. Another option is to cook the beans, make them into a puree, then add to your recipe. This requires a reduction in the liquid in the recipe and some experimenting, but does eliminate the bitterness.

- Coarser flours require more xanthan gum.

- If your grains are hard and do not mill finely enough, they can be pulsed in a food processor after milling to decrease the particle size and run through a sieve.

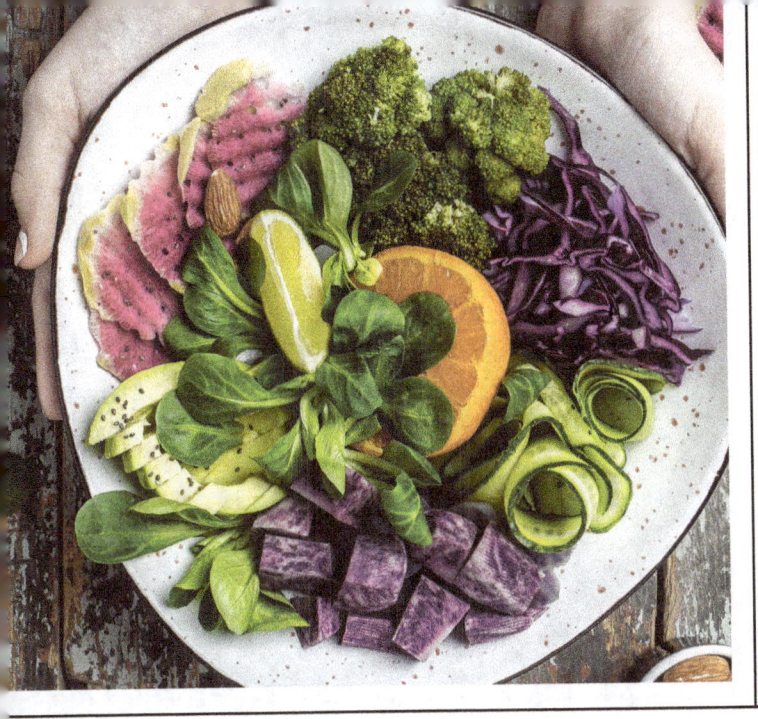

GLUTEN-FREE FOOD STORAGE

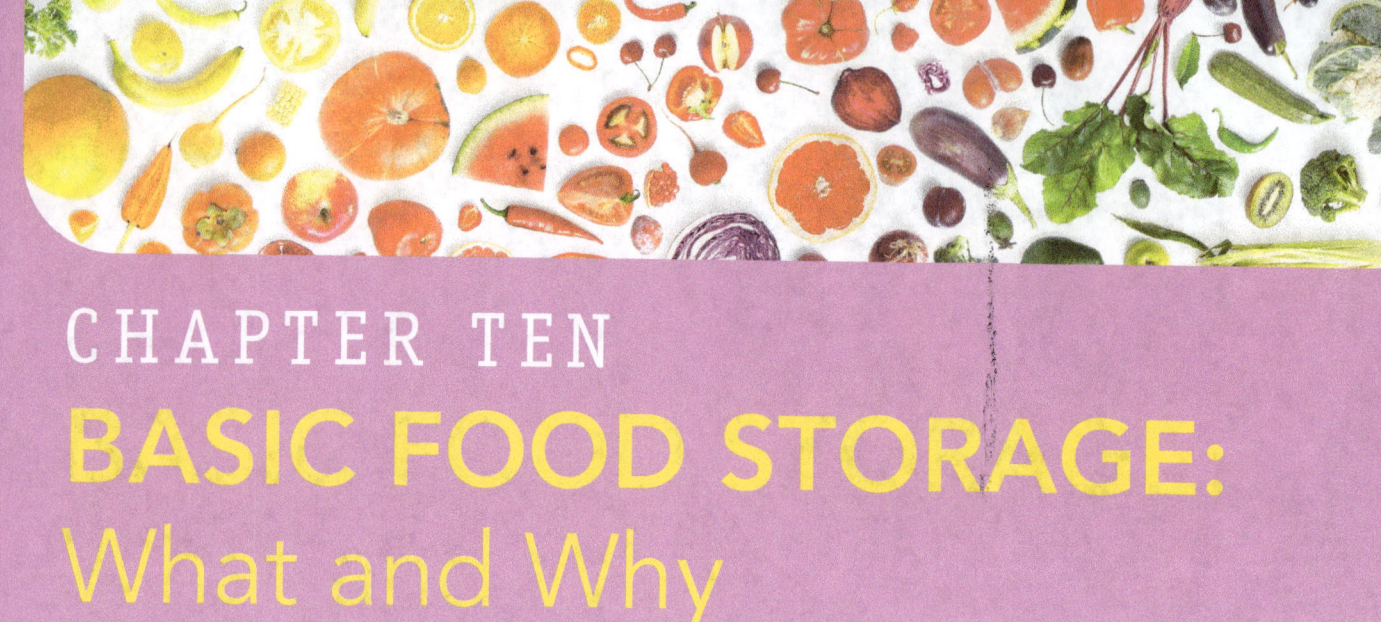

CHAPTER TEN

BASIC FOOD STORAGE:
What and Why

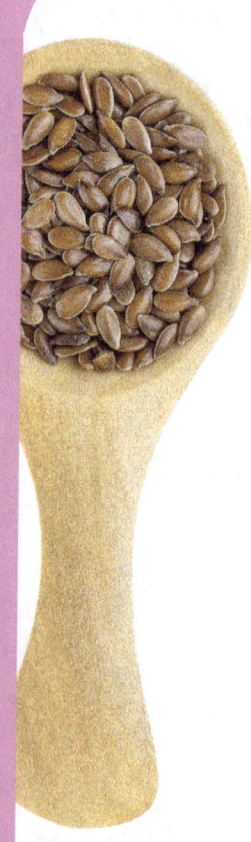

Why Store Food?

Humanity has been storing food for millenia. In earlier times, food storage was essential to survival and allowed communities to stay in one location rather than live a nomadic life. In hot, dry climates, food was dried. In cold climates, the frosty environment was used to freeze foods for future use. Over time other preservation methods were developed like pickling, curing, canning and fermenting. Storing food is still essential, but the locations of processing and storage have changed. With better storage technology, global markets, and better food supply chains, it has

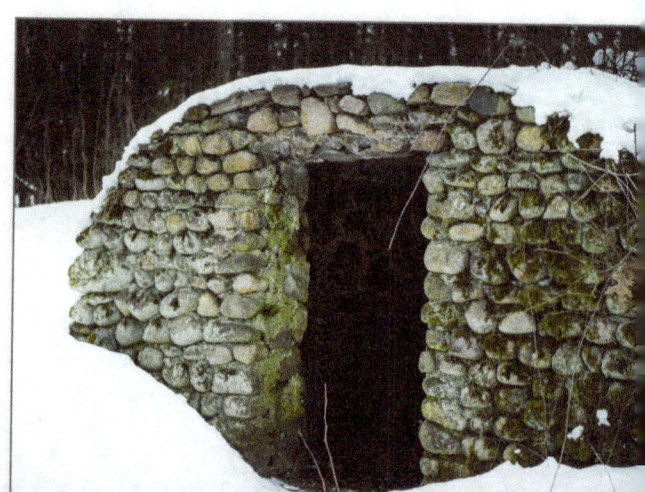

become easy to let others produce and store our food even though there are still modern advantages to storing food in your own home.

Those following a gluten-free diet often don't store food for several reasons. Gluten-free options are more expensive and less accessible than the glutenous ones. It is also difficult to know what to store since most food storage programs and suggestions focus on staple foods containing gluten. This section aims to level the playing field by teaching you why, how, and what to store. Having even a small supply of food has big advantages for saving time and money and preparing for the future in good times and bad.

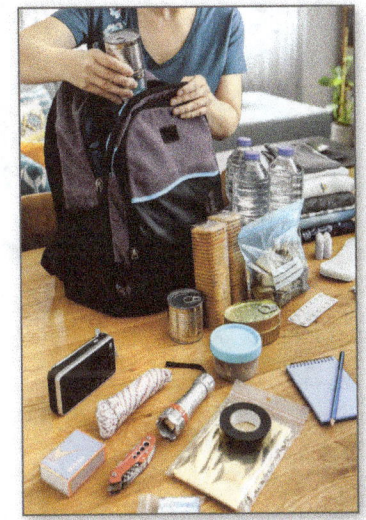

I grew up in a culture which espoused food storage. We were encouraged to have a supply of basic food, water, a 72-hour emergency kit and some savings. Home gardening was also encouraged. While these concepts were usually discussed in the context of natural disaster, that is not how these principles blessed most lives. The most common benefits were saving time and money, eating a more healthful diet, and helping people manage through unexpected financial problems like job loss or illness.

The value of storing food and other supplies hit home during the Covid-19 quarantine in 2020. I had used food storage to save money and time my entire life but when shortages arose, I wasn't worried. I had enough toilet paper, flour and yeast for myself and enough to share with others. My business however, was another story. In the beginning, I stocked up on ingredients just like I did at home. Then my accountant told me to limit money tied up in inventory. A valid point, but when the supply chains changed with Covid, I had some nail biting moments waiting for ingredients and packaging to fill orders. I also saw great volatility in prices I could have weathered with more supplies on hand. I now ignore my accountant and stock up.

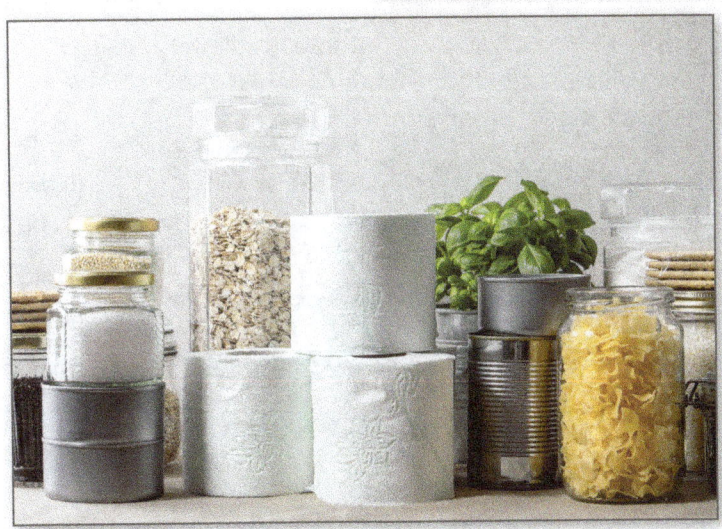

3 Types of Food Storage

The three types of food storage are 1) Emergency 2) Short term and 3) Long term.

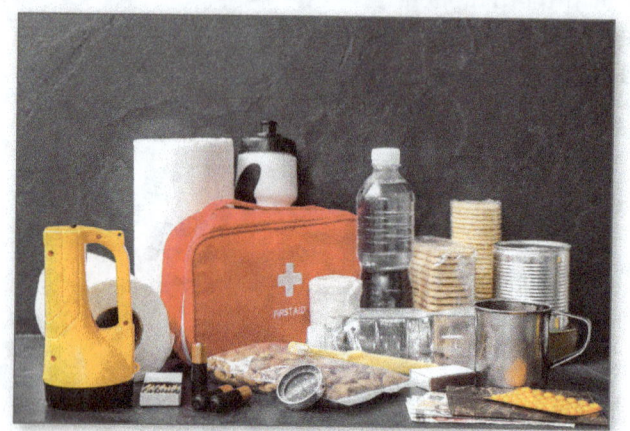

Emergency food storage is all about preparing for natural disasters such as storms, earthquake, floods, power outages or fire. These are foods suitable for a 72-hour or emergency evacuation kit designed to get you through until help arrives. Consider foods that are shelf stable, require little preparation and are compact. Every area of the world is prone to natural disasters of some sort. Start preparing for the one most likely in your area.

In addition to 72-hour kits, it is good to have a two-week supply of food for cases of shelter in place type emergencies. Choose foods that you like and know how to cook. This supply can be part of your short-term storage.

Short-term food storage is a 3-6 month supply of the foods and household items you normally consume. The everyday advantage of this storage is convenience and savings. Having a supply on hand reduces trips to the market and allows you to buy at lower prices.

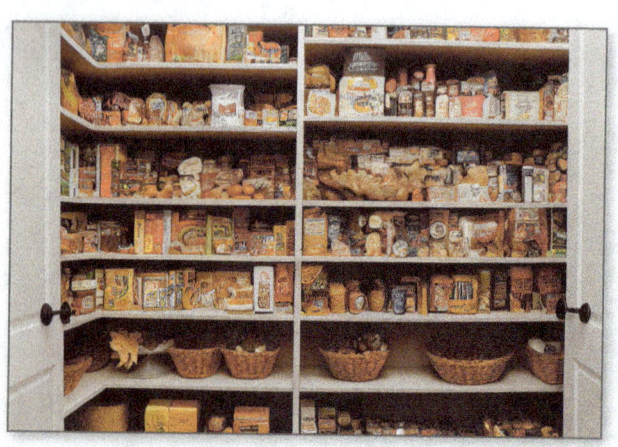

Building a short-term reserve helps prepare for unexpected events like recession, pandemics, or disasters in ways similar to having a rainy day fund. Food can be "banked". If your income was cut for some reason you could switch all remaining income to things requiring money and save cash by eating food you stored in better times. Having a store of goods and food insulates from the effects of supply disruptions from any source. Everyone was affected in some way by Covid price hikes and shortages, but consider who fared worst during this difficult time: people without reserves to cushion the impact.

Long-term food storage builds on short-term food storage by adding foods that have extended storability. The immediate advantage is that many foods which store well are also inexpensive and especially nutritious, like grains and beans. Having a supply on-hand encourages cooking and eating more healthfully. These products purchased in bulk also use less packaging and therefore fewer of the earth's resources.

These storage-hardy foods are important in preparing for longer lasting problems such as extended unemployment, global financial upheaval, drought or other natural disaster, supply chain problems, or war.

What Should I Include in My Storage/Preparedness Plan?

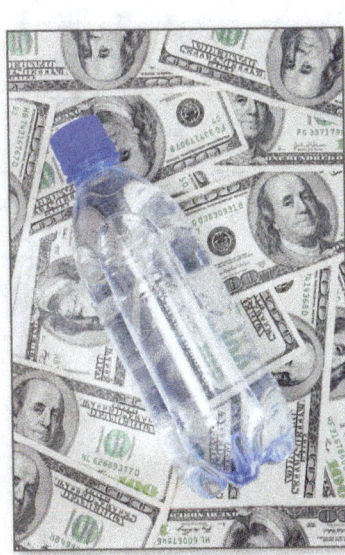

1. Water

2. Food

3. Money

4. Skills (I'll explain below!)

The list above includes more than food, because everyone needs other necessities in reserve to be prepared for future uncertainties. Since this is a gluten-free book, these other elements of personal preparedness will only be lightly touched on, but their importance should not be overlooked. Reserve resources of money and skills can lessen the severity of many problems and anyone who has unexpectedly lost water supply for a short time can appreciate the value of having some water on hand as well.

How do I Start?

Begin adopting the food storage/prepared lifestyle slowly with small, easy steps. Focus on short-term and emergency storage then progress to longer-term storage. Adapt to your own tastes and resource availability. An incremental but steady approach allows you to grow into skills and fit preparing into your budget of money and time. Start small and keep improving consistently. We have included a sample plan at the end of this chapter called "Developing a Plan of Your Own" to give ideas (p 133).

Emergency Storage & Preparedness

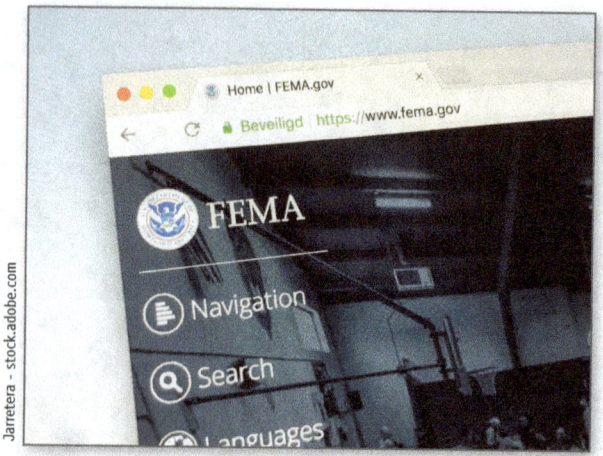

Jarretera - stock.adobe.com

A good source of information about emergency preparedness is the Federal Emergency Management Agency (FEMA) website FEMA.gov. Find their PDF on emergency food and water online[1]. FEMA recommends that a minimum of one gallon of water per person, per day, for two weeks should be stored for emergencies. Keep in mind this bare minimum only figures two quarts of water for drinking and two quarts for cooking and handwashing. Fortunately, it is easy to store emergency water. Commercially-bottled water or water from your tap in reused soda or juice bottles will work. FEMA's PDF gives more specific advice on how to do this.

State governments and extension services also frequently have disaster preparation guides on their websites which can give more specific information on the types of emergencies and resources in your area. The easiest way to find these resources is to Google emergency preparedness in your state.

The food for emergency kits should be small enough to fit easily in a backpack, shelf stable, provide enough calories, and be easy to

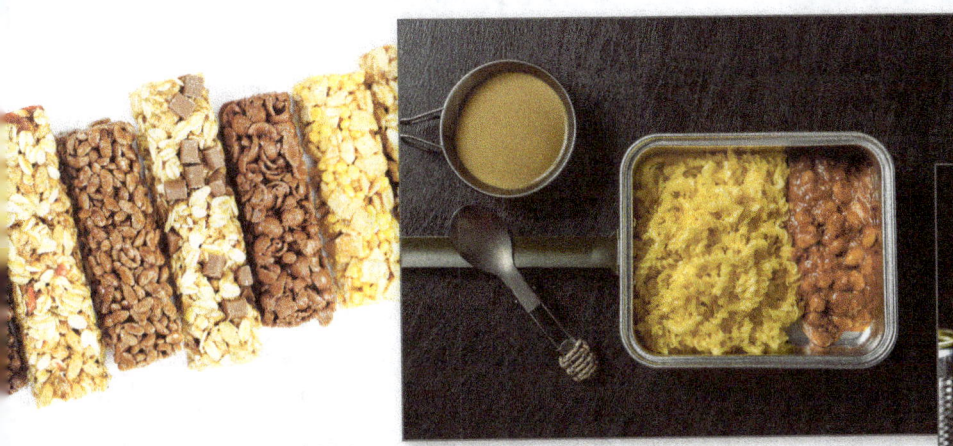

prepare.   Since this is
only a temporary food supply, don't worry about complete nutrition.
Foods like wrapped granola-type bars, dehydrated fruits and meals,
MREs (meals ready to eat), nuts, or canned goods with pull tops. The advantage
of canned foods is that they already have water in them, and clean water is often
scarce after disasters. The disadvantage is that they are heavy if you end up car-
rying your pack for long, might require a can opener, and are not as compact as
other foods.

　　　No one wants to eat bad-tasting or stale food so it's important to rotate
the food in your emergency kit. Plan a regular time once a year to eat the food
in your pack as if it were the only food you had, then replace it. This maintains
fresh food and provides a chance to see how much you really like the food
you selected. I have friends who chose an annual event as a cue to replenish
their packs. The first time they relied on their kit as their only food, they
discovered some of their choices had developed strange flavors and that
others were not as filling as they thought. The packs were refilled with
other foods, and when the next year came around they were much more
satisfied.

　　　A cash reserve is also helpful in emergencies. For natural disasters,
cash on hand will purchase needed items you were not able to store.
Small bills are preferable since sellers can't always make change. For

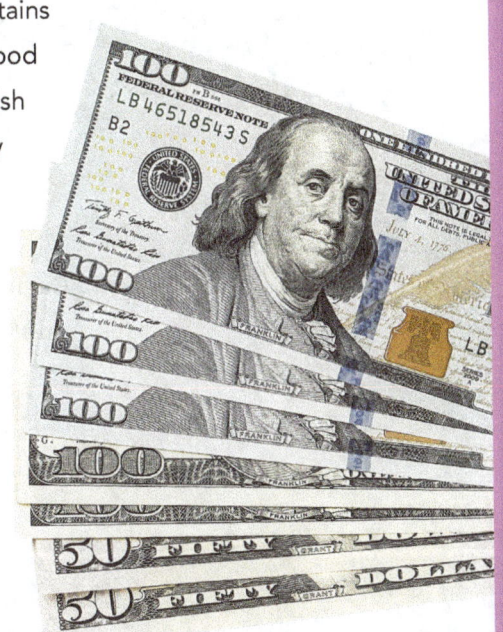

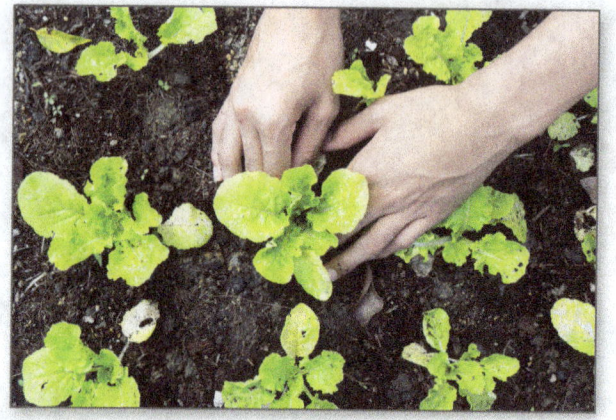

unexpected personal disasters like job loss, personal savings are invaluable to make it through the rough patch.

You may not consider building skills as something you need to "store," but skills can take the place of money. Anything you can do yourself is something you don't have to pay someone else to do or do without. You also need the skills to use any items or food you plan to use for emergencies. A disaster is a difficult time to learn new skills like how to cook in a solar oven or assemble a tent. There is no time for the learning curve. Skills are barterable. Skills like gardening and food preservation can help you build your food supply.

Additional Resources

Luther, D. (2015). The Prepper's Water Survival Guide. Ulysses Press.

National Celiac Association. Staying GF Safe in an Emergency Situation. https://nationalceliac.org/wp-content/uploads/2018/06/GFSafe.pdf

Ready.gov. (n.d.). Ready.gov. https://www.ready.gov/

Salsbury, B. (1995). Preparedness Principles: The Complete Personal Preparedness Resource Guide for Any Emergency Situation. Gold Leaf Press.

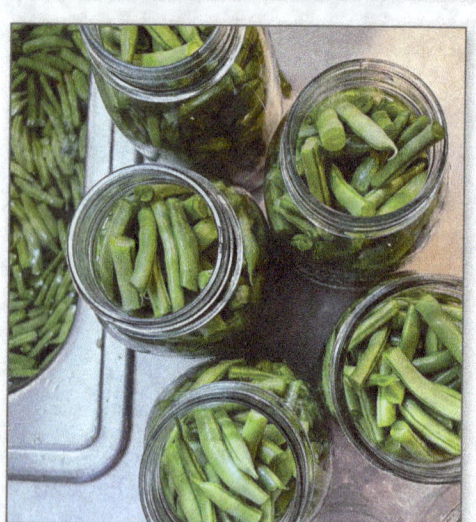

Short-Term Food Storage

The first step in short-term food storage is to store extras of the food you normally eat. *Store what you eat and eat what you store* is the primary rule for all types of food storage, but especially short-term storage. Watch for sales and buy extra. You can gradually build a three-month supply of this fast-moving storage, but if space and money are tight, buy one week's extra to begin with. Add non-food items you regularly use like detergent, toilet paper, and toothpaste. No lifestyle change is necessary, just a little more planning when grocery shopping.

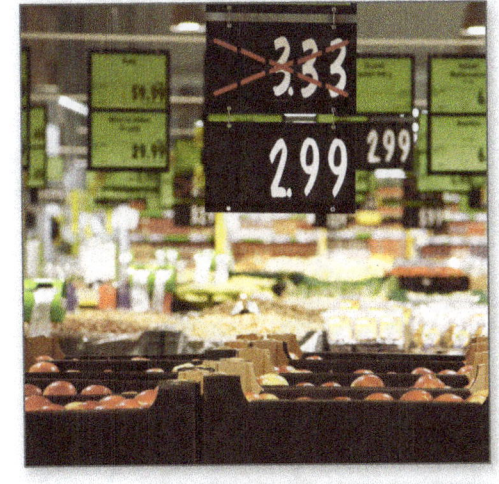

Step 1: Watch for sales on food, household, and personal items used routinely. Items don't have to be especially long-storing because they will rotate quickly.

Step 2: Buy extras on sale. You can estimate how much a three-month supply is by dating packages as they are opened and noticing when they are used up. This gives an approximate consumption rate to gauge usage for a week, month, or year's supply. When I tried this with my family, I discovered that we ate 1 lb of peanut butter each week. I needed 12 pounds for 3 months, or 52 pounds for a year.

As you buy items, write dates of purchase on each then place on the shelf behind older items for rotation. A first in, first out system will keep food from going bad before it is used.

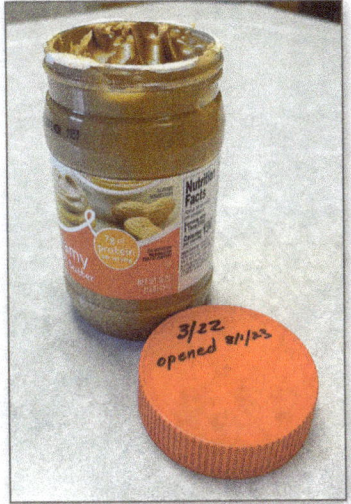

Step 3: Repeat.

Longer-Term Storage

Long-term food storage focuses on foods which store well and contain our basic macronutrients; in other words, nutrients our bodies need in larger volumes like protein, carbohydrates, fats/oils, and certain minerals including calcium, sodium, potassium and magnesium. Of course, we also need foods which contain micronutrients, nutrients our bodies require in small volumes like vitamins and other minerals, so long-term storage should store a variety of foods.

MACRONUTRIENTS

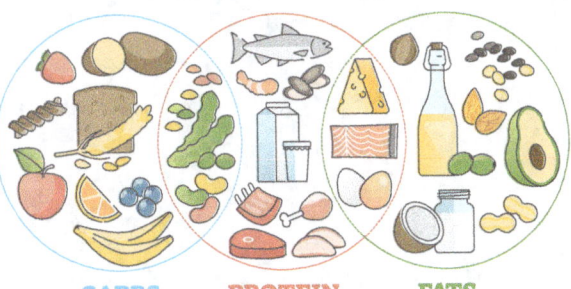

CARBS   PROTEIN   FATS

Unfortunately for the gluten free population, most food storage plans recommend using wheat and milk as foundational foods because they store well and cover macronutrient needs. To understand what foods will work in your gluten-free storage, let's start by examining why certain foods are recommended for long-term storage. If you know why foods are selected for storage you have power to choose foods that are appropriate for your dietary needs and still give your body what it needs.

Foods Commonly Found on Food Storage Lists and Why They're There

Grains

Why? Most whole kernel grains store well and contain protein, carbohydrates, minerals and vitamins, and some oils. They are also versatile. They can be cooked and eaten like rice, milled into flour for baking, or sprouted and eaten as microgreens for vitamins.

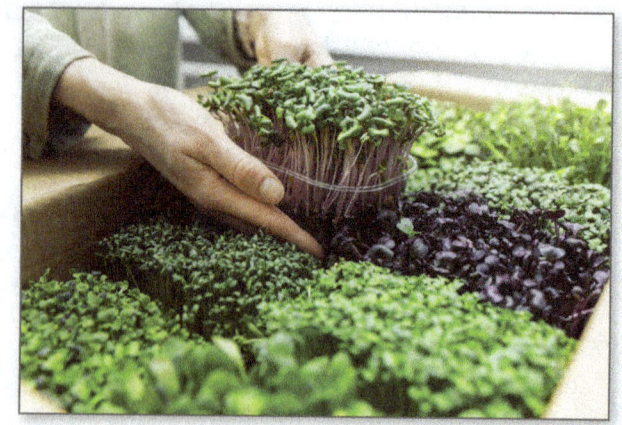

None of the gluten-free grain options store as long as wheat, but there are some good ones. If you plan to mill your own flour, you should store more of the grains in your flour blend vs. those you plan to eat cooked. Interestingly, there are more gluten-free grains that are complete proteins than other grains including: amaranth, buckwheat, quinoa and teff. Here is a short list of possibilities (see Chapter 5: Grains, Nuts and Seeds for more information).

Teff: Excellent storage life, tastes good, complete protein. Teff works best as flour or mixed with other grains. Cooked by itself it is porridge-like rather than rice-like.

Sorghum: Stores well, tastes good, and is high in complex carbohydrates. Milled together with teff, it tastes very much like wheat. It also has a fun texture when cooked. Note to home millers: Sorghum is hard to mill finely. Experiment to see if you like the texture of home-milled sorghum.

Quinoa: Stores well, easy to find, high protein, complete protein, works well as a rice replacement, easy to cook.

Oatmeal: Stores well (whole grain oats do not store as well), easy to use, tastes good, versatile, and readily available. It can be turned into flour in a blender and is a great texture improver for gluten-free baked goods.

Rice: Easy to purchase and cook. Can be milled into flour and almost everyone likes it. Though brown rice is more nutritious, the shelf life is significantly shorter than white rice.

Flour

Why? It's convenient, but once grain is ground into flour it loses vitamins quickly and is prone to rancidity. Flour is not really a long-term storage food and should be viewed as a short term/long term hybrid item. Store more flour than you would for short-term storage and less than truly long-term foods. Make sure flour is used and rotated frequently. Maximum storage volume should be a 6-12 month supply.

If you don't plan to mill your own flour, store 6 months to a year's worth of flour and keep it rotated. Each time you finish a bag, buy a replacement.

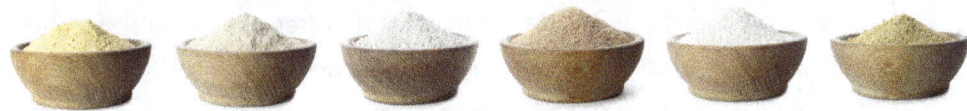

Powdered Milk

Why? It stores well and is high in protein and the minerals calcium and phosphorus. Milk protein (casein), like all animal sourced proteins, is high quality and contains all the essential amino acids. Milk can also supply vitamin B12 which is found only in animal-based foods. Another advantage in gluten-free cooking is that milk

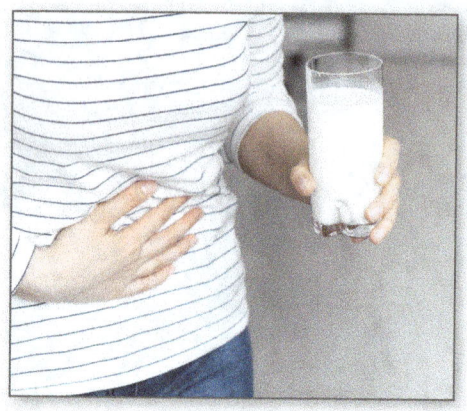

can function as a texture enhancer in baked goods and is easy to add to other foods as a nutrient booster.

What if you are dairy intolerant? Don't store it. The reason to store milk is for the nutritional value. Make sure the other foods you are storing and eating have complete proteins and the minerals milk provides. It does not matter if each of your protein sources is a complete protein by itself as long as the combination of proteins you eat contains all the essential amino acids. For instance, most combinations of grains and beans provide complete protein.

Fats or Oils

Why? Our bodies need fats and oils for a host of functions including cell membranes, hormone production, and transport of fat soluble vitamins (along with many other functions). Fats and oils are also important in making your food taste good, improving texture and providing calories. I am a strong believer that food should be enjoyable, especially in hard times or disasters.

Storage conditions for oil are very important. Poorly stored oils turn rancid quickly. Rancidity happens when oils degrade through an oxidation reaction that gives a musty smell and flavor. Have you ever eaten an old nut that tastes like paint? If so, you already know the flavor of rancidity. Light, heat, water and contamination increase the rate oils turn rancid. Store in dark, cool, places in original

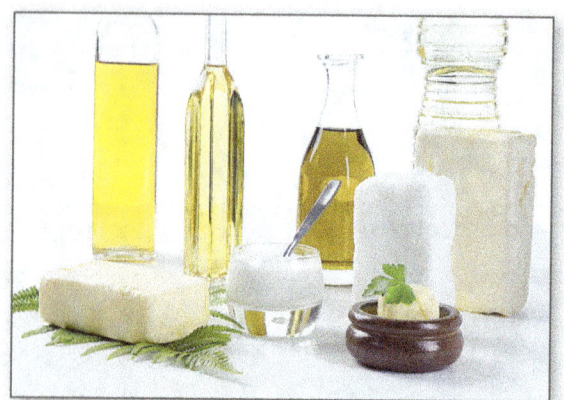

containers. Opening containers and transferring oils to others can introduce more oxygen and the possibility of contamination.

Highly-processed oils store longer than less refined oils because they have fewer impurities to start the oxidation reaction. Have you ever noticed that soy oil labels do not claim soy as an allergen? This is because they are processed to remove all traces of the soybean except the oil for shelf life purposes. Processors want the longest possible shelf life.

Why do some food storage recommendations suggest storing so much shortening for a fat source? Oils solid at room temperature like shortening and coconut oil store longer than oils which are liquid at the same temperature. Modern shortenings are not as stable as those produced previously because they are now trans fat free, but they still have a good storage life. Store the oils you like and use regularly. If you use shortening, store it. If not, don't. Don't store any food just because it is on a food storage list. You can also count peanut butter as a dietary fat source and it is easy to rotate and keep fresh.

Sugar/Sweeteners

Why? Sugar lasts almost indefinitely if it remains dry, and is a source of pure carbohydrates. During good times we are accustomed to thinking of simple carbs as bad because we eat too many. If you are storing food for extended famine or other catastrophic events, calories are very important. Sugar is also valuable in turning other basic storage items into delicious dishes which add variety and palatability to what otherwise might be a boring diet.

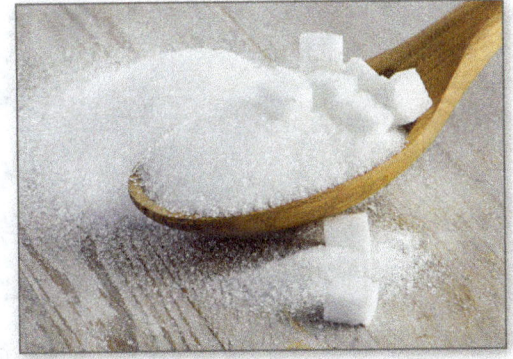

If you grow a garden or fruit trees and plan to preserve your harvest by home canning or freezing, plan on storing more sugar. Sugar added in processing improves the final product taste and functions as a preservative. Note: Stored sugar can develop an off smell, however, this does not indicate it is spoiled. The taste, nutritional value, and function remain the same. If this happens, taste a pinch and you will be convinced.

If you are not a big sugar user, other sweeteners can be stored as well. Honey has a very long shelf life, but darkens and grows stronger in flavor over time but remains safe to eat. Honey crystalizes and becomes hard over time, but is easily melted in warm water. For this reason, I suggest storing honey in quart mason jars. They contain a manageable amount of honey and jars can be placed in a pot of warm water to melt.

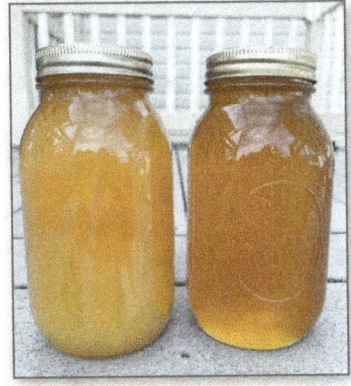

Lighter honey on the left is crystalized. Honey on the right is liquid.

HOW TO MELT (DECRYSTALIZE) HONEY

Place your container of honey in a pan of water and turn the stove on low or place in a slow cooker on warm. Water should be between 95-105° F. Since this is about body temperature, water feels slightly warm to the touch. You can also use a thermometer. Leave until the honey is completely melted. Do not allow pan to evaporate dry.

Once melted will it recrystallize? Yes. If any crystals remain, new crystals form easily around the old crystals.

Can I melt honey in plastic containers? Yes. Plastic containers will not melt because the temperature is so slow. Containers like half filled honey bears may float. In

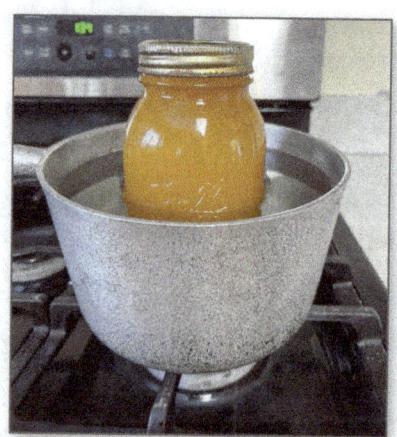

this case, weight the top with something small like a can.

Can I melt a big container of honey? If you have stored honey in 5 gallon buckets or metal cans it can also be melted. Place the whole container in a large pot to melt. If the bucket top is easy to remove, honey can be scooped out and placed in jars to be melted. Either way, it's a pain. Try not to store honey in any container larger than 1 gallon.

Can I melt honey in the microwave? It's generally a bad idea. Microwaves do not heat evenly so parts of your honey will cook rather than melt. Plastic also melts well in the microwave.

Canned Goods

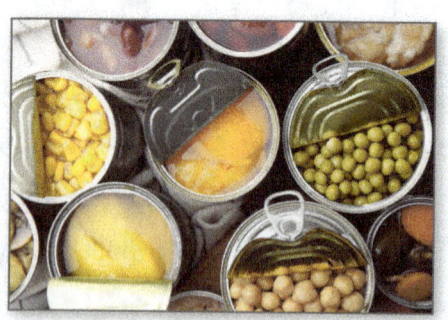

Why? Canned goods have multiple years of shelf life and are a good way to store foods with high vitamin content like fruits and vegetables. You can also store convenient premade foods like chili, soups, spaghetti sauce, and pasta dishes like ravioli. Meat also comes in canned varieties and is a good source of complete proteins and vitamin B12. Canned foods are part of both short- and long-term storage.

Dried Foods/Pasta

Why? Dried foods have a long storage life and are a way to store foods which have high vitamin and mineral content like fruits and vegetables. Dried foods also have less weight and require less storage space than their wet versions. Gluten-free pasta is also a dried food that lasts well and adds variety to your carbohydrate sources. Dried meat can be a good storage item for protein and variety as well.

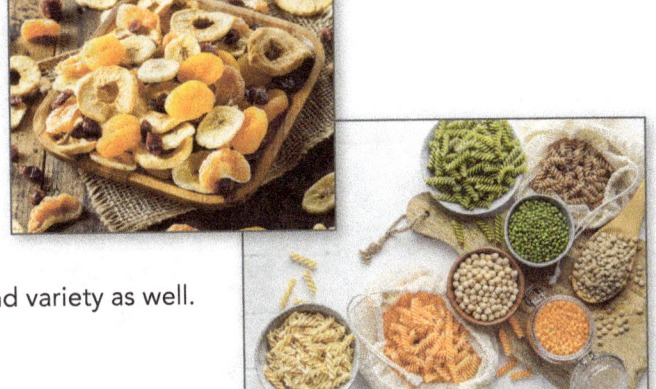

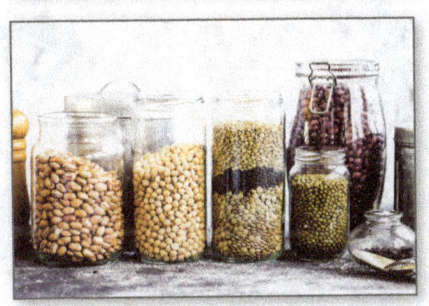

Beans

Why? Beans store well and are nutritious with high protein and fiber. Beans are inexpensive and readily available in the grocery store and in bulk. They are incredibly versatile too. Cooked beans can be mashed up and used as a shortening replacement in baked goods. Dry beans can be sprouted to become a fresh vegetable for salads or soups, or ground into flour to improve nutrition and texture of gluten-free bread. My favorite bean flour to include in gluten-free bread is chickpea/garbanzo bean. It is packed with folate and has the most mild flavor of readily available beans.

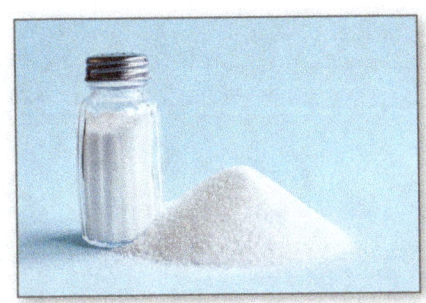

Salt

Why? Your body needs this essential nutrient. We can't live without it. Besides, who wants to eat food without salt? Not me. Salt can also be combined with sugar to make an oral rehydration solution to treat diarrhea. Recipes can be found through a web search.

Miscellaneous Flavorings and Baking Aids

Why? Bad-tasting or poorly-textured foods are miserable to eat. Think about what makes your food taste good and makes your baking work. The previously suggested long-term storage foods are unpalatable without them. To know what to store, take a look at what is in your kitchen cupboard: baking powder, soda, yeast, xanthan, psyllium, herbs, spices, bouillon, extracts. Storage needs are highly variable between people because of differing tastes and cooking patterns. Below are some to consider and include as needed.

Spices and herbs don't generally have long shelf life but they don't spoil either. Flavor decreases slowly over time. The more whole the herb or spice is, the slower it loses flavor. For instance, whole cumin retains flavor longer than ground cumin. Whole spices can be ground in a mortar and pestle at cooking time. Reducing temperature, light and oxygen exposure will decrease flavor loss as well.

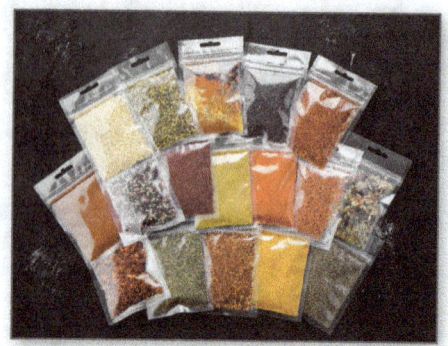

If you are really serious about storing herbs long term, buy them sealed in mylar packets with oxygen absorbers and keep them cool. I buy whole herbs when I can, and keep one package in my kitchen and an extra in my cool basement storage room. Consider what volume you use when purchasing. For instance, I bought a small bottle of cayenne pepper 15 years ago. I use it occasionally. Its heat has decreased over time, but I simply add more to recipes. I had an adequate storage supply in my kitchen cupboard without storing any extras.

Leaveners give rise to your baked goods by creating gas bubbles to expand dough. The two types of storable leaveners are chemical and biological. Examples of chemical leaveners are baking soda and baking powder used for quick breads like muffins, pancakes and biscuits. These leaven with bubbles produced by a chemical reaction. Yeast, the most common biological leavener, is a single cell fungus which gives off carbon dioxide as it metabolizes sugar and is a living, or biological, leavener.

Baking soda is sodium bicarbonate and reacts with acidic ingredients in your recipe like buttermilk, vinegar, fruit or cocoa to produce gas bubbles. Without such an acid, recipes do not leaven. The rule of thumb for recipes is ¼ tsp per 1 cup of flour.

Storing extra baking soda is a good idea because you can't produce it yourself and it can be used to create homemade deodorizer, toothpaste, soap in sponge baths and various other cleaning products.

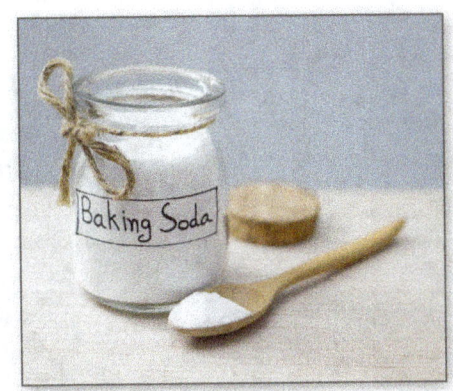

Baking soda has a published storage life of 3 years, however, it can be stored for much longer without losing potency if stored in a cool (40-70 degree), air tight, moisture proof container. Since soda absorbs moisture readily, the cardboard boxes from the grocery store are very poor long-term storage containers, especially if you live in a humid climate. The larger plastic bags from warehouse stores, airtight plastic buckets, or metal cans are much better.

To test potency of stored soda, mix one cup hot water with one tsp vinegar then add one teaspoon of soda. Alternatively you can mix 1 tablespoon of either vinegar or lemon juice and ¼ tsp soda. The mixtures should react quickly and give robust bubble formation.

Baking powder contains baking soda plus a weak acid. Since it contains the acid, your recipe does not need to contain an acidic ingredient, but this also means that the components of baking powder will react with themselves over time and has a much shorter shelf life than baking soda. The published storage is 18 months. Like baking soda, it must be stored in good conditions especially in regards to moisture. Once you open baking powder, make sure it is in an airtight container which does not absorb moisture from the environment.

There are two types of baking powder: single acting and double acting. Single acting starts to react as soon as it is hydrated. It does not need heat to start working. Double acting begins to react when liquid is added to the recipe, with additional components that don't react until they are heated. I prefer double acting because I like the nice extra "oven spring" I get with double acting baking powder.

You can also make your own baking powder with baking soda by mixing 1 part baking soda, 2 parts cream of tartar, and 1 part cornstarch. This will not be double acting baking powder so your batter should go in the oven right away.

Yeast comes in several types: fresh, instant active, and active dry yeast. Fresh has a very short shelf life and must be kept in the refrigerator. Both dry and instant have reasonably long shelf life if stored properly: low temperature, moisture, light and oxygen. Unopened packages of dry yeast have printed out dates of two years; amazing since they are living organisms which are essentially in a suspended metabolic state. The unopened package shelf life is extended by a year by freezing or refrigerating. Manufacturers recommend using yeast within 4-6 months of opening but this time can be extended through refrigeration or freezing. When returning opened yeast to the fridge or freezer make sure it is in an airtight container so it does not absorb moisture and become activated. Yeast doesn't spoil, but loses potency as the organisms age and die.

Individual yeast cells

IS MY YEAST STILL GOOD?

If you have old yeast and wonder if it is still good there is a simple test suggested by Red Star® yeast.

In a liquid measuring cup, dissolve 1 tsp sugar in ½ cup warm water. Water should be slightly warmer than body temperature (110 to 115) but NOT hot. Overly hot water can kill yeast.

Add one packet or 2 ¼ tsp yeast and stir until no yeast granules remain on top.

In ten minutes the yeast should have foamed up to the 1 cup measuring line with a rounded top. This indicates full activity. Lesser growth indicates diminished activity.

If the test shows no activity in your yeast, discard it. If it demonstrates decreased activity, you have options.

Option 1: Dissolve the yeast for your recipe in warm water with a little sugar and allow it to grow and divide. As the yeast is hydrated and starts to metabolize sugar it multiplies.

Option 2: Use more yeast. For instance, if you are at half potency use twice as much.

These two options can also be combined.

Storage Items Unique to Gluten Free

Xanthan and other gums are a must-have in gluten-free storage if you are making your own flour because baked goods fail without them. These structure-building ingredients are vulnerable to supply chain interruption since they originate in faraway places and require specialized food processing to manufacture. The published storage length is two years, but can be stored almost indefinitely with good conditions. This means that you can store a bigger volume without worry. If you plan to bake bread or use whole grain flour, I also recommend storing psyllium husk. If well stored, this has a similar published shelf life of two years but most likely has a longer shelf life. I have stored psyllium for four years without any taste or function problems.

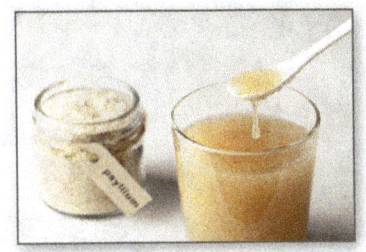

Starches are needed in much greater volumes in gluten-free storage if you plan to make your own flour. Store whichever starches you use in your regular flour blend. These can have a five-year shelf life if kept dry and pest-free, but will absorb moisture and smells if not properly stored.

WILL I BE MISSING NUTRIENTS?

If you had to eat solely from food storage you might miss some important nutrients, but there is an easy solution to cover the gaps: Take a vitamin plus mineral supplement daily. Most dieticians recommend celiac patients supplement anyway since gluten-free diets are frequently missing certain nutrients. A supplement with minerals also covers your calcium and phosphorus needs if you can't drink milk. Many also contain iodine.

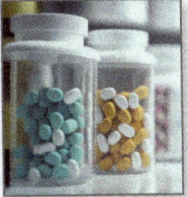

You may be wondering how vitamins could be part of long-term storage. The best way to store a supply is to use a rotation system like you would flour. Many vitamin tablets have a two-year shelf life. Look for bottles with the farthest out date you can find, then purchase two bottles and take one tablet daily. When one bottle runs out, begin the second bottle and buy another to replace the one you just finished.

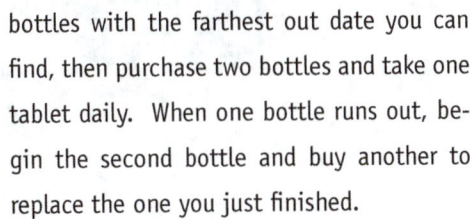

Gardening & Sprouting: Skills to Build

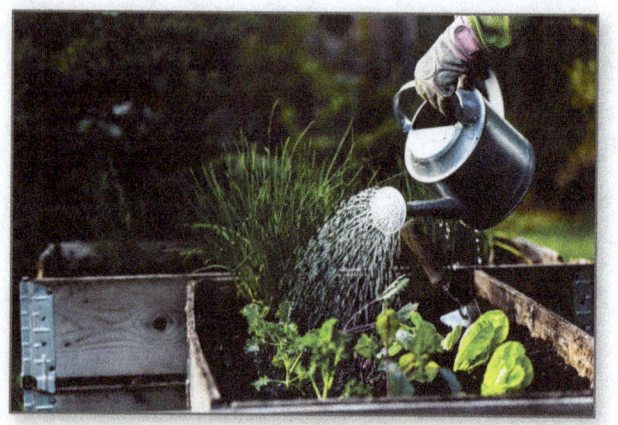

The joys of gardening include creating life, eating unbelievably good produce, and having extras to preserve for the future. I live in a community that encourages gardening and it is interesting to watch novice gardeners in the neighborhood. They are excited by their neighbors' beautiful gardens, but have disappointing results in their first few gardens. Expect a few failures as you go. Even seasoned farmers have crop failures. Like my neighbors, if you start small and learn you will soon be enjoying fresh vegetables yourself. It is amazing what one potted tomato or pepper can yield.

One of the best places to start is The Square Foot Gardening Foundation[2]. The square foot gardening technique was pioneered by Mel Bartholomew and is a very easy, step by step way to garden in small spaces and is particularly suited to novice gardeners. It also has a very high rate of success among beginners.

Sprouting seeds is another way to grow your own. It's a fast, easy way to produce vitamin, mineral and enzyme-rich foods in a few days and with only a small amount of shelf space. It is also a good way to use food storage grains. All you need is a mason jar, seeds, and a small piece of screen. Microgreen production is also a sprouting process where sprouts are allowed to grow longer before using. Popular seeds to sprout are broccoli, mung beans, alfalfa, peas, lentils and grains. If sprouting gluten-free grains, avoid sorghum as it can generate high levels of cyanide when soaked and sprouted. A quick internet search will yield all the necessary instructions to begin sprouting.

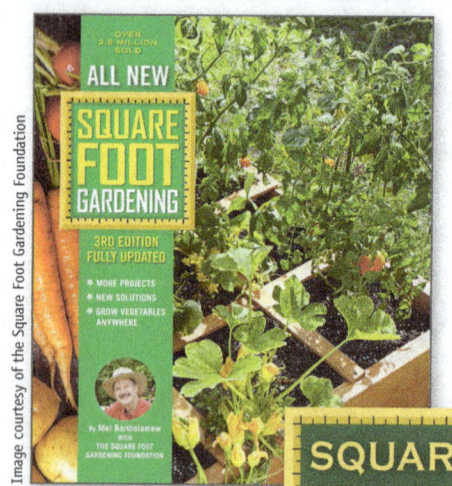

Additional Resources

Grant, B. L. (n.d.). How Many Vegetables per Person per Year? Gardening Know How. Retrieved May 10, 2023, from https://www.gardeningknowhow.com/edible/vegetables/vgen/how-many-vegetables-per-person-per-year.htm

Utah State University Extension. (n.d.). Gardening basics. Retrieved May 9, 2023, from https://extension.usu.edu/yardandgarden/gardening-basics

Storing Seeds

I had always heard that seeds stored in low oxygen environments, e.g. with oxygen absorbers or carbon dioxide, would not sprout. As I researched, I found contradictory information about seed storage and started looking for research that could definitively answer the question. I found the answer in research done at Wageningen University in the Netherlands[3]. Their study found improved germination rates in seeds stored in low-oxygen conditions. Storing seeds

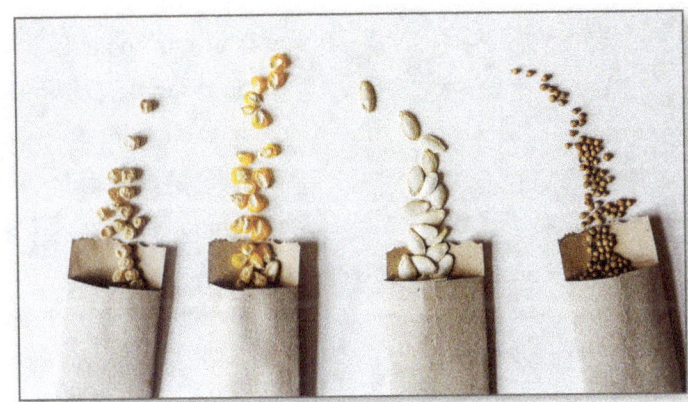

with oxygen absorbers in mylar pouches or mason jars in cool dark places is best.

Developing a Plan of Your Own

Over the years I have helped several people develop food storage plans that were definitely not one-size-fits-all. Budget, space, time, and how much cooking you are willing to do play heavily into every plan. Those I helped begin storing food ranged from a single mom on a tight budget to an affluent woman who hated to cook and had a picky family. The single mother started buying a few extras when things went on sale. She proudly reported her progress as her storage grew and she saved money.

The woman with the larger budget is still a work in progress. We started with a discussion of her priorities. Her top priority was disaster and long-term storage. We reviewed FEMA's emergency water storage suggestions. She already had the minimum but wanted more. I referred her to sources of different storage containers to come up with the following changes.

In ordinary times, about half the family's dinners are made from on-line meal kits. If times were to get bad, she wanted to continue with pre-made meals, so she purchased freeze-dried meals to store. The home includes a large pantry, and she stores extra ingredients she regularly uses in cooking. There was room to store more of those ingredients, so we increased her supplies. She was also storing some simple, common longer-storing items like rice, flour and sugar, baking aids, and oil. Her storage needed more of almost all of those things, especially the oil. She also confessed that she did not like rice, so we made a plan for her to store quinoa instead. This has good storage life and the family will actually rotate through it.

The take-home message from these examples is to experiment with what might work at this point in your life. Make progress by picking one easy, doable step and starting there. The plan and suggestions below may not fit your circumstances, but they should help you with ideas and an example of how to think through the process of making your own plan.

Beginners and Small Households

To buy: Start building a three-month supply of the shelf-stable or frozen food you regularly eat as items go on sale (items will vary by individual). It is also wise to buy extra non-food items that you use regularly like cleaners and toilet paper.

Specific basics to store (only if you will use them):

- Gluten-Free flour or components to make your own
- Rice, white and brown. Brown rice does not store as well so make sure you don't purchase more than you will eat in six months to a year
- Gluten-free pasta
- Canned or frozen fruits and vegetables
- Tomato sauce/paste
- Peanut butter
- Oatmeal
- Sugar, it stores forever unless it gets wet

Skills to develop/practice:

- Expand home cooking skills like learning to season food well. Knowing which herbs and spices to add to staples like rice, beans and pasta brings increased variety and enjoyment to your diet.
- Develop a repertoire of five or six recipes that you don't mind making and your family likes. Always keep ingredients for these recipes on hand.
- Write a purchase date on food. Use the oldest first.
- If you're able, plant a few vegetables like tomatoes and peppers in a pot.
- Write dates on packages when opened to determine your rate of consumption.

When I first started living on my own, my home storage consisted of one bucket each of flour, sugar and rice along with cases of canned goods we regularly ate. We also purchased a small freezer and used it for meat, bread and frozen vegetables that were bought during sales. We grew tomatoes and peppers in window boxes at our apartment.

Intermediate Experience

To buy: Continue to build a three- to six-month supply of foods you regularly eat and non-food products you use often. Add in foods that will store longer and have high nutritional value such as beans and whole grains. Purchase required tools as you learn new food production/ storage skills as needed, e.g. garden equipment and food storage containers.

Specific basics to store (if you will eat them):

- Flour (or ingredients to make your own blend)
- Gluten-free oatmeal
- Canned or dried fruits and vegetables
- Sugar
- Pasta
- Beans
- Oil
- Whole grains

    Store whichever whole grains you will eat. However, if you are just starting with whole grain cooking, consider quinoa and millet. They are easy to find and purchase and can be interchanged with rice and are cooked the same way. These grains will store for about two years at room temperature. Millet has the added benefit of being the most easily digestible grain.

Skills to develop/practice:

- Experiment with cooking beans and different whole grains. Find recipes you enjoy and start regularly cycling these into meals.
- Learn to make gluten-free bread. The no-fail bread recipe on p. 251 is a good place to start.

- Expand or start a garden, and improve your gardening skills, if you have space to do so.
- Use the information gleaned from writing dates on packages to determine what a six-month or one-year supply is for you.
- Learn to make your own baking mixes to save time.

As I progressed to the intermediate stage, I increased my cooking abilities, started making more bread, and stored more flour, sugar and canned goods. I also moved from an apartment to a townhouse and hid tomatoes and herbs among the plants in the flower beds and grew vegetables in pots. I also started buying peaches from a local farm and bottling them myself.

Advanced/Larger Households

To buy: Continue to use and replace items in your quickly-moving everyday storage as they go on sale. Acquire a one-year supply of longer-storing grains, beans and canned goods. Expand storage of non-food necessary items. Acquire any tools and supplies needed for skills you develop, e.g. garden tools, canning supplies, grain mills.

Specific basics to store:

- Foods on the above lists
- Additional Beans
- Garden Seeds

    My personal approach to storing seeds is to buy double garden seeds one year, and plant half. The next year I buy enough for that year's garden, but plant the previous year's seeds. Store seeds in a cool, dry, dark location and date the packages. Seed packets can be placed in mason jars or mylar pouches and kept in cool dark places. Adding an oxygen absorbing pack can further increase storage times.

Specific grains to store: This will be a personal preference, but the list below are my suggestions because they have broad appeal, long shelf life, good nutrition or are easy to find and use. Your list may be different and will be affected by whether you are milling grain for flour (see our section on home flour milling and grain sections—pg. 104-111).

- Quinoa: Stores well, high protein content and quality, easy to find for purchase, high in iron and calcium. When used as flour, the flavor can be too strong for some people's taste, but I sometimes add it at a 2% level to improve nutrients and flour performance.

- Sorghum: Great flavor, high in complex carbohydrates, performs well in baked goods, has a pleasing texture in salads and stir fry. Long shelf life. Flour made of a mix of sorghum and teff creates a very wheat-like flavor.

- Oatmeal: Easy to find, makes quick breakfast, high-quality fiber. Can be milled into oat flour in a blender.

- White and Brown Rice: Easy to find, well liked, inexpensive (remember, brown rice has a shorter storage life).

- Teff: Very long shelf life, tastes great, performs well in baked goods. It's a nutritional powerhouse, high in quality protein and minerals, good in cooked grain cereal blends and as a component of flour.

Skills to develop/practice

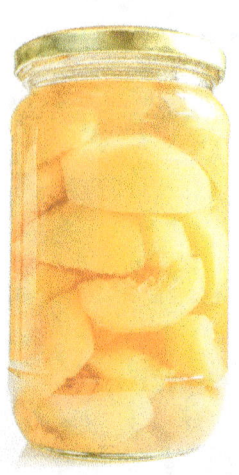

- Continue to improve gardening skills

- Learn to preserve your harvest, e.g. canning, drying, freezing. Local extension offices are a great resource for this. They hold classes and offer other printed information

- Mill your own flour (see our home flour milling section on pages 104-111 to determine if you want to do this or not)

- Continue to expand your cooking and baking skills

As my resources and skills grew over the years, our family expanded our gardens, planted fruit trees and berries and preserved a significant portion of our harvest. For a time, I made all the family's bread but this stopped when I started a business and had less time. My menus changed as life changed but the lifestyle is still in place.

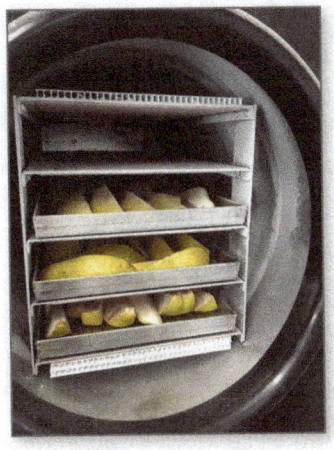

Pears in the freeze dryer.

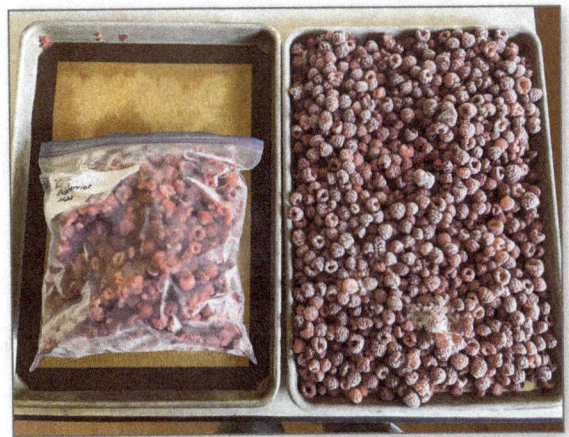

Tray frozen raspberries packaged for the freezer.

We always knew that our approach to food could be used to prepare for emergencies but the wisdom of this became apparent during the quarantine of Covid-19. Because I had purchased and stored a few extras, we never ran out of anything we needed. I even had enough to share with the neighbors. I ended up sharing toilet paper with my college-age children's friends, yeast with a neighbor and potatoes for a funeral luncheon. It was a good feeling to know I did not have to panic and could help others because I had built a reserve.

Additional Resources

U.S. Department of Health & Human Services. (n.d.). Food safety in disaster or emergency. Retrieved May 2, 2023, from https://www.foodsafety.gov/keep-food-safe/food-safety-in-disaster-or-emergency

Utah State University Extension. (n.d.). Food Storage: Preserving and preparing. Retrieved May 2, 2023, from https://extension.usu.edu/preserve-the-harvest/files/Food-Storage-Booklet.pdf

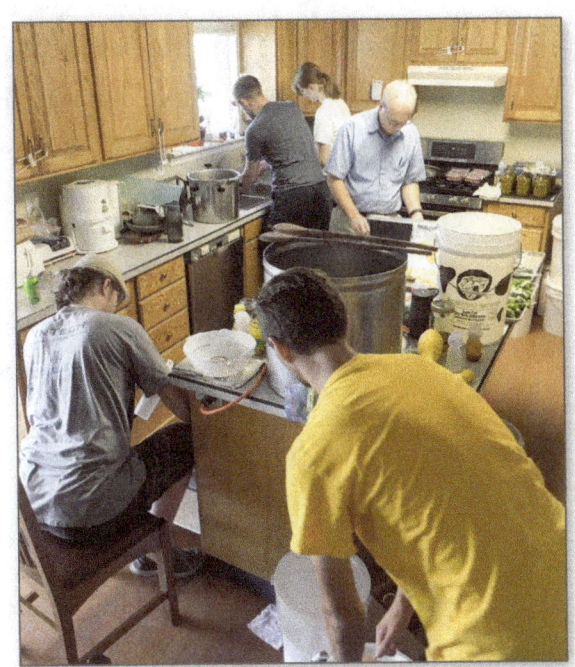

The Huffman Family preserves the harvest.

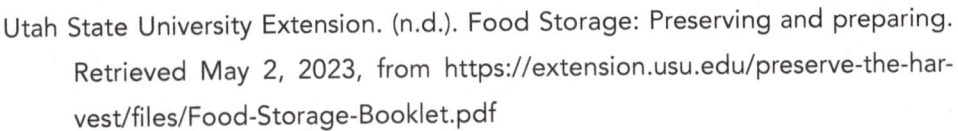

How Much Food Should I Store?

No one can answer this question but you, because needs are highly variable. Use what you learned from dating packages to find the amount of food your family ate in one week or month, then multiply by the number of weeks or months of storage you desire.

Online food storage calculators are also available. Plug in the number of adults and children in your house and the number of month's storage you want and it provides numbers in basic categories. ProvidentLiving.com has a good, basic long-term storage calculator. Keep in mind that the totals generated assume cooking from scratch and the categories are broad. For instance, the grain category contains flour and pasta as well as whole grains. The numbers produced by the calculator can also make food storage seem overwhelming. Don't worry about that, it is more important to take the first steps. One month's storage is much better than no storage. Start small, choose a shorter time frame, and work up to it.

No food storage calculator will tell you how many items unique to gluten free living, like xanthan gum, you will need to store, but you can figure this easily. Suppose you decide you need 100 lbs of flour and you plan to blend your own. Since xanthan is about 2% in flour, you would need to store 2 lbs. If your flour recipe contains 50% rice flour, you would need to store 50 lbs, and so on for other ingredients.

Additional Resources

ProvidentLiving.com. (n.d.). Food storage calculator. Retrieved May 4, 2023, from https://providentliving.com/preparedness/food-storage/foodcalc/

Where Can I Store Food?

Food storage can take up a lot of space so get creative. Pantries and basement under-stair closets are obvious choices, but also look at underutilized spaces like the tops of closets and under beds. Buckets and cans can form support for plywood shelves. Garages and crawl spaces can work if they maintain a good temperature. If not, move other non-perishable storage items to those spaces then store food in the space that was freed up. Food can be hidden under tables that have skirts or behind couches. A quick internet search can show ideas that have worked for others to spark your imagination. One of the sites I like is <u>Fav Family Recipes</u>[4]. This site shows pictures of places to put food that don't require building or buying much.

Table made from barrel of food and plywood.

How Long Will My Stored Food Last?

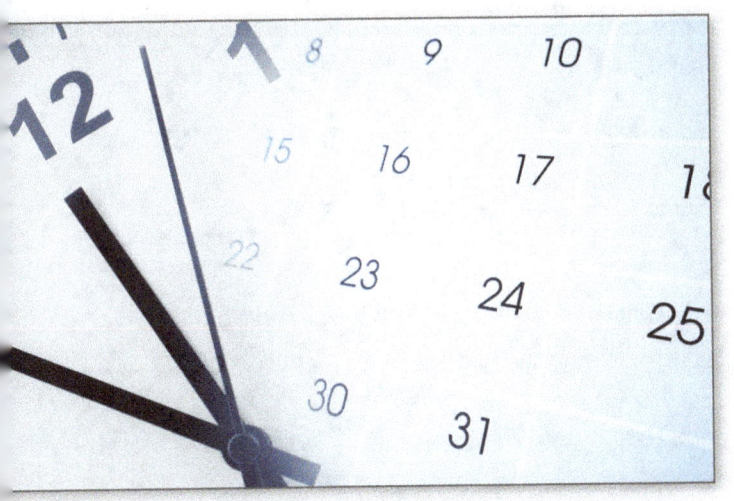

I hate that question for two reasons: (1)There is little scientifically validated shelf-life information specific to gluten free basics and (2) storage times are HIGHLY dependent on storage conditions.

WHAT CAN THE CHURCH OF JESUS CHRIST OF LATTER-DAY SAINTS TEACH ABOUT SHELF-LIFE?
(AND WHY IT'S USEFUL TO MEMBERS AND NON-MEMBERS ALIKE!)

A lot, actually. The Church of Jesus Christ has been encouraging self-reliance and food storage since the mid-1800's. This evolved over time, and The Church enlisted experts at Brigham Young University to figure out what storable foods a person would need to eat to survive for a year. What they came up with is the backbone of most long-term storage recommendation lists: wheat, powdered milk, rice, oils, sugars, and so forth. They also developed a chart of how much of each item to store per person, per year. The Church later opened home storage centers which sold recommended storage commodities packaged in number 10 metal cans with the oxygen removed. These Home Storage Centers are open to all, regardless of church membership.

In the last decade, Brigham Young University revisited the shelf-life question with testing. Researchers requested donations of canned staples that had been stored for 20-30 years. Tests showed the nutrient content was remarkably high and that people found the taste acceptable. Amazing! Well-stored food, i.e. low oxygen, light and temperature (stored mostly in Utah basements) tasted better and maintained nutrition much longer than anticipated. See chart below.

The official Church website[5] has excellent information about long term storage and a chart of how much to store based on this research.

Food	Storage Time
Dried Apple Slices	30 years
Beans (Black, Pinto, Great Northern)	30
Carrots	10
Non-Fat Dry Milk	20
Oatmeal	30
Dry Minced Onion	30
Potato Flakes	30
White Rice	30
Sugar	30

The moral of the BYU research is to use the principles of increasing shelf life to the best of your ability.

Another lesson is that food does not lose all nutrition at the end of its ideal storage time, so don't discard it just for being past date. No one has tested gluten-free grains, starches and gums in the same way as wheat, but the storage principles hold true for all food.

I found these factors at work for all the foods I tried to pin a storage time down for. For instance, I found dry bean shelf life ranges given between 2 years and 30 years. I also noticed that some sources reporting long storage times had tested canned dry beans. It turns out that the better your storage conditions for beans, the longer they remain fully hydratable.

Uncertain storage length for your particular conditions is a strong reason to incorporate storage foods into your diet regularly. You will learn experientially how long food remains palatable, or better yet, will never reach unpalatability by using the first in, first out system.

[1]Federal Emergency Management Agency. (2004). Food and Water in an Emergency. https://www.fema.gov/pdf/library/f&web.pdf

[2]Square Foot Gardening. (n.d.). Square Foot Gardening. Retrieved May 13, 2023, from https://square-footgardening.org/

[3]Wageningen Seed Science Centre. (n.d.). Low oxygen seed storage. Retrieved May 2, 2023, from https://www.wur.nl/en/research-results/projects-and-programmes/wageningen-seed-science-centre-1/research-topics-projects/research-topics-wssc/seed-technology/low-oxygen-seed-storage.htm

[4]Fav Family Recipes. (n.d.). Food Storage Tips: Where to Store Food. Retrieved May 6, 2023, from https://www.favfamilyrecipes.com/food-storage-tips-where-to-store-food/#:~:text=Store%20food%20in%20a%20cool,will%20protect%20food%20from%20moisture.

[5]The Church of Jesus Christ of Latter-day Saints. (n.d.). Longer-term food supply. Retrieved May 3, 2023, from https://www.churchofjesuschrist.org/topics/food-storage/longer-term-food-supply?lang=eng#2.

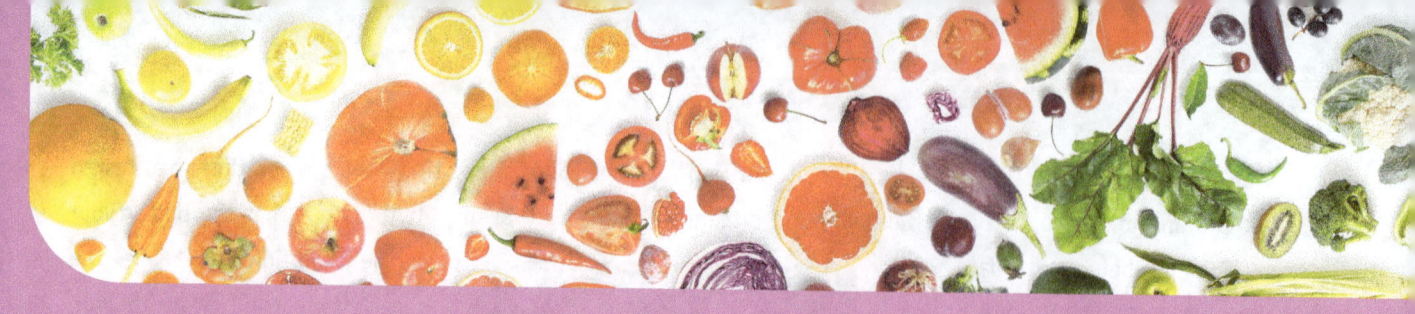

CHAPTER ELEVEN

How to STORE FOOD

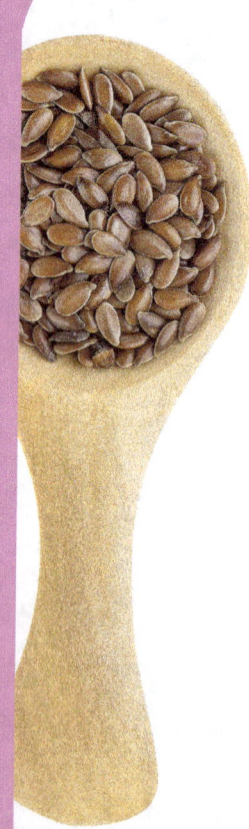

FOOD STORAGE MAKES YOUR LIFE EASIER BY BUILDING A RESERVE. Unexpected things happen to everyone, but having a reserve cushions the severity. From saving frequent trips to the store, to unexpected job loss or illness, to preserving your life after a natural disaster, food storage can be an important resource. For food storage to serve you well it should be nutritious, taste good and be something you like to eat even after it has been stored. There are two important keys to this: rotate food through storage, and store food in good conditions.

Use the FIFO System When Storing Food

All food in storage should be rotated using the First In First Out system. The FIFO system equates to using the oldest food item you have

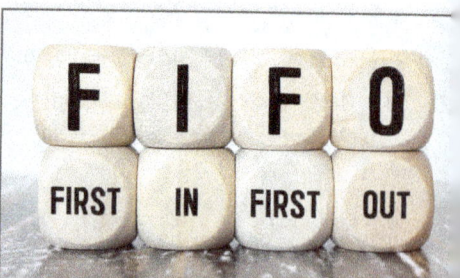

first to ensure food is eaten before it spoils. This is where writing the date on foods makes a big difference. Add new items to the back of the shelf and use items from the front of the shelf.

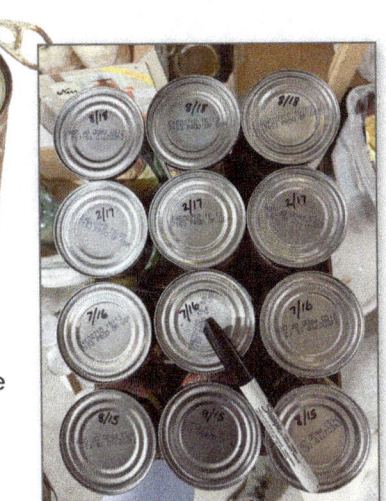

Food begins to degrade as soon as it is harvested or produced, so the core idea of food storage is to reduce spoiling, nutrient and flavor loss, and extend the time it can be eaten. The shelf life determines how much you can store, and how long you can store it. Understanding which forces speed food degradation enables you to maximize shelf life.

Quality vs. Safety

Stored food can be safe to eat without being good to eat. Most package dates are quality dates rather than safety dates and food is safe to eat for much longer periods. For instance, canned food sealed without bulging, rusting, or other damage is likely safe to eat, but may be so old that the contents are unpalatable. Foods with high oil content, like peanut butter and seeds, degrade faster so expiration dates are shorter. Highly-perishable foods, like meat or milk, employ dates that are meant to ensure food is not consumed spoiled. Other foods, like sugar, have a decades-long shelf life when stored properly.

Manufacturers of dry, packaged food base their recommendations on whether food will look good and still have excellent flavor at the end of the prescribed time. Most are palatable and nutritious much longer. A past-date dry or canned food should not be automatically thrown out. The questions to inform your decision of whether to toss or keep are: **is it safe, does it taste good, and can I afford not to eat it?**

A friend of mine was faced with this decision when her husband lost his job. She had no income and a houseful of children. She used her old food storage which contained a lot of rancid rice. It still had some nutrition, and they had to eat it. She found that adding vinegar to the water before cooking eliminated the rancidity and it sustained the family until they found employment again. It was still safe and she couldn't afford not to eat it. Fortunately, she found a way to make it palatable.

Factors that Influence Shelf Life

Not all factors that degrade food can be controlled, but understanding the environmental factors that speed food degradation will help you optimize storage and packaging choices. The factors that reduce shelf life are:

- Light
- Temperature
- Oxygen
- Moisture
- Pests such as rodents or insects

Light causes compounds in food to react and oxidize more quickly. This can degrade flavor compounds and vitamins especially. Have you ever wondered why beer is packaged in brown bottles, or olive oil in green? It is to reduce the light that degrades them. In the case of beer, UV light changes the bitterness of the hops. Olive oil becomes rancid quickly when exposed to light.

You can reduce light exposure in a number of ways. When you buy or repackage food to store, choose materials that block light or store the food in a dark room, cupboard or box.

Temperature increases or fluctuations speed up the rate of chemical change and influence microbial growth in food. Look for places to store food that are cool and without wide temperature swings. It may not be possible to store food in a truly cool place in your space, but do your best. Avoid hot places like garages and furnace rooms.

The shelf life of food decreases by half for each 10° Celsius. For instance, suppose a food has a shelf life of 2 years at 5° C. That food will undergo the following pattern of storage length changes:

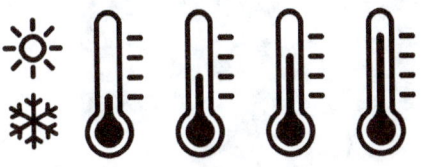

5° C (41° F) = 2 years

15° C (59° F)= 1 year

25° C (77° F)= 6 months

35° C (95° F)= 3 months

45° C (113° F)= 1.5 months

This highlights just how important temperature is and why freezing is an effective storage method. Temperature affects the chemical degradation as well as the microbial degradation. Food spoilage microbes are not killed by freezing, but do not grow or grow more slowly so store high quality food.

Oxygen oxidizes. This chemical reaction destroys nutrients and causes off flavors like rancidity. Oxygen is removed from food through processes like canning, vacuum sealing, and oxygen absorbing packets. Look for packaging that is airtight and fill your containers as full as possible. Completely filling the container or squeezing air out of soft-sided packages reduces the amount of oxygen available to react with your food. Food can also be sealed with a home vacuum sealer.

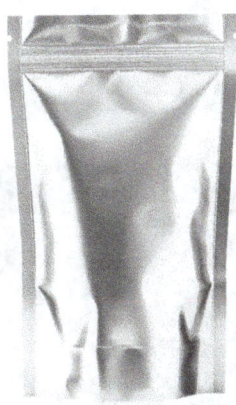

Oxygen absorbing packets are very easy to use and work well to remove oxygen from packages of dry foods. These packets allow oxygen and moisture to enter the packet and react with the iron powder inside. The chemical reaction of oxidation (rusting of iron) binds the oxygen inside your sealed packaging and continues to absorb until all the iron has reacted or there is no more oxygen in the container, whichever comes first. Since air is about 20% oxygen, packaging may not look completely vacuum sealed. The nitrogen from the air remains but does not deteriorate the food. Placing oxygen absorbers inside a package that will be vacuum sealed is unnecessary.

Tips for Using Oxygen Absorbing Packets

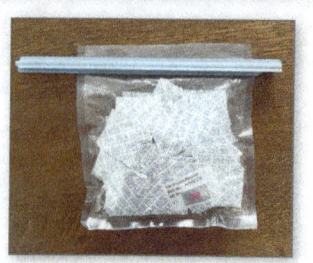

Because packets continue to absorb oxygen, you must reseal your container of packets quickly after opening. You can do this with a special clip, a heat sealer (including an iron or flat iron), or by putting them in the smallest mason jar they will fit into and screwing on the lid. If you do not have enough absorbers left to fill a jar, the empty space in the jar can be filled with rice. The mason jar should be unchipped along the upper sealing surface and have a new lid which has been boiled to ensure complete sealing.

Packets should be soft. Hard or crunchy packets have already been used up by oxygen exposure and must be discarded.

Oxygen absorbing packets (or O2 absorbers) come in a range of sizes measured in cubic centimeters, or cc. This is an indication of how much each oxygen the packet can absorb. Sizes range from 30 to 2,000 cc but are most commonly seen in 100 and 300 cc sizes.

Choose a container that your food can completely fill to decrease the number of O2 absorbers needed. Ideally, the volume of your food should fill the container. Containers with a lot of air space at the top or food with shapes which cannot be tightly packed like macaroni will require more O2 absorbers.

Get everything else prepped before opening the O2 absorbers. Fill your containers. Have all sealing equipment out. When it is all set up, add your packets to the food, seal up unused packets, squeeze as much excess air out of your food container as possible then seal. Assembly lines also work well for packaging efficiently.

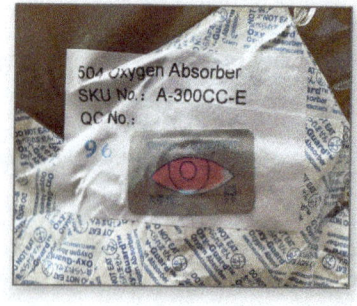

When you purchase O2 absorbers, the package includes an oxygen indicator, a small red paper-like dot. If this is red or pink the package is oxygen free. Blue indicates exposure to oxygen. This will turn blue when you open a package, but when resealed quickly will return to pink or red. This indicates that the remaining packets are still working.

O2 absorbers are unnecessary in vacuum-packed foods.

Use the chart below to determine how many packets are needed for your application. You may need more absorbers than listed depending on open space within your container.

CONTAINER	DENSELY PACKING FOODS Grains, Flour		LOOSELY PACKING FOODS Beans, Pasta
5 or 6 gallon bucket	100 cc	20	25-30
	500 cc	4	5-6
	1000 cc	2	3
	2000 cc	1	2
Use the same number of absorbers if using a mylar bag inside bucket			
2 gallon mylar	100 cc	10	15-20
	500 cc	2	3-4
	1000 cc	1	2
	2000 cc	1	1
1 gallon mylar	100 cc	3-4	4
	500 cc	1	1
	1000 cc	1	1
	5000 cc	1	1
Pint jar or bag	100 cc	1	100 cc 1
Quart jar or bag	200 cc	1	200 cc 1

Moisture. All life, including bacteria and mold, requires water to survive. Foods low in water or water activity (water can be bound by other ingredients in food like sugar which makes it unavailable for organisms) last longer and have a wider range of safe storage conditions. Very wet foods must be canned, pickled or frozen; while dry foods like pasta, beans and grains can be stored at room temperature or below as long as they are kept dry. Foods should be stored in packaging that prevents contents from becoming wet or absorbing humidity from the air.

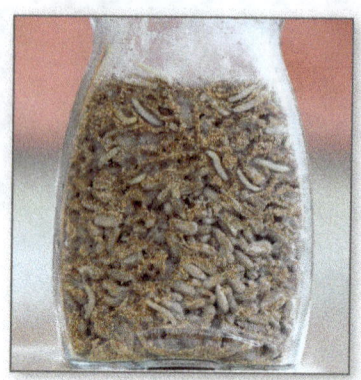

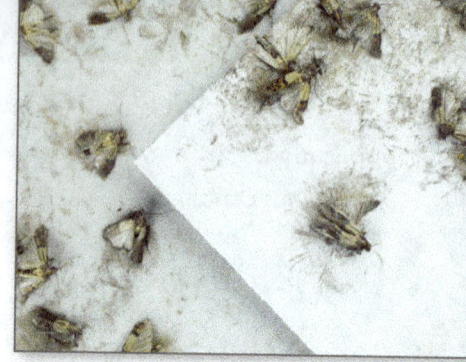

Indian meal moths on trap.

Pests should be controlled by careful selection of food for storage. Do not store food that is already known to be contaminated with insects. Package food in containers that are resistant to insects and rodents. Pests require oxygen to live and eliminating oxygen from packaging is also an effective insect control.

If you find an infestation of insects, discard all food that is visibly infested. Food that could be exposed but is not showing signs of infestation can be frozen to kill eggs and larva. Use traps specific to the insect you have a problem with like Indian meal moths. For rodent problems, use rodent-resistant containers and traps.

Tips for Storing Food in the Freezer

Freezers are a great way to store food both for convenience (like frozen entrees and pre-chopped vegetables) and for keeping food like meat and vegetables close to their original flavor and nutrition. The freezer can also increase shelf life of light- and temperature-sensitive foods like nuts and flours that lose nutrients or turn rancid quickly. Knowing a few things about how freezing works and how to prep food can make a big difference in food quality.

What is Freezer Burn?

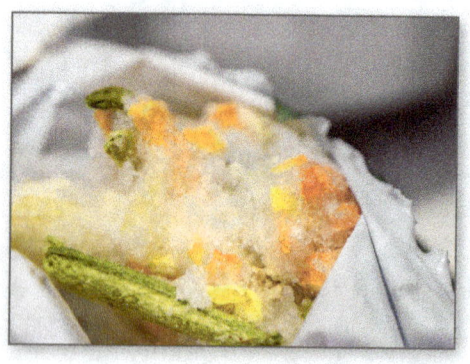

What people call "freezer burn" is actually dehydration. When placed in a freezer, the water in food freezes. Food contains a lot of water, but the air inside your freezer is very dry. When ice is exposed to dry, cold air, it sublimates. Sublimation is a solid (ice in this case) changing directly to a vapor, similar to evaporation which is a liquid changing to a vapor state. When cold, dry air surrounds a food, water migrates from inside the food to the outside where it is refrozen, leaving ice crystals on the outside and making the food hard and dry.

Keeping the Air Out

Keeping the air out is an absolute necessity to prevent or delay freezer burn. There should be no air space between the package and the food being frozen. If using lidded plastic freezer containers, leave only enough head space to allow expansion during freezing.

Vacuum sealing systems are ideal for freezer packaging because bags are not gas permeable and the process pulls the packaging directly onto the surface of the food by removing air. Foods with liquids like soups or juicy vegetables and fruits can be difficult to seal with the vacuum system since water or juice can be pulled into the area to be sealed, preventing a good seal. Solve this by filling bags then freezing before vacuum sealing.

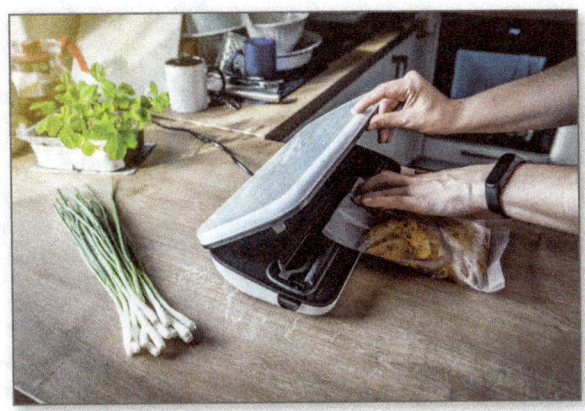

Vacuum bags have one side that is not smooth. This keeps the sides from closing off while you are removing the air. If you want to use mylar bags instead, there is a great hack and demonstration at Back Pack Hack on Youtube[1].

In place of a vacuum sealer, you can wrap food tightly in plastic wrap followed by another layer such as foil or freezer paper to get your sealed surface directly onto your food. You can also place plastic wrapped food into zippered freezer bags and remove as much air as possible. This method won't preserve food as long, but is quick and easy for short term freezing of items like muffins. If you know you will use an item quickly, you can be less vigilant about the container. For instance, I skip the wrapping step for cookies or cookie dough because my boys will eat them all before they have a chance to get freezer burned. They also don't contain a lot of water, which helps too.

Meat packaged in styrofoam trays with plastic wrap is very susceptible to freezer burn and should be repackaged. It is also possible to wrap the entire package tightly with foil then cover tightly with plastic wrap, or use one of the other options above.

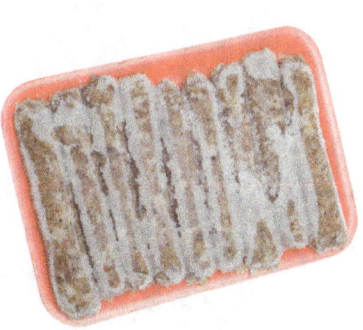

Liquids like broth will automatically fill in completely to the sides of your container so air space is less of an issue.

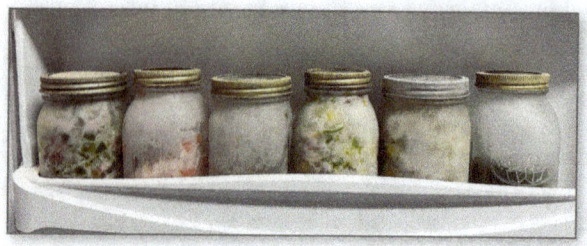

Mason jars are also great freezer storage containers. They do not allow gas exchange and keep strong smells like onion from being absorbed by other food in the freezer. Leave enough headspace to allow for expansion during freezing to avoid bottle breakage. Some vacuum systems can also be used with mason jars. If vacuum sealing a mason jar, freeze first and then seal to avoid expansion breakage. Bottles may also break through thermal shock. Do not place hot jars directly into the freezer or thaw frozen bottles in very hot water.

Freezer Temperature

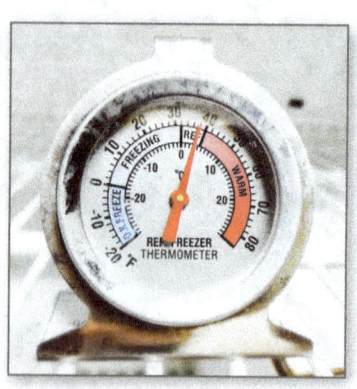

Use a freezer thermometer to find the setting that keeps your freezer at 0° Fahrenheit. Don't overfill or underfill your freezer. Already frozen food helps freeze new additions quickly, but an overfilled freezer can prevent the needed air circulation for freezing and over-tax the condenser. Keep vents clear and allow air space around shelves to keep air circulation and efficiency high.

Cool food before freezing. When unchilled or warm food is placed in a freezer it warms the food around it. Freezing items flat is one strategy to keep contents cool. Food in flatter packages freezes more quickly, and can fit more in the freezer. I freeze foods which contain liquid in freezer bags on a cookie sheet. Once frozen I remove the cookie sheet and they stack easily.

Fast freezing has the added benefit of creating smaller ice crystals than slow freezing. Small ice crystals do less damage to the structure of the food being frozen which improves the texture when thawed. This is especially noticeable when freezing fruit or vegetables. Addition of sugar to fruits can also improve freezing quality. For more instructions of freezing fruits, check out this article from University of New Mexico Extension[2]. Instructions for freezing vegetables can be found in a PDF from National Center for Home Food Preservation[3].

Food Storage Containers

The best food storage container for you varies based on type of food, length of intended storage, available space, and usage rate. If you use up a food quickly, large containers may be a good option. If usage rate is low, small packages might be best. Whatever your needs, the key is reducing the factors that destroy food quality in the container you choose. Containers should shield from moisture, light, heat, oxygen and pests. Several of the most common types of food storage containers are described below along with advantages and disadvantages.

Foil or Mylar Pouches

These pouches are also called laminate pouches because they are made of layers of material, typically including food-safe plastic polyethylene and a thin foil layer.

Advantages:

- Excellent barrier to oxygen, moisture, and light
- Available in many sizes and with resealable zippers. Sizes range from an 18" x 28" bag that fit five-gallon buckets to several inches
- Variable sizes allow packaging in volumes appropriate for your personal usage rate
- Found online and in camping and emergency supply stores

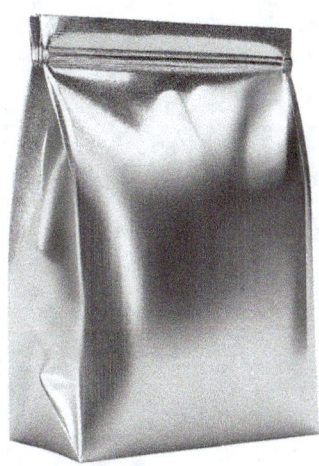

Disadvantages:

- Not rodent proof. Note: packages may be stored in rodent-proof containers such as lidded plastic buckets
- Small packages take up more space than larger ones for the same volume of food.
- Single use container. Not reusable or recyclable

- Must be sealed with a heat sealer. This can also be accomplished with a flat iron for hair styling

Glass Canning Jars with Two-Piece Lids

Advantages:

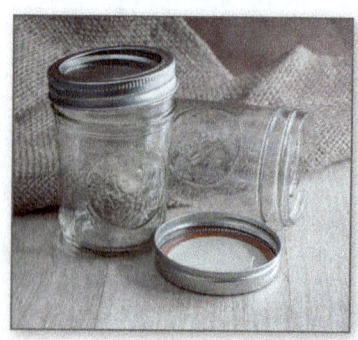

- Widely available in grocery and other stores
- Does not deteriorate or react with food
- Can be used in the freezer or on the shelf
- Does not allow oxygen to enter. Oxygen may be removed using an oxygen absorbing packet, vacuum sealer with bottle attachment, or through home canning processes for fresh fruit and vegetables
- Rodent proof
- Reusable for years and fully recyclable

Disadvantages:

- Does not block light. Note: this can be overcome by storing in a dark place or inside a box
- Can break or chip if dropped or mishandled
- Requires a lot of storage space

Plastic Bottles

PET or PETE, short for Polyethylene Terephthalate, a food grade plastic, bears a number 1 recycle symbol. It is rigid and strong with antimicrobial properties which make it good for food storage. It's commonly used for soda bottles and peanut butter jars.

PLASTICS BY THE NUMBER: IS THIS FOOD GRADE?

The terms "food grade" and "food safe" are not synonymous. Food grade can indicate two things. First, that the material is safe to eat (e.g. food-grade table salt vs non-food-grade de-icing salt). Second, to describe a material which comes in contact with food, like plastic containers. Food safe means using a food-grade material in ways that do not leach chemicals into the food or otherwise make it unsafe. For instance, some plastics are safe to store foods in (food grade), but not safe to heat foods in (food safe).

Generally, plastic numbers 1, 2, 4, and 5 are food grade. Recycle numbers 3 and 7, polyvinyl chloride (PVC), and polycarbonate are produced with BPA or Bisphenol A and are not considered food grade. Number 4, low-density polyethylene, is flexible and is used for bread bags and plastic wrap. Number 5 is used for rigid, single-use plastics like yogurt cups. Plastics 1 and 2 are the best and most accessible for home storage (see pages 154-156).

PET bottles for storage should have a screw-on lid with a plastic seal rather than a foam or paper lid seal. To test for airtightness, hold the sealed bottle under water and press on it. Bubbles will come out if it is not airtight.

Advantages:

- Convenient to open and use
- Can be reused
- Oxygen can be removed using an oxygen removing packet
- Inexpensive if reusing bottles originally purchased containing other foods or beverages. For instructions on how to do this, see <u>The Provident Prepper</u>[4].

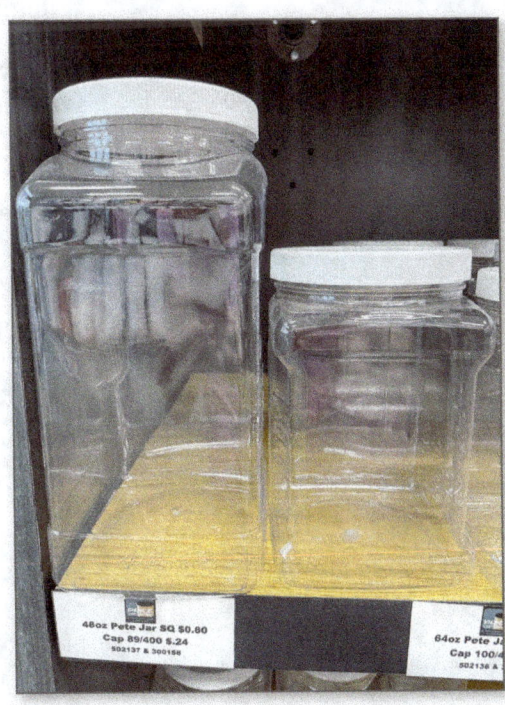

Disadvantages:

- Not a light barrier
- Slowly allows oxygen to enter. Best for medium term storage (one or two years)
- Not suitable for foods with a high oil or water content

Metal Cans

Cans are used to store wet or dry foods. Wet food in cans has a shorter shelf life than dry canned foods.

Advantages:

- Near zero oxygen transfer rate
- Stores dry foods such as grains and powdered milk with little nutrient loss for many years
- Many staples can be purchased pre-canned for long-term storage
- Recyclable
- Rodent proof

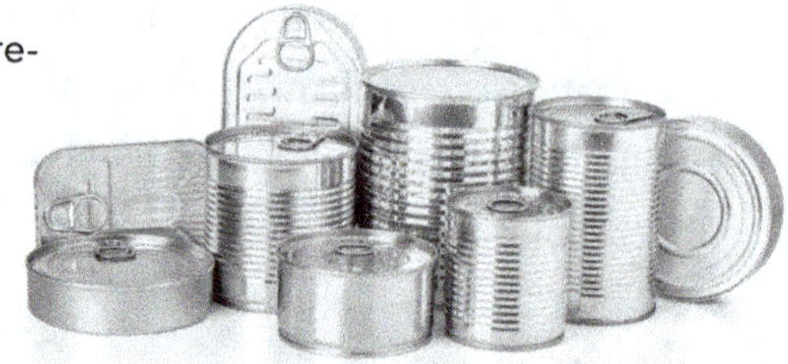

Disadvantages:

- Requires special equipment to can at home
- May rust if stored in a humid environment
- Not resealable

Plastic Buckets

Plastic buckets come in varying sizes and are made of high-density polyethylene plastic (HDPE) recycle number 2. These are generally food grade, but may not be if they were dyed with non-food safe dyes or previously contained a non-food item. If you are buying new buckets, the supplier will be able to tell you whether it is food grade. Press-on lids with gaskets are best for long-term storage because they are airtight. Gamma lids, or screw top lids, are convenient but not as airtight. If you like the convenience of a gamma lid you can store with a gasketed lid then replace with a gamma lid once the bucket is opened for use.

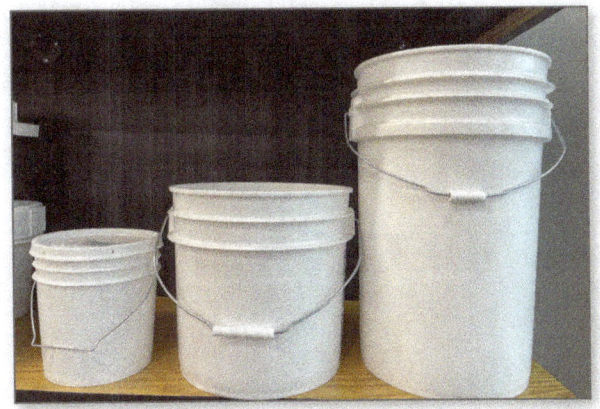

Buckets may be reused if they held food previously. Sourcing used buckets at bakeries, restaurants, or food manufacturers can save money. Keep in mind that plastic is slightly porous and can absorb and later release what it previously held, such as flavors or chemicals. Buckets which held paint, chemicals, and so forth, are not safe for food. Always check used lids to make sure they are still air-tight. Replace with new lids as needed. There is no point removing oxygen from a bucket that leaks air.

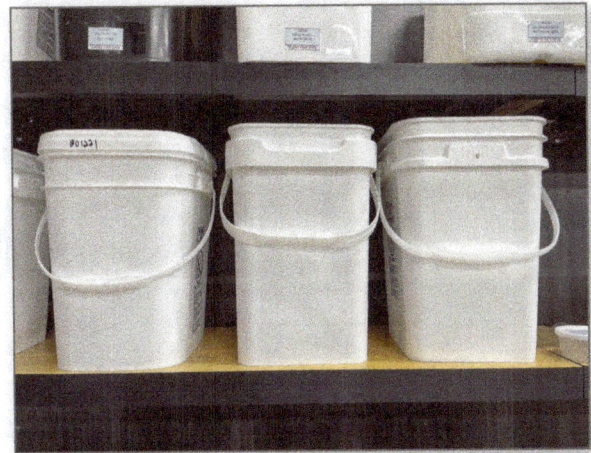

For ideal bucket storage, use a mylar-type bag and oxygen absorbers inside the buckets. Another reason to consider using a lining bag is that stacked buckets can rupture in a fall during an earthquake. For this reason, buckets with a thickness of 90 mil are recommended for stacking rather than 70 mil buckets. If using plastic bags inside a bucket, make sure the bag is food grade. Garbage bags are not food grade.

Advantages:

- Oxygen enters at a slow rate (even with an airtight lid). Stores food well for five years, generally

- Can store large quantities of food, about 30 lbs

- Easy to find and inexpensive. Watch for sales at farm or hardware stores

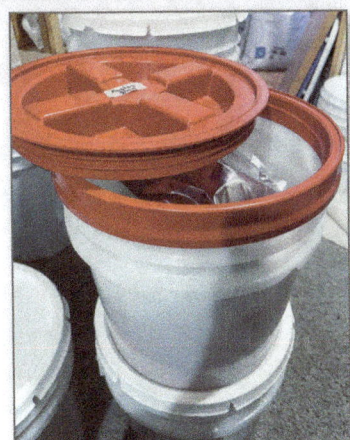

Bucket with gamma lid

- Available in square or round shapes to fit your space

- Are stackable

- Some come with handles for easy moving

- Reusable, though some lids are not and must be replaced

- Work well to store food in other smaller packaging, such as mylar bags

- Rodent proof

Disadvantages:

- Large, choose a size that you can lift and move alone

- Heavy, depending on what is inside

- Opening frequently to remove small amounts of food introduces oxygen and degrades the storage environment for the remaining food. Mylar bags within buckets can be resealed to prevent oxygen entering. If doing this, cut the smallest functional whole to remove food and quickly reseal

[1]Back Pack Hack. (2016, September 30). DIY Emergency 100 Hour Candles [Video]. YouTube. https://www.youtube.com/watch?v=fCgsbiTdnDA

[2]University of Minnesota Extension. (n.d.). How to Freeze Fruit for Best Flavor. Retrieved May 10, 2023, from https://extension.umn.edu/preserving-and-preparing/how-freeze-fruit-best-flavor#apricots-425261

[3]Andress, E. L., & Harrison, J. A. (2006). Freezing Vegetables. National Center for Home Food Preservation, University of Georgia. Retrieved May 10, 2023, from https://nchfp.uga.edu/publications/uga/uga_freeze_veg.pdf

[4]The Provident Prepper. (n.d.). Packaging dry foods in plastic bottles for long-term food storage. Retrieved May 12, 2023, from https://theprovidentprepper.org/packaging-dry-foods-in-plastic-bottles-for-long-term-food-storage/

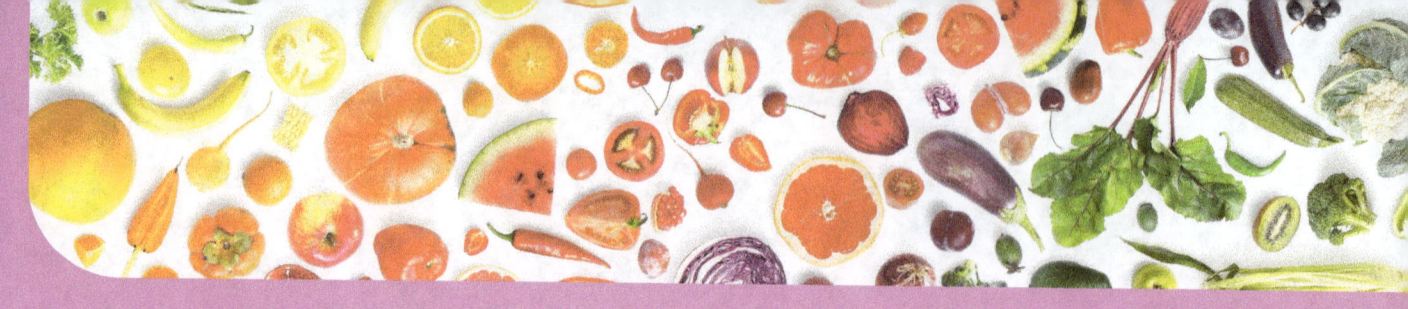

CHAPTER TWELVE
WHERE TO BUY
Food Storage

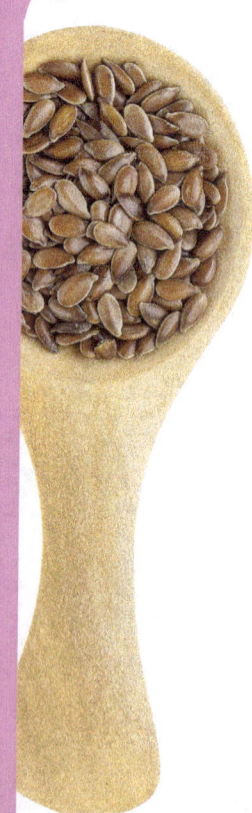

Where Can I Purchase Food for Storage?

Food for storage can be purchased from many local places you already shop. In fact, your short-term storage will almost always come from stores you frequent since it is food you are already buying and eating. When building a longer-term reserve, it is helpful to buy some foods in bulk. Bulk food can be less expensive, especially commodities like flour, beans and grains—but make sure you do the math because this is not always true. Since businesses and websites change and resources differ by region, strategies for finding bulk foods, as well as sources, will be covered in this section.

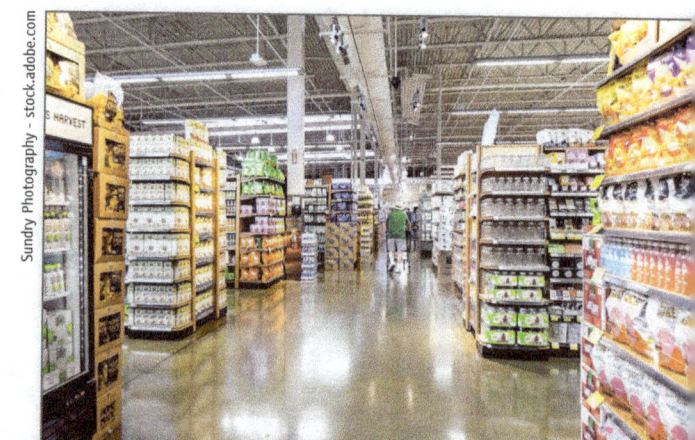

Sundry Photography - stock.adobe.com

Warehouse Clubs

Warehouse Clubs like Sam's Club or Costco often carry food in larger sizes and multipacks at a discount. They also have large sizes of basic items like sugar, oil, rice, and beans. Be sure to compare unit prices like cost per pound. For instance, I have found that sugar is actually cheaper at WalMart than at Sam's.

Costco Business Centers, which cater to small businesses, are a great resource if there is one near you. These stores sell food, cooking equipment, cleaning and office supplies in packaging and types appropriate for businesses. Regular members are allowed to shop at these centers as well as business customers. The Business Center in my state carries 25 lb bags of Bob's Red Mill gluten-free flour cheaper than I have seen anywhere, ever.

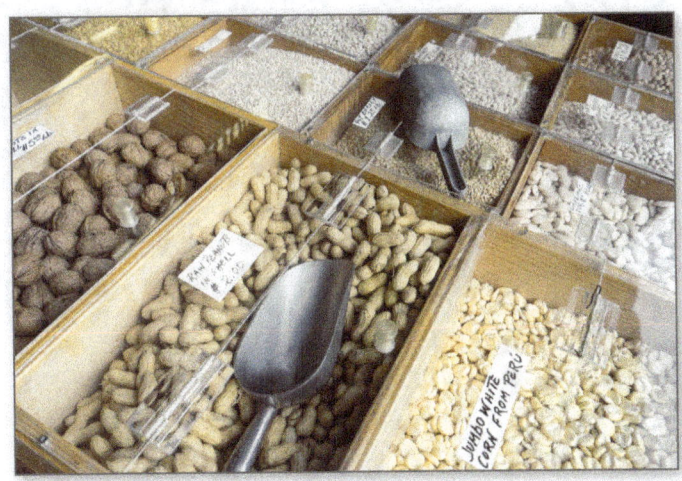

Stores with Bulk Bins

Those with food allergies and intolerances are usually counseled to avoid bulk food aisles because of possible cross contamination problems. However, these stores buy in bulk packaging then fill bins, which means they can sell you an unopened box or bag. If you see an item in the bins you want, talk to the manager about buying the bag. The items the store has in bulk are also a clue to what the store might be able to order. Related food items may not be carried in the store, but be available by special order from the store's distributors.

WinCo is an example of a store chain in the West and Midwest that carries a large array of bulk items, from gluten-free flours to candy and many types of beans. Additionally, they carry bulk dog food, pet treats, birdseed, and bulk teas. Some of the items in WinCo's bulk department are ingredients I use in my company and know the wholesale price of. I found prices of these items to be very competitive.

Find local bulk stores in your area by searching on Google for "bulk food stores near me" or "bulk food stores in (name of your city)," and you will soon come up with stores that carry bulk foods near your home. You may find local, family-owned shops that carry gluten-free bulk items.

Asian Markets/Restaurant Supplies

Many Asian foods are gluten free so it makes sense to check out your local market or Asian restaurant supply store. They can be a good source for bulk tapioca flour, rice in many varieties, and rice flour. They also have bean varieties seldom found in a traditional grocery store like soy and mung.

Home Storage Centers

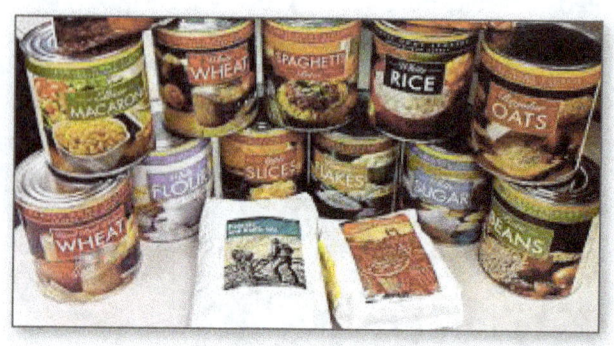

The Church of Jesus Christ of Latter-Day Saints operates home storage centers throughout the United States which sell basic foods packaged for storage. Not all items fit gluten-free storage needs but there are items like dried onions, carrots, apples, and instant potatoes which do. Oxygen absorbing packets are available from their online shop as well. The volunteer staff can answer other food storage questions you might have. Membership is not required to purchase. Visit the Church website for further information[1].

Bakeries that Mill Flour

Bakeries that mill their own flour buy grains in bulk. Even chain bakeries like Great Harvest are locally owned and sometimes willing to sell bags of grain. Most of the grains these bakeries buy are not gluten free, but they can sometimes order grains that are, and they know grain suppliers in the area. You can call or visit the store, although I find it most helpful to visit the store during non-busy hours of operation. In-person communication generally yields more information.

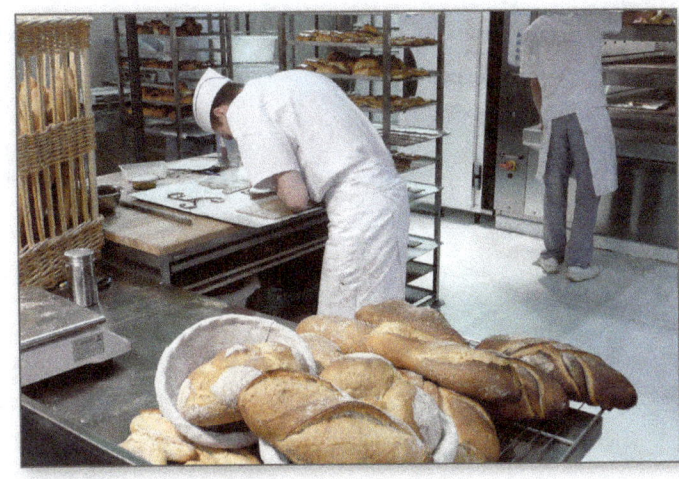

I usually say something to the effect of, "I'm looking for a source for a few bags of grain for home food storage. Do you ever sell bags of grain? No? Do you know where else I might try? Is there someone around that sells grain wholesale? Can you please point me in the right direction?"

Honeyville Inc.

Honeyville sells grains, bakery ingredients and a food storage line of products. They carry a large selection of gluten-free flours and grains in bulk and sell to businesses and consumers. These can be purchased online[2] or picked up at their warehouses (Utah, California, Arizona).

Rainy Day Foods

Rainy day foods is based in Southern Idaho and sells bulk commodities and food packaged for food storage. Food can be ordered online[3] or by phone and can be picked up if you live within driving distance. They are more consumer-friendly than Honeyville for local pickup.

Online Stores that Offer Gluten Free Foods

Webstaurant[4] is an online restaurant supply that sells a number of gluten-free flours in 25 lb bags. The prices are good, but shipping can be expensive (though I have found their shipping rates to be comparable to other businesses). Shipping rates go down significantly for large orders that can be shipped on a pallet. If you have a big family or friends that will order with you, this can be a good source.

NuLife Market[5] is a high-quality source of sorghum grain and flour. They sell to consumers and businesses. The sorghum is high quality and grown and processed for human consumption. As a bonus it is grown by a family with gluten-free members so they never grow it in fields that have grown gluten-containing crops.

The Teff Company[6] is the oldest and biggest grower of Teff in the United States. They offer bulk and smaller packaging of teff and teff flours on their website. They also have a number of good recipes on their sites.

Gluten Free Prairie[7] specializes in oats and oat flour. The oats are certified gluten free and are grown and processed by a gluten-free family. Products are available in bulk or consumer-sized packaging.

Azure Standard[8] is an organic food company that sells mostly organic in bulk and delivers food to drop points around the country. You meet the truck and pick up the order. Small orders can also be shipped via UPS or USPS. Check online to find the closest drop point for you. You may also start a drop point of your own.

Nut Garden[9] is based in Utah and sells bulk seeds, including quinoa and nuts. They also sell nut meals like almond. If you live in Utah, local pickup is available, otherwise items can be shipped. Many of the items carried can be found in grocery store bulk bin sections so compare prices before ordering.

Sage and Plow,[10] formerly Alpine Food Storage, has a wide range of bulk grains, dried fruits, beans and storage products. They offer bulk orders at set drop points similar to Azure Standard. Currently drop points are only in Utah and Idaho. There is also a new store front in American Fork, UT.

[1]The Church of Jesus Christ of Latter-day Saints. (n.d.). Provident Living. https://providentliving.churchofjesuschrist.org/?lang=eng. Retrieved May 10, 2023.

[2]Honeyville Inc. (n.d.). Home page. Retrieved January 23, 2024 from https://www.honeyville.com

[3]Rainy Day Foods. (n.d.). Home page. Retrieved January 23, 2024 from https://www.rainydayfoods.com

[4]WebstaurantStore. (n.d.). Gluten-free foods. Retrieved May 1, 2023 from https://www.webstaurantstore.com/57613/gluten-free-foods.html

[5]Nulife Market. (n.d.). Home page. Retrieved May 1, 2023 from https://nulifemarket.com/

[6]Teff Company. (n.d.). Home. Retrieved May 5, 2023, from https://teffco.com/

[7]The Gluten-Free Prairie. (n.d.). Home. Retrieved May 3, 2023, from https://www.glutenfreeprairie.com/

[8]Azure Standard. (n.d.). Drop point locator. Retrieved October 11, 2023 from https://www.azurestandard.com/drop-point-locator/

[9]The Nut Garden. (n.d.). Retrieved May 5, 2023 from https://www.thenutgarden.com/

[10]Sage and Plow. (n.d.) Home page. Retrieved March 13, 2024, from https://sageandplow.com/

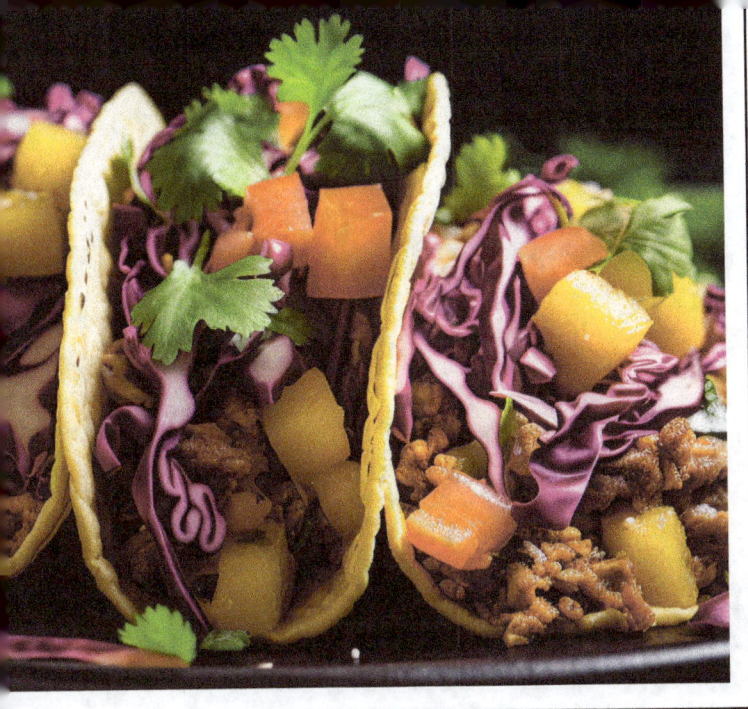

RECIPES

BLENDER OAT PANCAKES

(From *USU Extension*)

BREAKFAST

INGREDIENTS

1⅓ C Milk

1 tbsp Apple Cider Vinegar

1½ tbsp Olive Oil

2 tsp Vanilla Extract

2 C GF Rolled Oats

2 tsp Baking Powder

½ tsp Baking Soda

¼ tsp Sea Salt

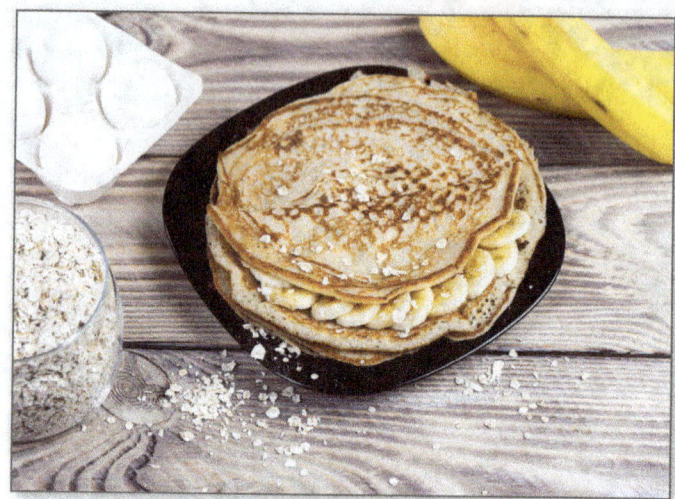

INSTRUCTIONS

Place all ingredients in a blender or food processor and blend on high until completely smooth. Heat a griddle on medium heat; lightly grease with oil or non-stick cooking spray. Drop batter on the griddle, about ¼ C per pancake. After multiple bubbles appear on the surface of the pancake, flip and cook for an additional 30-60 seconds. The pancake batter thickens as it sits. You may need to add additional milk toward the end of cooking to thin the batter. Serve with your favorite pancake toppings.

Substitute the milk with eggs (for additional protein), applesauce, pumpkin, or mashed banana for flavor, and add frozen blueberries, chocolate chips, or nuts while cooking the pancakes as you so desire.

Utah State University Extension. (n.d.). Recipes. Retrieved May 22, 2023, from https://extension.usu.edu/nutrition/recipes/index

BANANA BREAD WAFFLES

(From *USU Extension*)

INGREDIENTS

⅓ C Teff Flour

⅓ C Sorghum Flour

⅓ C Brown Rice Flour

¾ C Tapioca Starch

2 tbsp Coconut Sugar

2 tsp Baking Powder

½ tsp Xanthan Gum

1½ tsp Cinnamon

¼ tsp Nutmeg

½ tsp Salt

2 Very Ripe Bananas

¼ C Oil

1 tsp Vanilla Extract

1¼ C Almond Milk

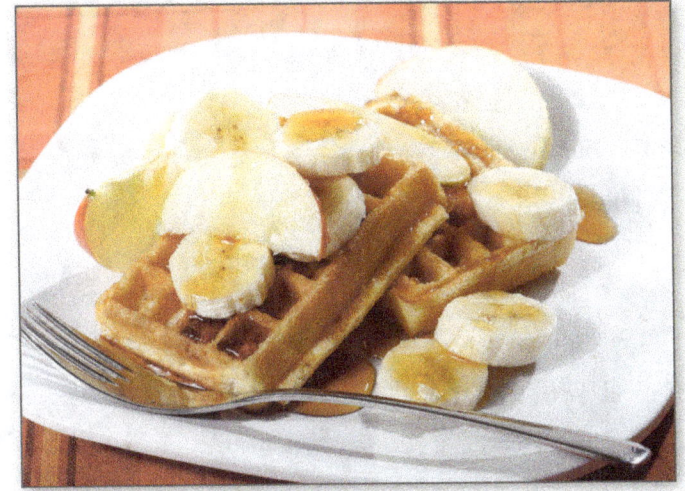

INSTRUCTIONS

Preheat the waffle iron. Combine dry ingredients in a large bowl and set aside. In a medium bowl, combine bananas, oil, vanilla, and milk. Add mixture to the dry ingredients and mix until just combined. Use a pastry brush to oil the top and bottom of the waffle iron. Ladle batter onto the iron and cook.

TEFF PANCAKES

INGREDIENTS

1 ½ C teff flour

2 tsp baking powder

2 tbsp brown sugar

½ tsp salt

½ tsp cinnamon

2 eggs

1-1¼ C buttermilk

3 tbsp oil or melted butter

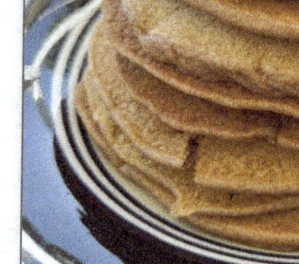

INSTRUCTIONS

Mix the dry ingredients together in a bowl, then add in wet ingredients and stir until well blended. Prepare skillet or griddle by preheating to medium heat. Pour ¼ C batter on prepared griddle and cook until bubbles appear and pop. Flip and cook an additional 30-60 seconds.

Delicious served with fresh strawberries and/or bananas. For more variety try adding ¼ C blueberries or mini chocolate chips to the batter.

DARK CHOCOLATE TEFF PANCAKES

(Adapted from *Grain Power: Over 100 Delicious Gluten-Free Ancient Grains & Superblend Recipes*)

INGREDIENTS

2 C teff flour

⅓ C unsweetened cocoa powder

4 tsp baking powder

¼ C white sugar

½ tsp salt

2 large eggs

1¼ C milk

¾ C water

¼ C melted butter

2 tsp vanilla extract

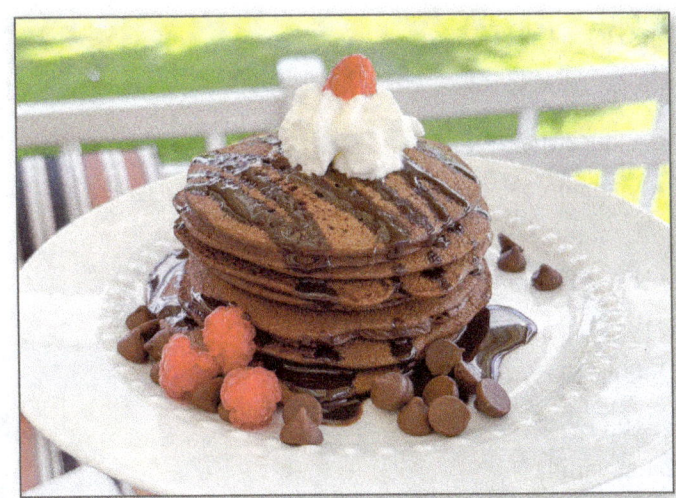

INSTRUCTIONS

Mix the dry ingredients in a large bowl. Whisk together the wet ingredients in a separate bowl then combine with the dry ingredients. Preheat a skillet or griddle to medium heat then pour ¼ C batter on griddle and cook until bubbles appear and pop. Flip and cook an additional 30-60 seconds.

Note: If you would like milkier chocolate pancakes, add 2 Tbsp sugar and increase the vanilla. Also tastes great with Hershey's Chocolate syrup.

Green, P., & Hemming, C. (2014). Grain Power: Over 100 Delicious Gluten-Free Ancient Grains & Superblend Recipes. Penguin Random House.

MOLASSES SPICE GRANOLA

(Adapted from *Grain Power: Over 100 Delicious Gluten-Free Ancient Grains & Superblend Recipes*)

INGREDIENTS

2 C rolled oats

½ C buckwheat groats

¾ C combo of pumpkin seeds and sunflower seeds

½ C millet

2 tbsp teff grain

2 tbsp amaranth seeds

½ C maple syrup, honey, agave, or corn syrup

2 tsp molasses

2 tsp vanilla

3 tbsp chia seeds

2 tsp cinnamon

⅛ tsp ground ginger

⅛ tsp nutmeg

½ tsp salt

½ C raisins or dried cranberries

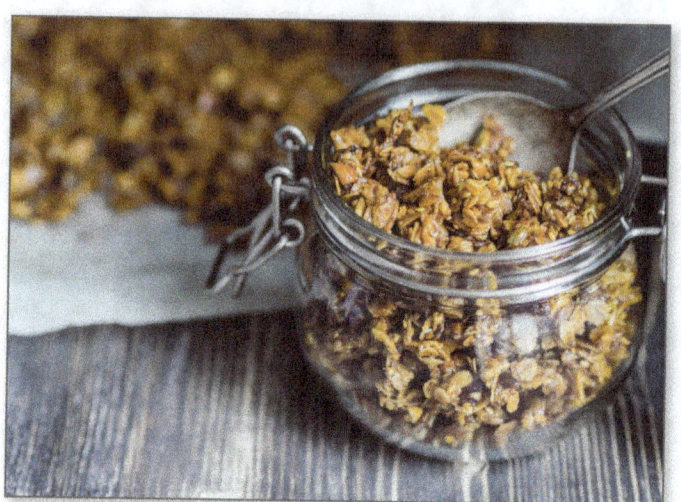

INSTRUCTIONS

Preheat the oven to 225° F and line a large baking sheet with parchment. Combine the grains and seeds in a bowl and set aside. In a small bowl or measuring cup, mix together the maple syrup (or sweetener of choice), molasses, vanilla, chia seeds, cinnamon, ginger. Nutmeg and salt. Pour liquid mixture over the dry mixer and stir until well combined. Pour on the baking sheet and bake for 1 hour, stirring every 20 minutes. Remove from the oven and cool completely. Stir in the raisins and store in a sealed container.

COCONUT BUCKWHEAT GRANOLA

(From *24 Carrot Life*)

INGREDIENTS

2 C raw buckwheat groats

2 C unsweetened flaked coconut

2 tsp ground cinnamon

¼ tsp salt

¼ C agave (or honey or other syrupy sweetener)

2 tbsp melted coconut oil

2 tbsp brown sugar

1 tsp vanilla extract

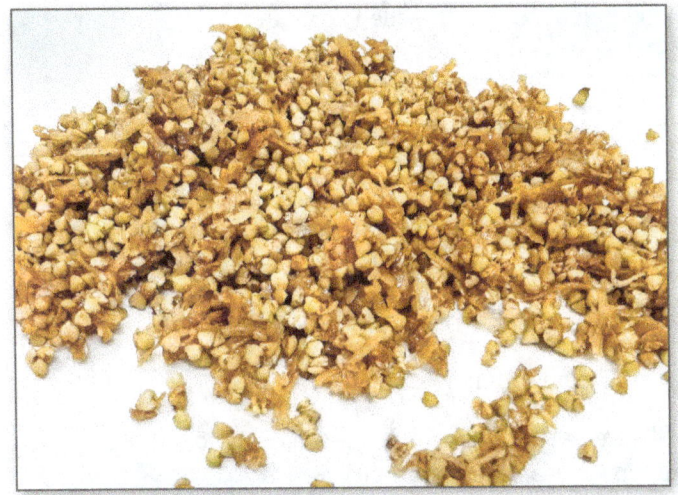

INSTRUCTIONS

1. Preheat the oven to 325° F.

2. Add groats through salt to a medium bowl and whisk to combine completely.

3. Add honey through vanilla extract to a small glass bowl and mix until completely combined.

4. Add wet ingredients to the dry mix and toss to incorporate.

5. Spread the mixture evenly on a large baking sheet and bake for 20 minutes, or until golden brown.

6. Let cool completely before storing in an airtight container at room temperature.

24 Carrot Life. (2014, November 12). Coconut Buckwheat Granola. Retrieved May 18, 2023, from https://24carrotlife.com/2014/11/12/coconut-buckwheat-granola/

BREAKFAST PORRIDGE ADDITION IDEAS

Slivered almonds, shredded coconut, chocolate chips

Orange segments, dried cranberries, honey

Peaches, sprinkle of cardamom and cinnamon, pistachios

Raisins, cinnamon, diced apples or applesauce, walnuts

Bananas, strawberries and shredded coconut

Chia, hemp, ground flax

Slivered almonds, walnuts, pecans, sunflower seeds, poppy seeds, pumpkin seeds

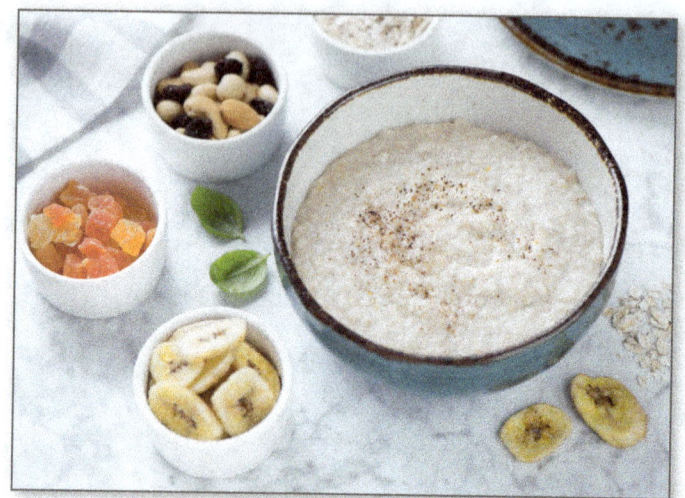

QUINOA SALAD

(From *Cookie and Kate*)

INGREDIENTS

1 C uncooked quinoa, rinsed in a fine-mesh colander

2 C water

1 can (15 oz) chickpeas, rinsed and drained, or 1½ C cooked chickpeas

1 medium cucumber, seeded and chopped

1 medium red bell pepper, chopped

¾ C chopped red onion (from 1 small red onion)

1 C finely chopped flat-leaf parsley (from 1 large bunch)

¼ C olive oil

¼ C lemon juice (from 2 to 3 lemons)

1 tbsp red wine vinegar

2 cloves garlic, pressed or minced

½ tsp salt

Freshly ground black pepper, to taste

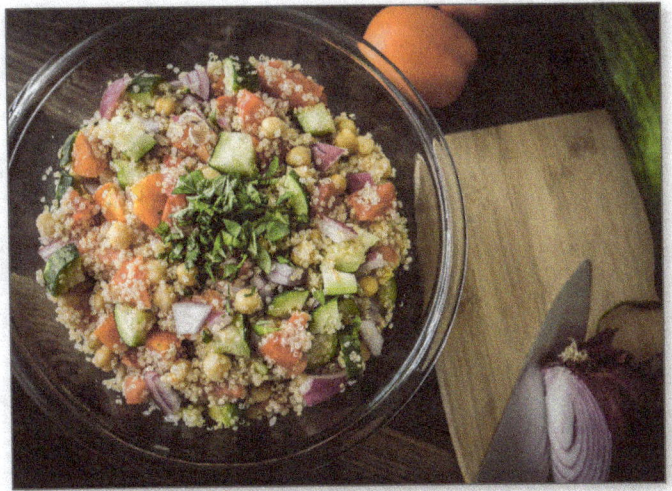

INSTRUCTIONS

To cook the quinoa: Combine the rinsed quinoa and the water in a medium saucepan. Bring the mixture to a boil over medium-high heat, then decrease the heat to maintain a gentle simmer. Cook until the quinoa has absorbed all of the water, about 15 minutes, reducing heat as time goes on to maintain a gentle simmer. Remove from heat, cover, and let the quinoa rest for 5 minutes, to give it time to fluff up.

In a large serving bowl, combine the chickpeas, cucumber, bell pepper, onion and parsley. Set aside.

In a small bowl, combine the olive oil, lemon juice, vinegar, garlic and salt. Whisk until blended, then set aside.

Once the quinoa is mostly cool, add it to the serving bowl, and drizzle the dressing on top. Toss until the mixture is thoroughly combined. Season with black pepper, to taste, and add an extra pinch of salt if necessary. For best flavor, let the salad rest for 5 to 10 minutes before serving.

This salad keeps well in the refrigerator, covered, for about 4 days. Serve chilled or at room temperature.

Cookie and Kate. (n.d.). Best Quinoa Salad Recipe. Retrieved May 18, 2023, from https://cookieandkate.com/best-qui-noa-salad-recipe/

QUINOA FRUIT SALAD

INGREDIENTS

½ C quinoa

1 C water

1 C sliced strawberries

1 mango, peeled and diced

2 mandarin oranges, peeled, segments cut in half width-wise

1 banana sliced

1 tbsp fresh lime juice

1 tbsp honey

2 tbsp shredded coconut

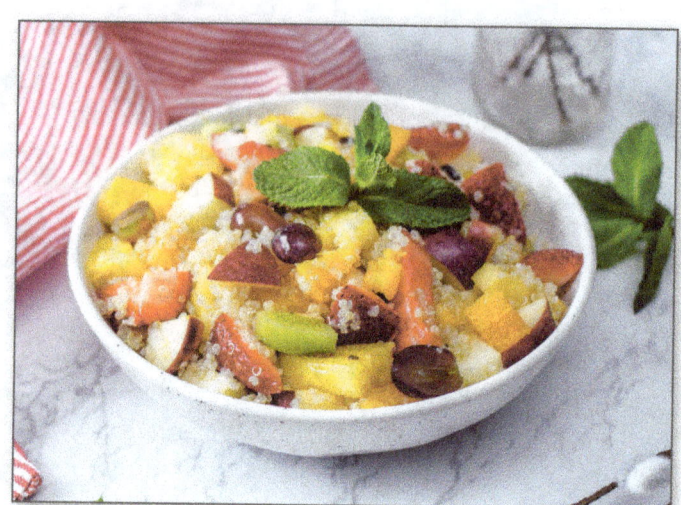

INSTRUCTIONS

Bring quinoa and water to a boil, reduce heat to a simmer, cover and cook for 15-20 minutes until the quinoa is tender and water is absorbed. Remove the lid and fluff with a fork and set aside to cool. When quinoa is cool, mix sliced fruit and quinoa together. Stir lime juice and honey together until well mixed and drizzle over fruit mixture. Top with shredded coconut.

This recipe can be adapted to whatever fruit you have on hand. It is delicious using mixed berries, pears, or fresh pineapple. You can top with slivered almonds, toasted coconut, pistachios, or leave out toppings all together. Try swapping out the lime juice for pineapple juice, orange juice, or fresh lemon juice.

SALADS

SORGHUM KALE SALAD

INGREDIENTS

1 C sorghum

3 C water

½ small red onion, diced

2 green onions, diced

4 C baby kale or other leafy green (remove stems if
  using larger greens with tough stems)

3 tbsp lemon juice

3 tbsp olive oil

½ tsp salt

1 large clove of garlic minced or pressed

1½ tsp dijon mustard (yellow works, too)

1 tsp sugar

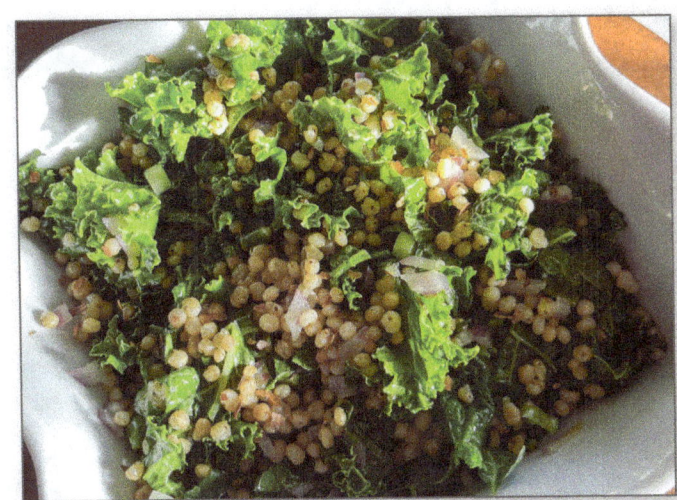

INSTRUCTIONS

Combine water and sorghum in a medium saucepan and bring to a boil. Reduce heat to a
simmer, cover and cook 50 minutes or until water is absorbed. When it is done, remove the
lid and allow it to cool 10 minutes then fluff with a fork. In a small bowl whisk together
the lemon juice, oil, salt, garlic, mustard and sugar. Combine the cooked sorghum, red and
green onions, dressing and kale in a bowl. Serve warm. If you want to serve it cold then
cool the sorghum after cooking and then combine the ingredients.

Serve alongside your favorite meat, or add shredded chicken or a can of drained/
rinsed white beans or chickpeas to make it a meal.

SORGHUM SWEET POTATO SALAD

INGREDIENTS

1 C sorghum

3 C chicken or vegetable broth (or water plus 3 tsp bouillon)

3 sweet potatoes

1-2 tbsp olive oil

¾ tsp cinnamon

¾ tsp cumin

¼ tsp garlic powder

½ tsp salt

½ C chopped cilantro or parsley

3 tbsp pumpkin seeds, optional (sunflower seeds or slivered almonds work)

½ C green onions, tops and bottoms diced

2 tbsp olive oil

Juice from 1 lemon

1 clove of garlic, pressed or finely minced

Salt and pepper to taste

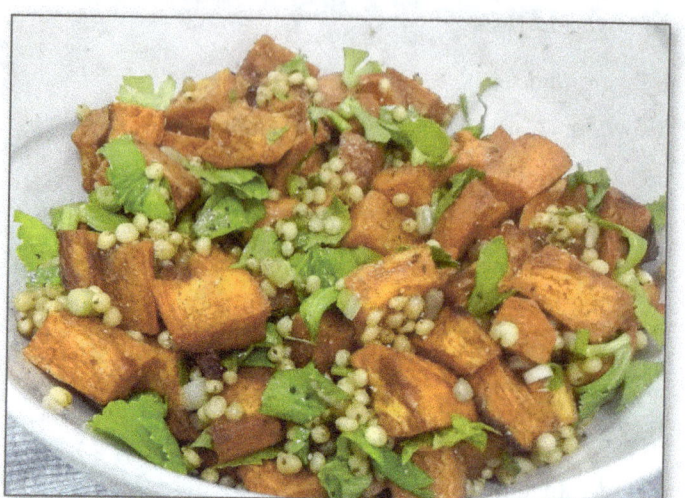

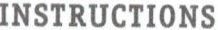

INSTRUCTIONS

Combine sorghum and broth in a medium saucepan and bring to a boil. Reduce heat, cover and simmer until water is absorbed and sorghum is cooked through- about 50 minutes. Meanwhile, preheat the oven to 425 then cube the sweet potatoes into ½" cubes, toss with 1-2 tbsp olive oil and cinnamon, cumin, garlic and salt. Arrange on a greased/parchment-lined baking sheet and bake for 30-40 minutes until potatoes are tender and browned.

To make the dressing combine 2 tbsp olive oil with the juice from 1 lemon and garlic.

When sorghum is finished cooking, combine it with the herbs, pumpkin seeds, and green onions. Stir in the dressing, season with salt and pepper, then toss with the sweet potatoes. Serve warm.

THAI PEANUT MILLET SALAD

(Adapted from *Cookie and Kate*)

INGREDIENTS

1 C millet (or quinoa)

2 C water

3 C purple cabbage shredded (green tastes great, too)

1 orange or red bell pepper, sliced

2 carrots shredded or sliced julienne-style

1 C fresh snap or snow peas

⅓ C green onions, chopped

½ C chopped cilantro

1 can mandarin oranges (optional)

⅓ C chopped peanuts (garnish)

Peanut sauce

¼ C smooth peanut butter

3 tbsp GF soy sauce or tamari

1 tbsp honey or agave

1 tbsp rice vinegar

1 tsp toasted sesame oil

1 tsp grated fresh ginger

½ lime, juiced (about 1 ½ tbsp)

⅛ tsp garlic powder

Pinch of red pepper flakes

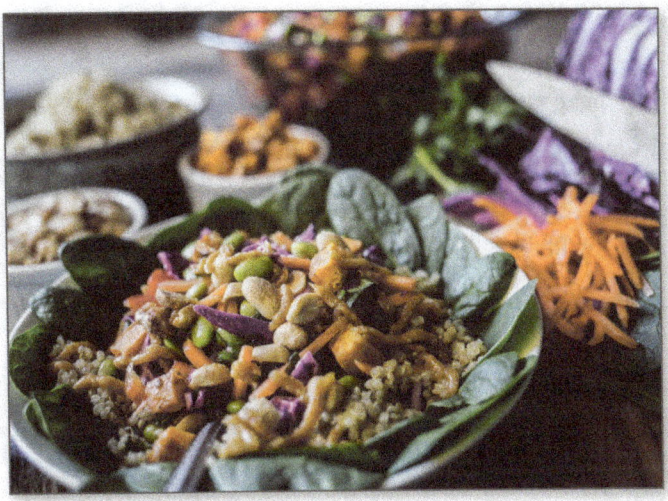

INSTRUCTIONS

Heat a medium saucepan over medium high heat and add the millet. Stir for 1 minute to lightly toast then add water, bring to a boil, reduce heat to a simmer, cover and cook for 15 minutes until tender and all water is absorbed. Set aside to cool. To make peanut sauce combine all ingredients in a jar. Secure with a lid and shake to combine. Add water to thin if desired.

To assemble salad combine cabbage, pepper, carrots, peas, onions and cilantro in a large bowl. Stir in cooled millet, then stir in peanut sauce. Garnish with chopped peanuts and mandarins if using.

Make it a meal by adding 2 C of diced or shredded chicken or a can of drained and rinsed chickpeas.

Cookie and Kate. (n.d.). Thai Peanut Quinoa Salad Recipe. Retrieved May 18, 2023, from https://cookieandkate.com/thai-peanut-quinoa-salad-recipe/

SALADS

FAVORITE CHICKPEA SALAD

INGREDIENTS

2 cans chickpeas, rinsed and drained, or 3 C cooked chickpeas

1 medium red bell pepper, chopped

½ C chopped fresh flat-leaf parsley (about ½ bunch)

½ C chopped red onion

½ C chopped celery

3 tbsp olive oil

3 tbsp lemon juice (from 1 to 1 ½ lemons), or more if needed

2 cloves garlic, finely minced

½ tsp salt

Black pepper, to taste

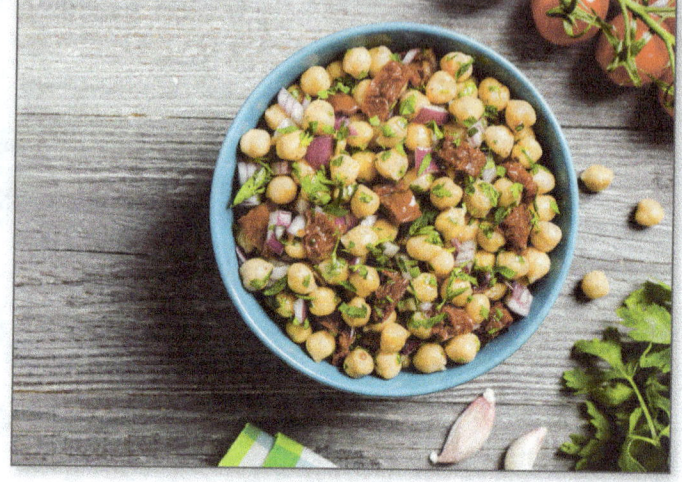

INSTRUCTIONS

1. In a medium bowl, combine all of the ingredients. Toss until combined. Taste and add additional lemon juice, salt, or pepper if necessary.

2. Tastes best if refrigerated 30 minutes to allow flavors to blend.

SALADS

GREEK CHICKPEA SALAD

(From *Spend With Pennies*)

INGREDIENTS

1 can chickpeas, drained and rinsed or 1.5 C cooked

1 ½ C cucumbers, diced

1 ½ C red bell pepper, diced

1 C cherry tomatoes, halved

½ C kalamata olives, pitted and halved

½ C crumbled feta cheese (omit if dairy free or use
    vegan version)

Dressing:

3 tbsp red wine vinegar

Juice from ½ of a lemon

½ tsp dijon mustard

½ tsp garlic powder

½ tsp dried oregano

¼ tsp salt

¼ tsp black pepper

¼ C olive oil

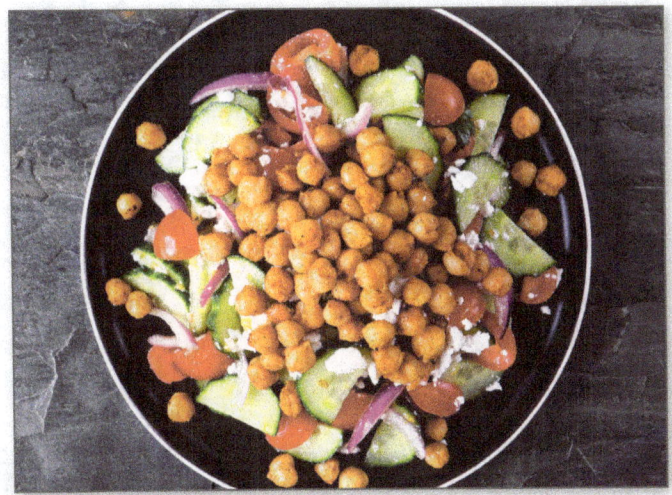

INSTRUCTIONS

1. Combine dressing ingredients in a bowl and whisk to combine.

2. Add drained and rinsed chickpeas to another bowl and add cucumbers, peppers, tomatoes and olives.

3. Pour dressing over chickpea mixture, stir and then refrigerate 30 minutes to allow flavors to blend.

4. Top with feta cheese when serving.

Spend With Pennies. (2022, March 21). Chickpea Salad. Retrieved May 18, 2023, from https://www.
spendwithpennies.com/chickpea-salad/

BLACK BEAN AND CORN SALAD/SALSA

INGREDIENTS

2 cans black beans, drained and rinsed or 3 C cooked

1½ C corn kernels fresh, frozen or canned

⅓ C red onion, minced

1 red bell pepper, diced

1 avocado, diced

1 jalapeno, minced

⅓ C fresh cilantro, chopped

1 tbsp olive oil

1 tbsp honey (optional, sugar works too)

Juice of 2 limes

1/2 tsp chili powder

1/2 tsp cumin

salt and pepper to taste

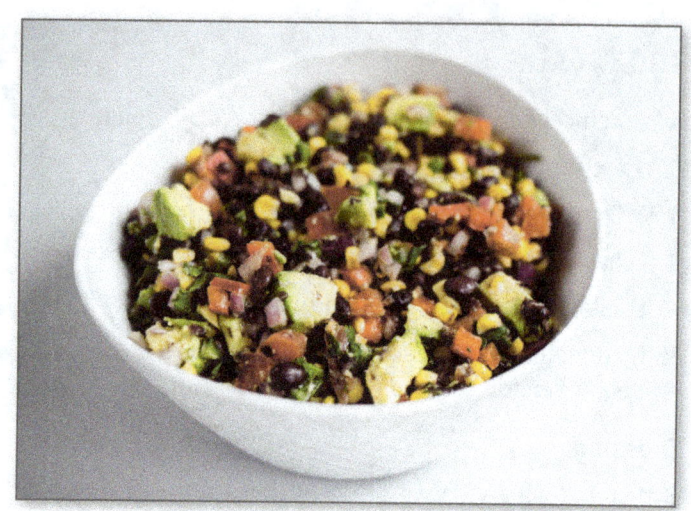

INSTRUCTIONS

1. Place the black beans, corn, red onion, red bell pepper, avocado and jalapeno in a large bowl.

2. In a small bowl, mix together the cilantro, olive oil, lime juice, honey, chili powder, cumin and salt and pepper.

3. Add dressing to black bean mixture and toss to coat. Refrigerate 30 minutes for flavors to blend.

4. Eat with tortilla chips or on its own.

SALADS

LENTILS AND BROWN RICE (MUJADARA)

(Adapted from *Cookie and Kate* and *Bon Appetit*)

INGREDIENTS

2 tbsp olive oil

2 tsp ground cumin

2 tsp ground coriander

¼ tsp cinnamon

5 C water

2 bay leaves

2 large cloves garlic

1¼ tsp salt

¼ tsp pepper

1 C brown rice

1 C lentils

½ C diced green onions

½ C chopped cilantro and parsley mix

¼ C raisins (optional)

Fresh lemon wedges for serving (optional)

Plain yogurt for serving (optional)

Caramelized onions

3 tbsp olive oil

2 large onions, halved and thinly sliced

Sprinkle of salt

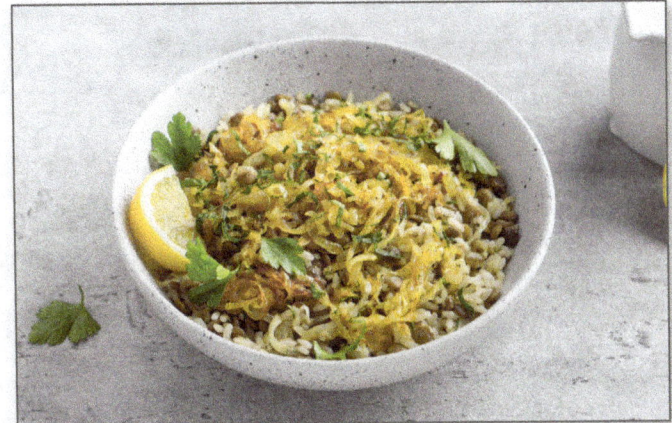

INSTRUCTIONS

Heat olive oil in a large saucepan or dutch oven over medium heat. Add cumin, coriander and cinnamon and saute until fragrant- about 30 seconds. Add the rice and salt and stir to coat in spices, then carefully pour in the 5 C of water. Add the bay leaves and whole cloves or garlic and bring to a boil. Reduce heat to a simmer and cover to cook for 10 minutes. Stir in the lentils, cover and return to a simmer for 20-25 minutes until liquid is absorbed.

Remove the lid and let the steam escape, then remove bay leaves, smash the garlics against the side of the pan and stir in with green onions, cilantro/parsley, and raisins. Top with caramelized onions when serving or gluten-free fried onions for a quick alternative. Traditionally eaten with plain yogurt and served hot or room temperature. Cold leftovers are also delicious!

While the rice and lentils are cooking, heat the oil in a heavy pan over medium high heat. Add the onions and stir to coat in the oil. Allow the onions to cook undisturbed for a few minutes until they start to brown at the edges. Reduce the heat to avoid burning if necessary. Sprinkle with salt and stir. Allow the onions to continue to brown, stirring as needed. Add water to deglaze the pan if it is getting too dry. Once the onions are a deep caramel color and getting crispy edges, turn off the heat and set aside for serving. To save time, make larger batches of caramelized onions ahead of time and store in the freezer to quickly spruce up many recipes.

Cookie and Kate. (n.d.). Mujaddara Recipe. Retrieved May 18, 2023, from https://cookieandkate.com/mujaddara-recipe/

Bon Appétit. (2014, January 27). Herbed Brown Rice Mujadarra. Retrieved May 18, 2023, from https://www.bonappetit.com/recipe/herbed-brown-rice-mujadarra

SIDE DISHES

SUPERBLEND GRAINS

(Adapted from *Grain Power: Over 100 Delicious Gluten-Free Ancient Grains & Superblend Recipes*)

INGREDIENTS

2 C water or broth

½ C quinoa

¼ C millet

3 tbsp buckwheat groats

1 tbsp amaranth or teff grains

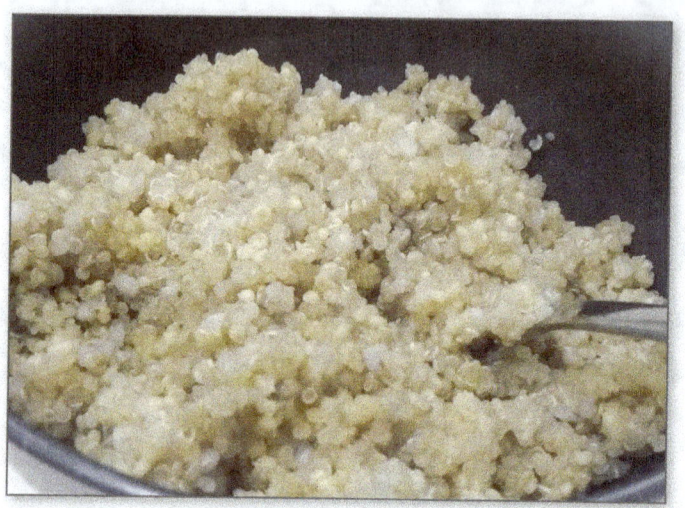

INSTRUCTIONS

Combine all ingredients in a medium saucepan and bring to a boil. Reduce to a simmer, cover and cook for 20 minutes. Remove from heat and fluff with a fork.

Any blend of these grains to equal 1 C grains will work when cooked for 20 minutes in 2 C of water.

Green, P., & Hemming, C. (2014). Grain Power: Over 100 Delicious Gluten-Free Ancient Grains & Superblend Recipes. Penguin Random House.

SIDE DISHES

FRIED BROWN RICE

(Adapted from *Gimme Some Oven*)

INGREDIENTS

3 tbsp butter, divided

2 eggs, whisked

2 medium carrots, peeled and diced

1 small white onion, diced

½ C frozen peas

3 cloves garlic, minced

salt and black pepper

4 C cooked and chilled brown rice (or try sorghum or buckwheat for another variety)

3 green onions, thinly sliced

3–4 tbsp soy sauce, or more to taste

½ tsp toasted sesame oil

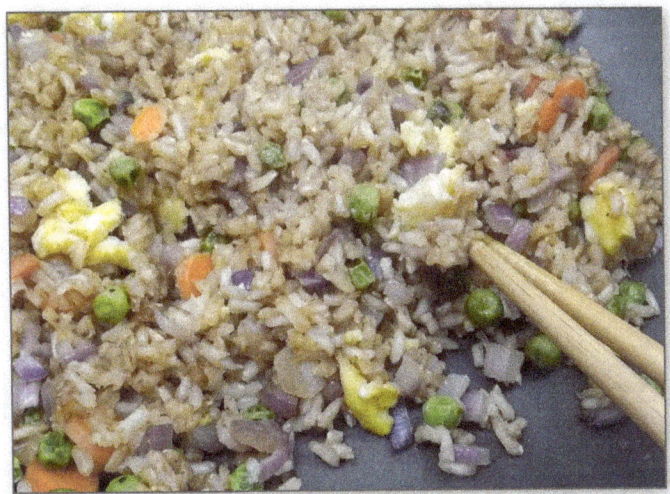

INSTRUCTIONS

Heat ½ tbsp of butter in a large sauté pan over medium-high heat until melted. Add egg, and scramble until cooked through. Remove egg to a separate plate.

Add an additional 1 tbsp butter to the pan and heat until melted. Add carrots, onion, peas and garlic, and season with a big pinch of salt and pepper. Sauté about 5 minutes or until the onion and carrots are soft. Increase heat to high, add in the remaining 1½ tbsp of butter, and stir until melted. Immediately add the rice, green onions, soy sauce and stir until combined. Continue stirring for an additional 3 minutes to fry the rice. Then add in the eggs and stir to combine. Remove from heat, and stir in the sesame oil until combined. Taste and season with extra soy sauce, if needed.

You could also use 1½ C frozen pea and carrot mix in place of the fresh carrots and frozen peas.

Gimme Some Oven. (n.d.). Fried Rice Recipe. Retrieved May 18, 2023, from https://www.gimmesome-oven.com/fried-rice-recipe/

HERB RICE

INGREDIENTS

2 C of broth or water with 1 tsp chicken or vegetable bouillon

1 C brown rice

1 tbsp butter

2 tbsp low-sodium soy sauce

1 tsp dried minced onion

½ tsp onion powder

¼ tsp dried basil

¼ tsp dried marjoram (can sub with oregano if you don't have marjoram)

¼ tsp dried thyme

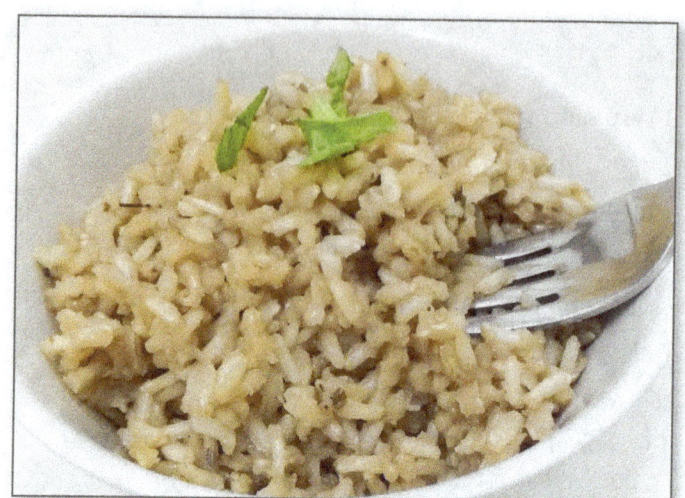

INSTRUCTIONS

In a saucepan bring broth (or water plus bouillon) and butter to a boil. Add remaining ingredients. Reduce heat and cover and simmer for about 40 minutes or until liquid is absorbed and rice is tender.

Try a quicker variation using quinoa, millet, or buckwheat in place of the 1 C of rice, and then simmer for 15-20 minutes. You could also use a combination of quinoa, millet, buckwheat, amaranth or teff for an interesting variety of texture and nutrition.

WHOLE GRAINS IN THE INSTANT POT: MASON JAR METHOD

Cook several varieties of whole grains at once using mason jars. Brown rice, sorghum, and oat groats all cook for about 22 minutes at pressure in the instant pot. Put 2 C of water in the pot of your pressure cooker and then the rack. If you have a 6 quart pot you can use pint jars, while an 8 quart cooker can fit pint or quart jars depending on the height of your rack. Fill each jar with up to ½ C grain and the appropriate amount of water (or other cooking liquid), plus a pinch of salt. Cover the jars with tin foil or a metal canning lid (does not need to be new, as its purpose is to keep water from dripping into the jar,) and place jars into the instant pot. Close the lid and set the vent to seal. Use the pressure cook setting for 22 minutes on high pressure. Allow to naturally release for 10 minutes and then you can quickly vent.

Brown rice ratio ½ C rice to ½ C water (can do up to ¾ C rice in pint jar)

Sorghum ratio ½ C sorghum to 1 C water

Oat groats

MEXICAN QUINOA SWEET POTATOES

(From *Simply Quinoa*)

INGREDIENTS

2 large sweet potatoes

1 tbsp olive oil

¼ C chopped red onion

¼ C chopped bell pepper

½ C frozen corn

½ C cooked quinoa

1 C canned black beans drained & rinsed

1 tbsp chili powder

1 tsp cumin

¼ tsp tsp garlic powder

½ tsp smoked paprika

Sea salt to taste

To Garnish:

1 avocado mashed

Tahini

Hot sauce

Cheese

Sour cream

Chopped cilantro

INSTRUCTIONS

Preheat the oven to 400° F. Place sweet potatoes on a baking sheet and prick with a fork. Place in the oven and bake for 40 minutes.

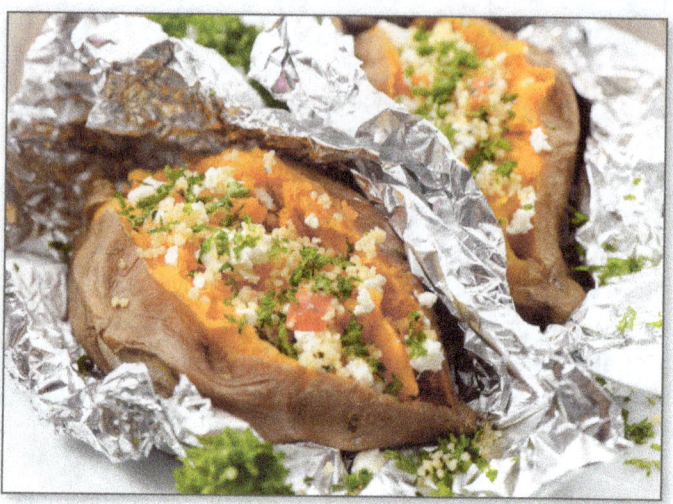

Meanwhile, heat the oil in a large skillet. Add the onion and pepper and saute until tender, about 5 minutes.

Add corn, quinoa, black beans and spices and cook 2 - 3 more minutes.

When sweet potatoes are fork tender, remove from oven and let rest for 5 minutes. Slice in half and place each half on a plate. Top with quinoa mixture, avocado and other optional garnishes. Finish with a sprinkle of cilantro and enjoy!

Meat version:

After sauteeing the onion and pepper for a couple minutes, add ½ lb ground beef and cook till no longer pink. Then add corn, quinoa, beans and spices (you may want to increase the spices 25%.

Any cooked whole grain can be subbed for the quinoa.

Simply Quinoa. (2018, August 30). Mexican Quinoa Stuffed Sweet Potatoes. Retrieved May 18, 2023, from https://www.simplyquinoa.com/mexican-quinoa-stuffed-sweet-potatoes/

SLOW COOKED VEGETARIAN BAKED BEANS

(Adapted from *The Simple Veganista*)

INGREDIENTS

1 medium onion, diced

1½ tsp smoked paprika

1 tsp garlic powder

1 tsp onion powder

1 lb (2 C) dried small white beans (navy or great northern), rinsed picked over

2½ C vegetable or chicken broth

½ C maple syrup (can substitute with ⅓ C brown sugar)

6 oz can tomato paste

¼ C apple cider vinegar

2 tbsp mustard

½ tsp ground pepper

2 bay leaves

½–1 tsp salt, or to taste

Small green bell pepper, diced - saute with the onion

Chop up ¼ lb bacon into small chunks and saute with the onion

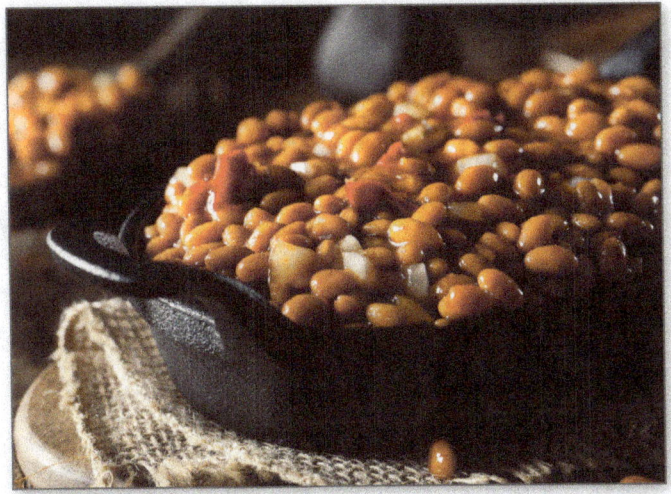

INSTRUCTIONS

1. Soak beans in 2 quarts of water overnight or do a quick soak by adding beans to a pot covered with 3 inches of water and bringing to a boil, boiling 3 minutes, removing from heat and then allowing to sit for an hour.

2. Drain and rinse the soaked beans.

3. Add all the ingredients except the salt to a slow cooker and stir to mix in the tomato paste. Cook on high for 8-10 hours. Stir every few hours and add extra water if needed. Add salt to taste after cooking. Add more maple syrup or brown sugar if you want sweeter beans.

4. This recipe can also be made in an electric pressure cooker—in the pot, saute the onion in a tbsp of oil for a few minutes. Add the paprika and garlic powder and cook another minute then add all the rest of the ingredients and stir to mix in the tomato paste. Pressure cook on high for 60 minutes.

*For extra heat add a minced jalapeno or ¼ tsp cayenne powder. You can also add a diced green pepper or ¼ lb chopped bacon for other variations.

Simple Veganista. (n.d.). Healthy Baked Beans (Instant Pot). Retrieved May 18, 2023, from https://simple-veganista.com/healthy-baked-beans-instant-pot/

SIDE DISHES

RED BEANS

INGREDIENTS

1 tbsp olive oil

½ medium onion, diced

½ green pepper, diced

1 stalk of celery, diced

2 cloves garlic, minced

1 C water or chicken/vegetable stock

2 cans drained kidney beans

1 tsp thyme

¼ tsp paprika

¼ tsp smoked paprika

⅛ tsp cayenne

⅛ tsp rubbed sage

⅛ tsp fennel

⅛ tsp black pepper

Salt to taste

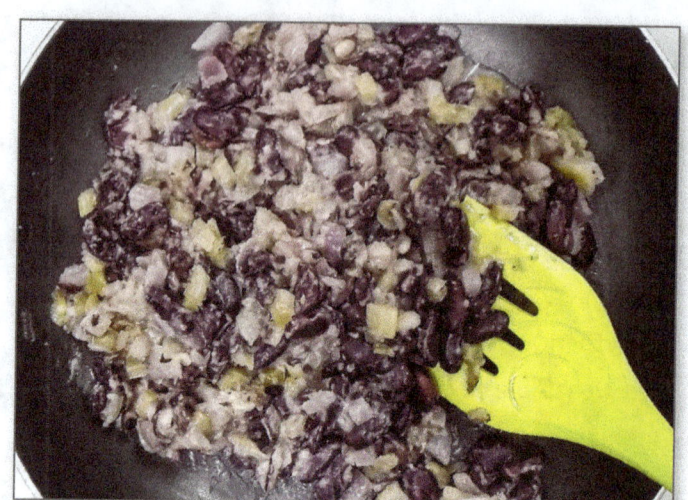

INSTRUCTIONS

Saute onion, pepper, celery and garlic in oil for about 5 minutes, add spices and stir for another minute.

Add in beans and water and let simmer for 15 minutes. Use a fork or potato masher to mash a portion of the beans to thicken the sauce and allow to simmer for another couple minutes. Serve with rice or sausage links.

SIDE DISHES

EASY REFRIED BEANS

(Adapted from *Cookie and Kate*)

INGREDIENTS

1 tbsp extra-virgin olive oil

½ C finely chopped yellow or white onion (about ½ small onion)

¼ tsp fine sea salt

2 cloves garlic, pressed or minced

½ tsp chili powder

¼ tsp ground cumin

2 cans (15 oz each) pinto beans, rinsed and drained, or 3 C cooked pinto beans

½ C water

2 tbsp chopped fresh cilantro

1 tbsp lime juice (about ½ medium lime), to taste

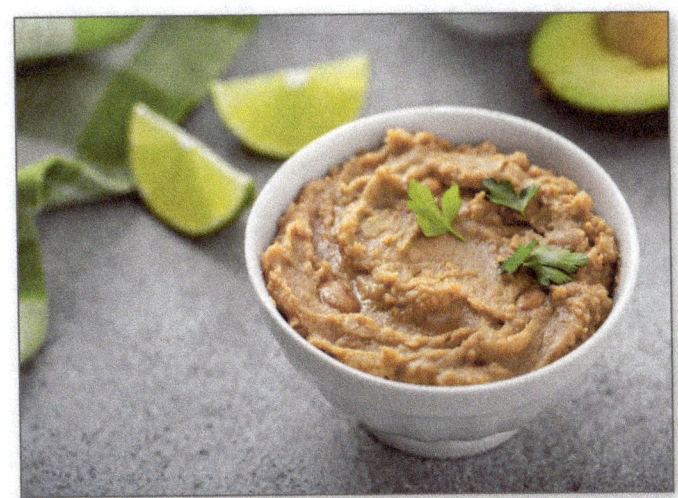

INSTRUCTIONS

In a medium saucepan over medium heat, warm the olive oil until shimmering. Add the onions and salt. Cook, stirring occasionally, until the onions have softened and are turning translucent, about 5 to 8 minutes.

Add the garlic, chili powder and cumin. Cook, stirring constantly, until fragrant, about 30 seconds. Pour in the drained beans and water. Stir, cover and cook for 5 minutes.

Reduce the heat to low and remove the lid. Use a potato masher or the back of a fork to mash up about at least half of the beans, until you reach your desired consistency. Continue to cook the beans, uncovered, stirring often, for 3 more minutes.

Remove the saucepan from the heat and stir in the cilantro and lime juice. Taste, and add more salt and lime juice if necessary. If the beans seem dry, add a very small splash of water and stir to combine. Cover until you're ready to serve.

Note: You can change up the type of bean you use according to your preference.

Cookie and Kate. (n.d.). Easy Refried Beans Recipe. Retrieved May 18, 2023, from https://cookieandkate.com/easy-refried-beans-recipe/print/28453/

CRISPY BAKED FALAFEL

(Adapted from Cookie and Kate)

INGREDIENTS

1 C dried chickpeas, rinsed, sorted and soaked overnight (not canned or cooked)

¼ C + 1 tbsp extra-virgin olive oil

½ C roughly chopped red onion

½ C fresh parsley

½ C fresh cilantro

4 cloves garlic, chopped

1 tsp salt

½ tsp black pepper

½ tsp ground cumin

¼ tsp ground cinnamon

INSTRUCTIONS

1. Preheat the oven to 375° F and pour ¼ C olive oil in a rimmed baking sheet and spread around to coat the bottom of the pan.

2. In a food processor, combine the soaked and drained chickpeas (uncooked), onion, parsley, cilantro, garlic, salt, pepper, cumin, cinnamon, and 1 tbsp of olive oil. Process for about a minute until smooth- the chickpeas should still give it some texture but it should not be chunky.

3. Scoop out about 2 tbsp at a time of mixture and form into small patties about ½ inch thick and lay in the oiled baking sheet. Can also form larger patties to use like a burger.

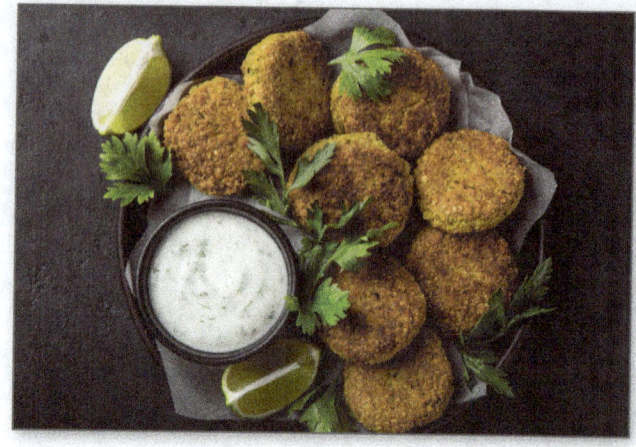

4. Bake for 25 to 30 minutes, flipping the patties halfway through baking. The falafels should be golden brown when finished.

5. Serve on salads, in sandwiches or wraps with other toppings, or with a dipping sauce for an appetizer or snack. Goes great with tomatoes, cucumber, red onion, greens, etc.

Tahini Lemon Sauce for Falafel

½ C tahini

Juice of 1 lemon- about 3 tbsp

1 clove garlic - several cloves of roasted garlic also work

1 tsp salt

½ tsp black pepper

¼ tsp cumin

3-4 tbsp water

Whisk together all the ingredients except the water. Add water to thin to desired consistency. Let flavors meld for 20-30 minutes then taste and adjust seasonings if needed. Drizzle on sandwiches, salads or use as a dipping sauce.

Cookie and Kate. (n.d.). Crispy Falafel Recipe. Retrieved May 18, 2023, from https://cookieandkate.com/crispy-falafel-recipe/

SIDE DISHES

SMOKY AMARANTH CORN CHOWDER

(Adapted from *Whole Grains for a New Generation*)

INGREDIENTS

1 tbsp olive oil

½ diced onion

½ red bell pepper diced

1 rib celery diced

2 tbsp chopped celery leaves

½ tsp smoked paprika

1 tsp chili powder

2½ C vegetable broth or water

⅔ C uncooked amaranth

2 C sweet corn kernels (from 2-3 cobs or frozen)

1 sweet potato, peeled and diced

Salt and pepper to taste

Fresh basil or cilantro

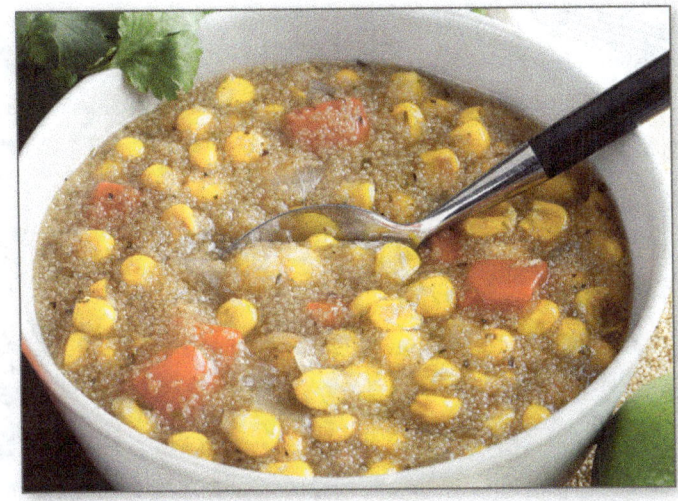

SOUPS

INSTRUCTIONS

In a 3-quart saucepan, heat the oil over medium high heat and saute onion, bell pepper and celery until tender, about 5 minutes. Add the celery leaves, paprika, chili powder, broth, amaranth, corn and sweet potato. Bring to a boil, then lower heat and simmer until the amaranth grains are translucent and the sweet potato is very soft, about 20 minutes. Season with salt and pepper and serve with fresh basil or cilantro. 4 servings.

Krissoff, L. (2012). Whole Grains for a New Generation: Light Dishes, Hearty Meals, Sweet Treats, and Sundry Snacks for the Everyday Cook. Stewart, Tabori & Chang

INSTANT POT VEGETABLE AND RICE SOUP

INGREDIENTS

1 tbsp olive oil

1 large onion (oz), chopped

3 garlic cloves, minced

1-inch fresh ginger, grated

1 lb (3 C) red (or white) potatoes, chopped

3 medium carrots (12 oz), chopped

10 oz (2½ C) French green beans, trimmed and cut into 2-inch pieces

4 celery sticks (7 oz), chopped

1 C dry brown rice

2 tbsp tomato paste

1 tbsp dried parsley

1 tbsp dried basil

1 tsp dried rosemary

1 tsp dried thyme

4 C vegetable broth

2 C water

Salt and pepper, to taste

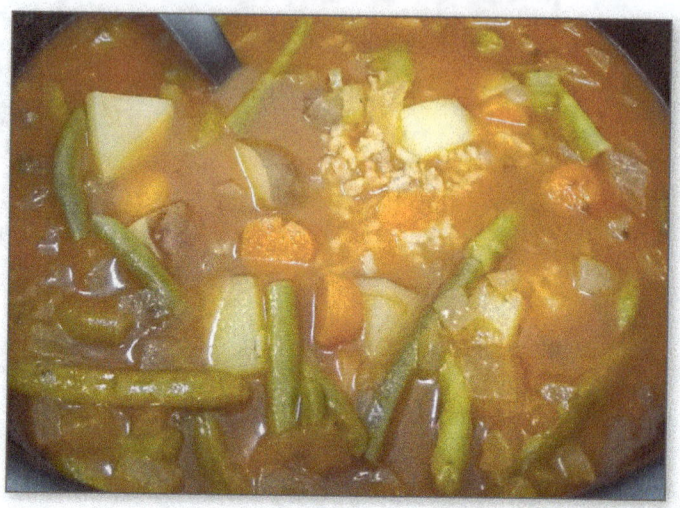

INSTRUCTIONS

1. Set the Instant Pot to "sauté". Pour a tbsp of olive oil into the pot and add the onion, stirring until soft and brown, about 4-5 minutes. Add in the garlic and ginger and stir for another minute.

2. Press "cancel" to turn off the Instant Pot. Add the remaining ingredients into the pot, starting with the vegetables, then rice, tomato paste, herbs, and top with the vegetable broth and water.

3. Season generously with salt and pepper. Give the ingredients a good stir to distribute the ingredients throughout the pot. The liquid should just cover the top of the ingredients. Add more broth or water if necessary.

4. Seal the Instant Pot and cook at high pressure ("manual"/"pressure cook" function) for 18 minutes. After the stew is ready, allow natural pressure release for 10 minutes before a quick pressure release to completely depressurize (until floating valve drops).

5. Taste for additional salt and pepper and top with chopped green onions if you like.

AFRICAN PEANUT STEW WITH CHICKPEAS

(Adapted from *Making Thyme for Health*)

INGREDIENTS

1 tbsp olive oil

1 onion, finely chopped

1 jalapeno, cored and finely chopped

4 garlic cloves, minced

2 tbsp fresh ginger, peeled and minced

2 tsp cumin powder

¼ tsp cayenne

3 tbsp tomato paste

1 large sweet potato, peeled and chopped into 1-inch cubes

½ C creamy peanut butter (unsweetened is best but sweetened works)

4 C vegetable or chicken broth

1 C water

1-2 cans chickpeas, drained or 1½-3 C cooked beans

1 bunch collard greens or kale, stems removed and roughly chopped

Salt to taste

fresh cilantro, cooked brown rice or other whole grain, roasted peanuts and lime juice for serving

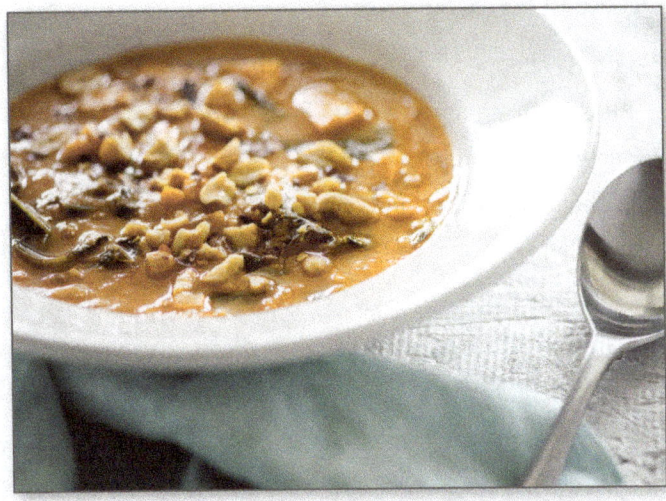

INSTRUCTIONS

1. Heat the olive oil over medium heat in a large pot. Add the onion and saute until translucent, about 3 minutes then add the garlic, jalapeno, ginger, cumin and cayenne and cook 1-2 minutes.

2. Stir in the tomato paste then add the sweet potato, peanut butter, chickpeas, broth and water. Bring to a boil then reduce heat to a simmer, cover and cook for 15 minutes.

3. Add in chopped collard greens and then cover and cook about 10 minutes more or until the sweet potatoes and collards are tender.

4. Use the back of a spoon or fork and mash some of the sweet potatoes and chickpeas to help thicken the broth and simmer for a few more minutes. Salt to taste.

5. Serve warm over rice and garnish with cilantro, peanuts and lime juice.

*If you don't have sweet potatoes, carrots or red potatoes are good substitutes. White beans or kidney beans work well in place of chickpeas.

Making Thyme for Health. (n.d.). One-Pot African Peanut Stew. Retrieved May 18, 2023, from https://www.makingthymeforhealth.com/one-pot-african-peanut-stew/

LENTIL VEGETABLE STEW

INGREDIENTS

2 onions, chopped

2-3 C carrots, chopped

2 C celery, chopped

8 oz chopped mushrooms (optional)

1 tbsp thyme

2-3 bay leaves

2 quarts tomatoes, or 2 large cans (diced, crushed or pureed works)

2-3 quarts broth or water (Adjust depending on if you want it stew or soup)

2 C lentils

3 cloves garlic, minced

1 tbsp italian seasoning (optional, or add 1t each oregano, basil, marjoram, parsley)

Salt and pepper to taste

Chopped/shredded cabbage or other greens (optional)

Balsamic vinegar for serving

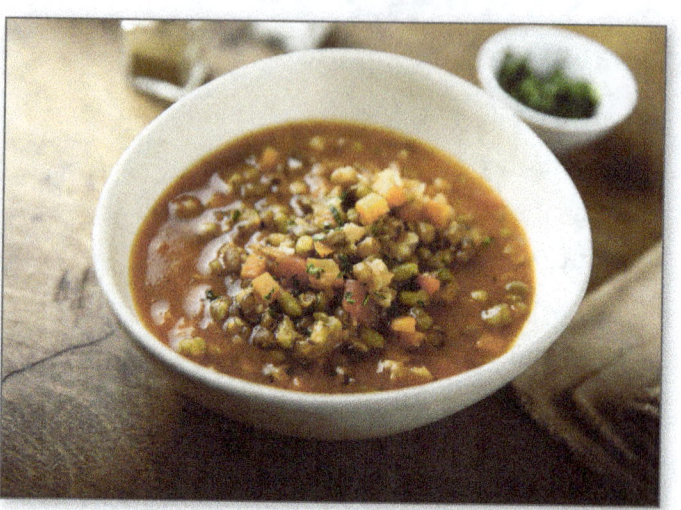

INSTRUCTIONS

1. This recipe makes a lot—cut in half if desired.

2. Saute onions 3-5 minutes, add other vegetables and saute till they start releasing water.

3. Add remaining ingredients and simmer until lentils and carrots are tender—about 30 minutes. Salt and pepper to taste. Turn off heat and stir in chopped cabbage. Drizzle with balsamic vinegar when serving.

*Can add whatever other vegetables you have on hand—potatoes, sweet potatoes, green beans, frozen peas, etc.

MUSHROOM LENTIL SOUP WITH KALE

(Adapted from *Plant and Vine*)

INGREDIENTS

1 C dry lentils, rinsed (brown or french green)

4 C vegetable broth, divided (chicken or beef broth work)

3 bay leaves

3 tbsp olive oil

1 yellow onion, chopped

1 lb mushrooms, quartered

8 cloves of garlic, finely chopped

¾ C water or stock for deglazing

1 tsp thyme

¼ tsp salt

½ C full fat canned coconut milk (or 1 can of light coconut milk, or ½ C cream or half n half if not dairy free)

3 C fresh kale, chopped (frozen also works, spinach, collards, or Swiss chard are great alternatives)

Salt and pepper to taste

Chopped green onions for topping (optional)

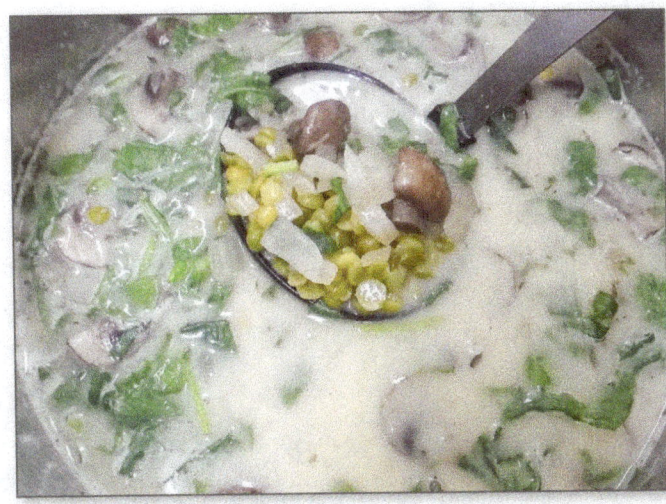

INSTRUCTIONS

1. Put lentils, bay leaves and 3 C of broth in a pot and bring to a boil. Once boiling, reduce heat to medium low, cover and cook for 20-25 minutes until the lentils are tender. Remove from heat and discard the bay leaves.

2. In a large pot, heat the oil over medium high heat, add the onion and saute for 3-5 minutes till the onion is soft.

3. Next add the mushrooms and salt and saute another few minutes until the mushrooms soften. Add the garlic and cook for another minute then add ¾ water or broth to deglaze the pan. Continue cooking until most of the water has evaporated.

4. Reduce the heat to medium low and add the last cup of broth, cooked lentils in broth, coconut milk, and kale. Simmer for a few minutes just until the kale begins to soften. Season to taste with more salt and pepper. Top with green onions if desired.

5. Delicious served on its own or over baked potatoes, mashed potatoes, rice, squash etc.

*Meat option—For meat version add ½ lb Italian sausage and saute with onions, or add 1 C diced ham in step 4, or garnish with cooked chopped bacon.

SPLIT PEA SOUP

INGREDIENTS

1 lb green split peas

1 large onion, chopped (about 1½ C)

1 C celery, diced

1 C carrots, diced

1 potato, diced

1 tsp salt

½ tsp pepper

¼ tsp marjoram

¼ tsp garlic powder

2 chicken bouillon cubes or 2 tsp bouillon paste

1 quart water (can sub water and bouillon for broth)

1 meaty ham bone or 1 C cubed ham or ½ lb chopped bacon, cooked

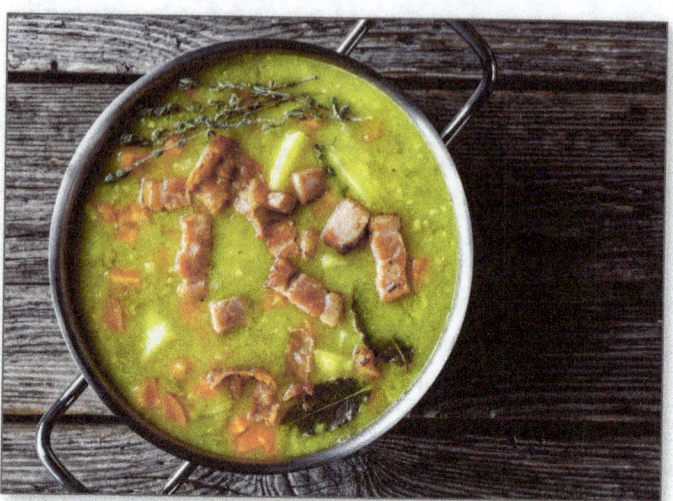

INSTRUCTIONS

1. Rinse the peas and then soak them overnight in several inches of water.

2. Drain the peas and add them to a stock pot or crock pot along with all the vegetables, seasonings and a quart of water. If using a ham bone add it to the pot, otherwise reserve the cubed ham for later.

3. Bring the soup to a boil and reduce to low and simmer for about 2 hours. If using a crockpot, cook on low for 5 hours. After the soup is cooked remove the meaty ham bone and use an immersion blender and puree to desired consistency. You can also blend in batches in a blender, but be careful with the hot mixture and be sure the lid has a vent for steam to escape.

4. If using ham on the bone, cut the meat off the bone and add it to the soup, otherwise add the cubed ham or chopped bacon.

COCONUT CURRY LENTIL AND SPINACH SORGHUM STEW

(Adapted from *Grain Power: Over 100 Delicious Gluten-Free Ancient Grains & Superblend Recipes*)

INGREDIENTS

1 tbsp oil

1 C chopped onion

½ tsp curry powder

½ tsp ground cumin

½ tsp ground coriander

3 tbsp tomato paste

1 lb dried yellow lentils or yellow split peas (green works, too)

4 C vegetable or chicken broth

2 C water

1 C coconut milk

½ chopped tomatoes

½ C sorghum grains

3 C chopped baby spinach

Salt and pepper to taste

INSTRUCTIONS

Heat a large saucepan on medium-low heat and add the oil. Cook the onion until it starts to soften, 5-7 minutes. Stir in the curry powder, cumin, coriander, and tomato paste. Heat for an additional minute. Stir in lentils, broth, water, coconut milk, tomatoes and sorghum. Simmer, covered for 45 minutes or until the lentils and sorghum are tender. Stir in spinach and heat until just wilted. Season with salt and pepper.

You can substitute an equal amount of quinoa or amaranth for the sorghum after the lentil mixture has simmered for 20 minutes.

Green, P., & Hemming, C. (2014). Grain Power: Over 100 Delicious Gluten-Free Ancient Grains & Superblend Recipes. Penguin Random House.

QUINOA CHILI

INGREDIENTS

2 tbsp extra-virgin olive oil

1 medium onion, chopped

1 large red bell pepper, chopped

2 carrots, chopped

2 ribs celery, chopped

½ tsp salt, divided

4 cloves garlic, pressed or minced

2 tbsp chili powder

2 tsp ground cumin

1 ½ tsp smoked paprika

1 tsp dried oregano

1 large can (28 oz) or 2 small cans (15 oz each) diced tomatoes with their juices

3 cans of bean of choice (15 oz)

1 (4 oz) can diced green chilis

1 C quinoa

4 C vegetable broth or water

1 bay leaf

⅓ C chopped fresh cilantro

1 to 2 tsp red wine vinegar or lime juice, to taste

Garnishes sliced avocado, tortilla chips, sour cream, grated cheddar cheese, etc.

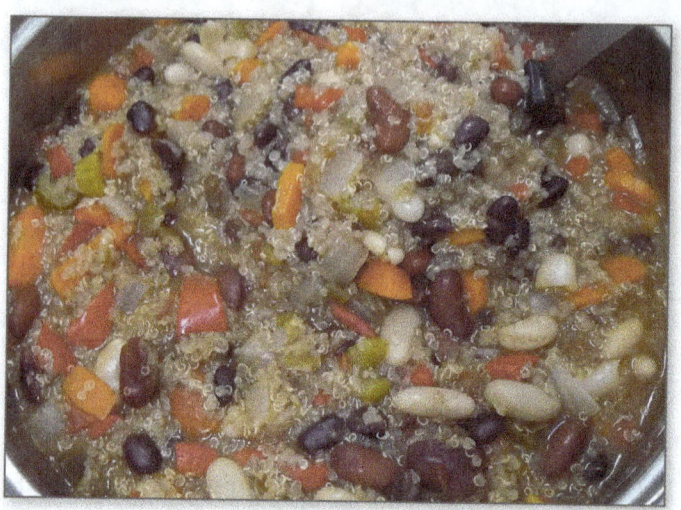

INSTRUCTIONS

Heat oil in a large stock pot then saute onion, bell pepper, carrots and celery and ¼ tsp salt until tender- about 7 minutes. Then add the garlic, chili powder, cumin, paprika and oregano and saute another minute until fragrant. Stir in tomatoes, drained beans, green chilis, broth, quinoa and bay leaf. Stir to combine and then simmer until quinoa is cooked and vegetables are tender- stirring occasionally, about 30 minutes. Remove the bay leaf and stir in cilantro and add vinegar/lime juice and more salt to taste.

Meat version: Reduce beans to 2 cans. Saute 1 lb ground beef or 1 lb cubed chicken with the onion and pepper until almost cooked through, then add the other vegetables and saute a few more minutes. Stir in spices and cook til fragrant then proceed with the instructions above. You could also stir in shredded rotisserie chicken at the end.

BLACK BEAN SOUP

(From *Our Best Bites*)

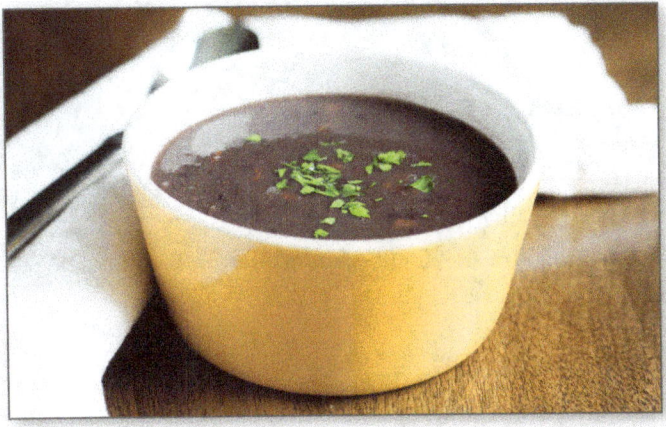

INGREDIENTS

1 tbsp olive oil

4 large cloves garlic, minced

2 carrots, diced

2 stalks celery, diced

1 medium onion diced

3 C cooked black beans* or 2 cans, rinsed and drained

1 (3½ oz) can diced green chilies

1 quart beef broth (vegetable works too)

3/4 tsp salt

1/8 tsp black pepper

1/2 tsp chili powder

1/4 tsp cumin

1/2 tsp dry oregano leaves

¼ tsp smoked paprika (optional, but great if using canned black beans. Omit if black beans were cooked from scratch with it already)

1 bay leaf

1 lime

Optional Toppings: sour cream, avocado, diced tomatoes, tortilla chips, grated cheese, chopped cilantro, etc.

INSTRUCTIONS

1. Using a large stock pot saute on carrots, celery, onion, and garlic in olive oil over medium-high heat for 4-5 minutes.

2. Next add the black beans, green chilies, broth, salt, pepper, chili powder, cumin, oregano, and bay leaf and stir to combine.

3. Simmer uncovered until the carrots are tender- about 20 minutes

4. Remove from heat and remove the bay leaf.

5. Using an immersion blender, puree the soup until it is totally smooth. Add the juice from the lime and stir in.

   *You can also use a regular blender and puree in batches if needed. Just be careful to avoid getting splattered with hot soup and be sure to remove the lid stopper so steam can escape.

6. Ladle into bowls and top with desired toppings. Serve with extra lime wedges.

   *For black beans: soak 1 lb beans overnight. Drain and rinse beans then put them in a pot and cover with several inches of water. Add 2 bay leaves, 1 quartered onion, several cloves crushed garlic and 2 tsp smoked paprika. Optional—If you have lard or fat rendered from bacon and ham add a heaping scoop to the pot for extra flavor. Bring the beans to boil then reduce to a simmer and cook until soft—about 2 hours. You can also cook the soaked beans in an electric pressure cooker for 5 minutes.

Wells, S. (2023, February 8). Black Bean Soup. Our Best Bites. Retrieved May 18, 2023, from https://ourbestbites.com/black-bean-soup/

PIONEER BEAN SOUP

INGREDIENTS

2 C mixed beans

7 C broth (chicken or vegetable)

1 ham hock (or 1-2 C cubed ham)

2 cloves garlic, minced

1 large onion, diced

3 carrots, diced

2 stalks celery, diced

1 bay leaf

1 (8 oz) can tomato sauce

1 tsp chili powder

Salt and pepper to taste

1 lemon

Topping suggestions: diced green onions, shredded cheese, sour cream

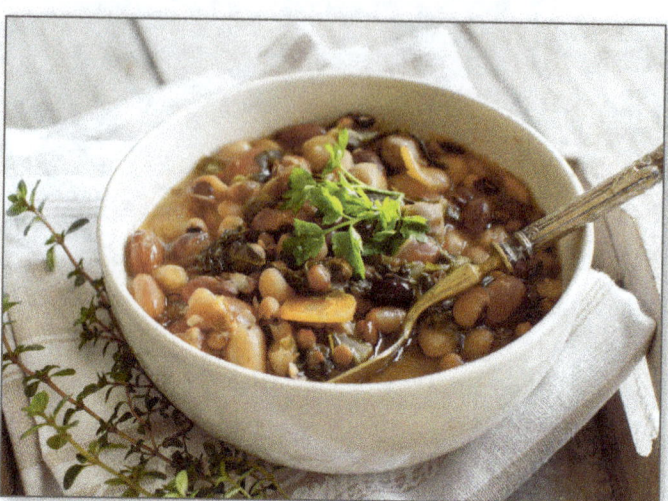

INSTRUCTIONS

1. Soak the beans overnight in water. When ready to assemble soup, drain and rinse beans.

2. Add the soaked beans, broth, ham hock, garlic, onion, carrots, celery and tomato sauce to a slow cooker and cook on high for 4-5 hours or low for 6-8. Alternatively, cook in a stock pot on the stove for 2-3 hours until the beans are tender.

3. Remove ham hock and bay leaf. Cut the meat off the bone, dice the meat then return it to the soup. Before serving add the juice of one lemon to the soup.

4. Top with green onions, cheese, or sour cream.

ROSEMARY GARLIC WHITE BEAN SOUP

(Adapted from *Budget Bytes*)

INGREDIENTS

2 tbsp olive oil

4 cloves garlic

3 (15 oz) cans cannellini beans or 4.5 C cooked beans

2 C vegetable (or chicken) broth

1½ tsp fresh rosemary, finely chopped or ½ tsp dry

¼ tsp dried thyme

1 pinch crushed red pepper

Pepper to taste (Freshly cracked is best)

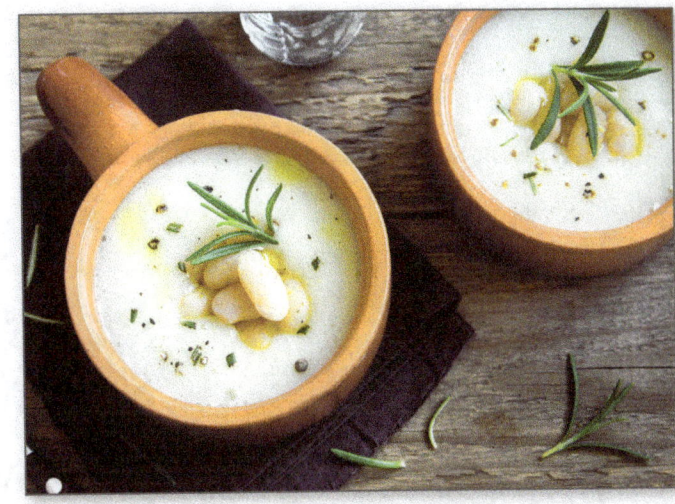

INSTRUCTIONS

1. Add one can of beans with its liquid to a blender and puree until smooth. Drain the other two cans of beans. If you are using cooked dried beans add 1.5 C of beans to a blender along with ½ C water and blend.

2. Heat the olive oil in a pot on medium heat, add the minced garlic and saute for about a minute until the garlic is fragrant.

3. Add the remaining ingredients and bring to a boil. Once boiling, uncover and reduce heat to medium low and simmer for 15 minutes, stirring occasionally.

4. If you want to thicken the soup more, use the back of a spoon or fork to mash beans slightly. Taste and add salt or pepper if needed.

Budget Bytes. (2019, September 7). Easy Rosemary Garlic White Bean Soup. Retrieved May 18, 2023, from https://www.budgetbytes.com/easy-rosemary-garlic-white-bean-soup/

MINESTRONE

INGREDIENTS

SOUPS

1 large onion, chopped

3 carrots, diced

3 stalks celery, diced

3 cloves garlic, crushed

3 quarts of broth (vegetable, chicken or beef)

1 tsp oregano

1 tsp basil

½ tsp thyme

½ tsp marjoram

12 oz green beans (frozen or fresh, but a can will work as well)

6 C cooked beans or 4 cans, drained (mix of chickpea, kidney beans, pinto, black or whatever you have on hand)

28 oz can crushed tomatoes (or 1 quart jar)

1 C gluten-free macaroni or other small pasta (can omit if desired)

Salt and pepper to taste

Red wine vinegar, balsamic vinegar, or lemon slices for serving (optional)

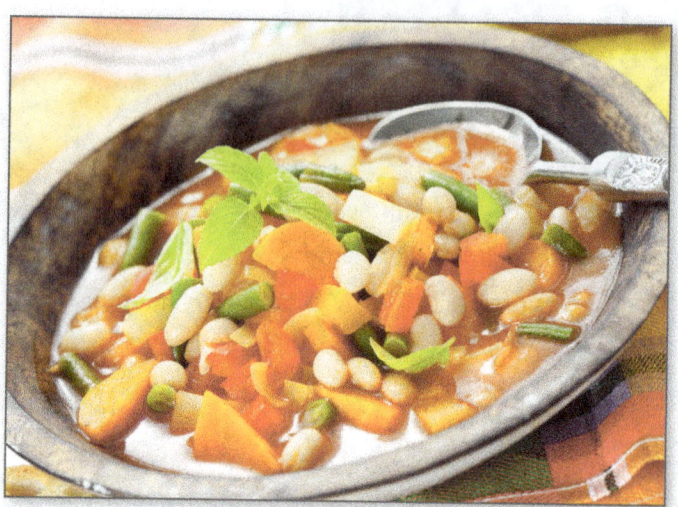

INSTRUCTIONS

1. In a large stock pot over medium heat, saute the onion until it starts to soften then add the garlic, carrots and celery and saute a couple minutes more until fragrant.

2. Add the broth, seasonings and beans then bring to a boil, reduce heat and simmer for 30 minutes.

3. Add the tomatoes and dry pasta and simmer for an additional 10-15 minutes or until pasta is al dente. Salt and pepper to taste. Alternatively, you can cook the pasta separately and add it at serving time so the pasta won't be overcooked in the leftover soup.

4. Serve with a splash of red wine vinegar, balsamic vinegar or a squeeze of fresh lemon juice.

TACO SOUP

INGREDIENTS

1 lb hamburger

1 onion, diced

1 large can stewed tomatoes

1 (8 oz) can tomato sauce

1 can corn, with liquid

3 cans beans, undrained (any type—black, pinto, kidney are colorful options), or 4½ C cooked beans with 1 extra C of water

1 package taco seasoning or homemade version*

Chopped cilantro, green onions, cheese, sour cream, avocado, tortilla chips for serving

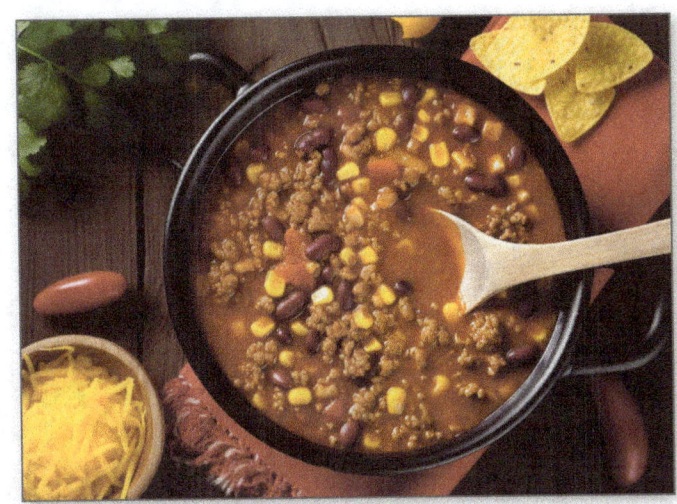

INSTRUCTIONS

1. In a soup pot, brown the hamburger with the onion until the meat is no longer pink.

2. Drain liquid off 1 can of beans and add the beans to the pot. Add the remaining ingredients including the 2 remaining undrained cans of beans.

3. Bring to a boil then reduce heat and simmer for 20 minutes. Garnish with grated cheese, sour cream, green onions etc.

Recipe for Homemade Taco Seasoning—equivalent to 1 packet

1 tbsp chili powder

2 tsp paprika

1 tsp kosher salt

1 tsp onion powder

1 tsp garlic powder

1 tsp ground cumin

¼ tsp cayenne pepper

WHITE CHICKEN CHILI

SOUPS

INGREDIENTS

2 C shredded rotisserie chicken, or ¾ lb boneless
  skinless chicken breasts

1 tbsp olive oil

1 medium onion, chopped

1 jalapeno pepper, seeded and chopped

4 garlic cloves, minced

2 tsp dried oregano

1 tsp ground cumin

1 (4 oz) can diced green chilis

1 can corn, drained or 1½ C frozen corn

3 cans white beans, rinsed and drained or 4½ C
  cooked beans

3 C chicken broth, divided

1½ C shredded cheddar cheese

Toppings: avocado, chopped tomatoes, chopped cilantro, sour cream, tortilla chips, chopped
  green onions, lime wedges

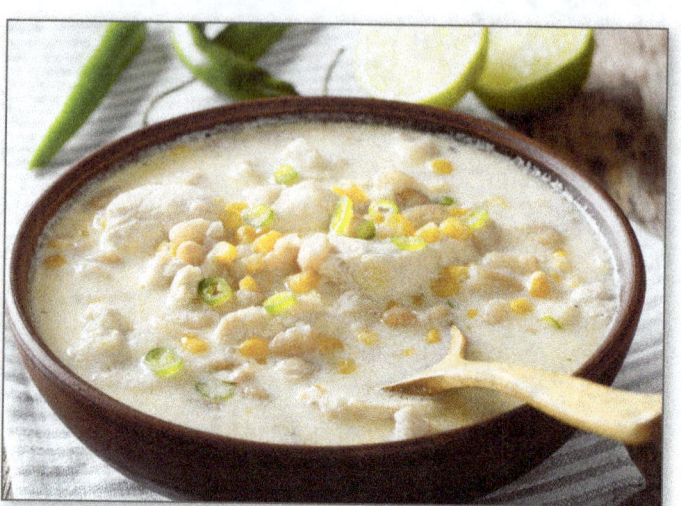

INSTRUCTIONS

1. If using boneless skinless chicken breast, chop into 1 inch chunks and season with salt, pepper and
   garlic powder. Saute over medium heat till the meat has browned and cooked through. Set aside.

2. Put one can of beans (or 1½ C cooked beans) and 1 C of broth into a blender and puree until smooth.
   Set aside.

3. In a large soup pot, heat the oil over medium heat and then add the onion and saute till it starts to
   soften. Add the jalapeno and garlic and saute another minute until fragrant.

4. To the pot, add the chicken, oregano, cumin, green chilis, corn, beans, pureed beans and remaining
   broth. Simmer for 15-20 minutes for flavors to blend.

5. Serve with shredded cheese and other toppings.

RED LENTIL THAI CHILI

(From *Isa Does It*)

INGREDIENTS

1 large yellow onion, diced

1 bell pepper, diced

1 tsp salt

3 cloves garlic, minced

1½ lbs sweet potatoes or carrots, diced

1 C red lentils (can use brown as well—they just don't break down as much)

4 C vegetable or chicken broth

2 tbsp chili powder

2 (15 oz) cans kidney beans, rinsed and drained (or 3 C cooked beans)

2 tbsp Thai red curry paste (Thai kitchen brand)

1 can coconut milk (lite works)

1 (28 oz) can crushed tomatoes or 1 quart tomatoes (diced or puree work)

½ C chopped fresh cilantro

Lime wedges

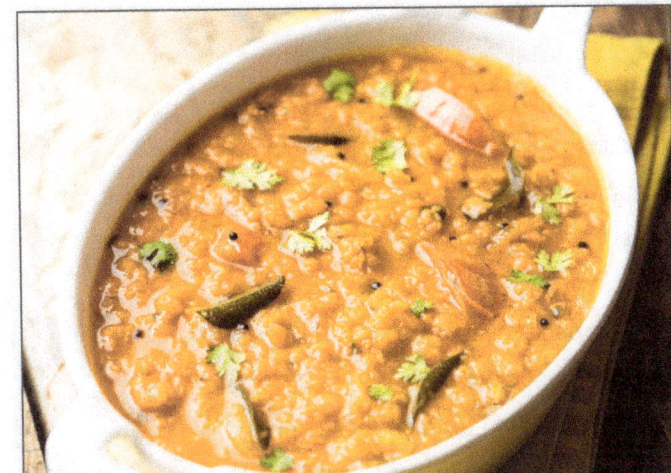

INSTRUCTIONS

1. Preheat a pot over medium heat and saute onion and bell pepper with a pinch of salt for 5-7 minutes. Add garlic and saute another minute.

2. Add the sweet potatoes, lentils, broth, chili powder and remaining salt. Cover and bring to a boil. Let boil for 15-20 minutes, stirring occasionally. When the lentils are soft and mushy and vegetables are tender, add the beans, curry paste, coconut milk, tomatoes and cilantro and heat through.

3. Taste and adjust seasoning, top with additional cilantro and lime wedges if desired. Eat as soup or serve over whole grains or vegetables.

Moskowitz, I. C. (2013). Isa Does It: Amazingly Easy, Wildly Delicious Vegan Recipes for Every Day of the Week. Little, Brown and Company.

AMARANTH AND BROCCOLI

INGREDIENTS

1 C amaranth

2 C low sodium chicken, vegetable or beef broth (or water plus 2 tsp bouillon)

1 medium garlic clove minced (or ½ tsp dry)

1 tsp fresh grated ginger (or ¼ tsp dry)

2 tbsp soy sauce

¼ C chopped green onions, tops and bottoms

Salt and pepper to taste

1 lb broccoli florets, fresh or frozen

2 tsp toasted sesame seeds (optional)

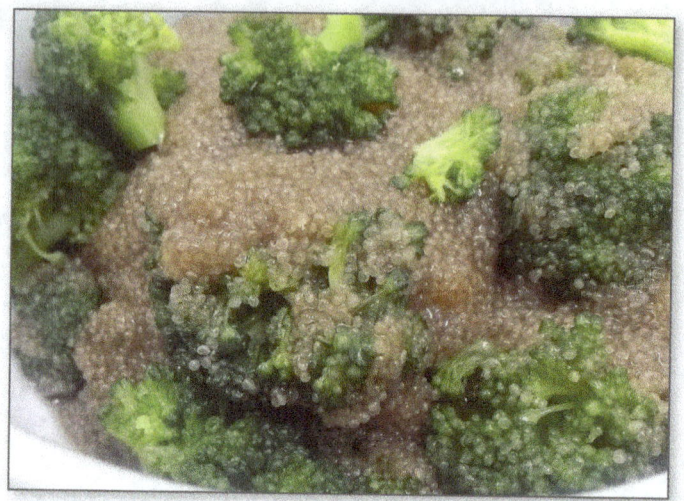

INSTRUCTIONS

Heat a medium saucepan on medium high heat and then add in amaranth. Toast the amaranth for about a minute, stirring occasionally so it doesn't burn. Pour in the broth, garlic and ginger, and bring to a boil, reduce heat to a simmer then cover and cook for 20 minutes till the water is absorbed. Meanwhile, cook the broccoli according to package directions if using frozen. If using fresh- bring an inch of water to a boil in a saucepan then add broccoli, cover and cook 7 minutes till just tender. When the amaranth is done cooking, stir in soy sauce then toss with green onions and broccoli, salt and pepper to taste, garnish with sesame seeds, and serve warm.

Feel free to substitute broccoli with cauliflower, peas, green beans, etc.

BUCKWHEAT COCONUT CURRY

(Adapted from *fullofplants.com*)

INGREDIENTS

1 tbsp coconut or olive oil

1 onion, finely chopped

2 cloves of garlic, minced

1 tbsp grated fresh ginger

¼ C cashews roughly chopped (or peanuts)

¾ C buckwheat groats

1 tsp ground coriander

½ tsp ground cumin

1 tsp turmeric

1 tsp smoked paprika

1 tbsp sugar

1 (14 oz) can coconut milk

2 tbsp soy sauce

¼ tsp sriracha (optional)

1 and ½ C water (add ½ additional C for a more soupy curry)

4 C spinach or other leafy green, finely cut

1 tsp lemon juice

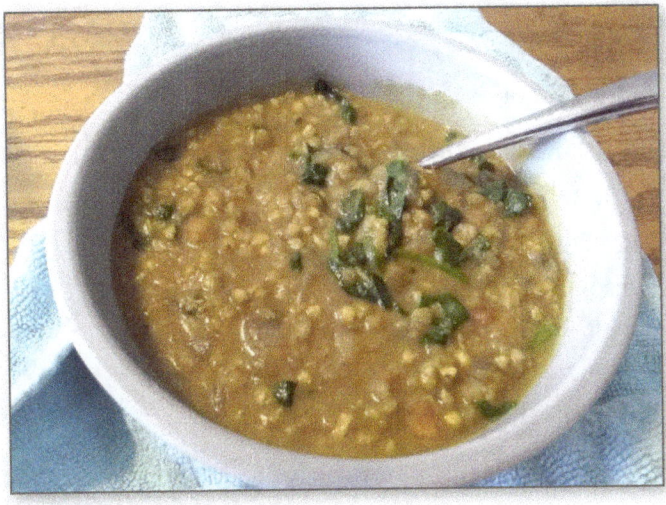

INSTRUCTIONS

Heat oil in a large skillet and saute onion, garlic and ginger until soft—about 7 minutes. Add buckwheat groats and cashews/peanuts and toast about 2 minutes being careful not to burn them. Add coriander, cumin, turmeric, paprika and sugar. Stir in soy sauce, coconut milk, water and hot sauce (if using) and bring to a simmer. Cover and cook for 20 minutes until buckwheat is tender. Add more water when cooking if needed. Remove from heat and stir in lemon juice and spinach. If you are using sturdier greens like kale you may want to let them cook with the buckwheat. Serve on its own, over steamed or roasted vegetables, or on top of another grain like brown rice.

Full of Plants (n.d.). Retrieved May 18, 2023. https://fullofplants.com.

CHICKPEA SALAD SANDWICH FILLING

(Adapted from *Minimalist Baker*)

INGREDIENTS

For the salad:

1 can chickpeas, rinsed and drained (1½ C cooked)

3 tbsp tahini (Mayonnaise works too if not egg-free)

1 tsp Dijon or spicy brown mustard

1 tbsp maple syrup, agave nectar, or honey

¼ C diced red onion

¼ C diced celery

¼ C diced pickle

1 tsp capers, drained and loosely chopped

¼ tsp salt

¼ tsp pepper

1 tbsp sunflower seeds (optional)

For serving:

Gluten-free bread, wrap or crackers

Mustard

Lettuce

Sliced tomato

Sliced red onion

Other sandwich toppings of choice

INSTRUCTIONS

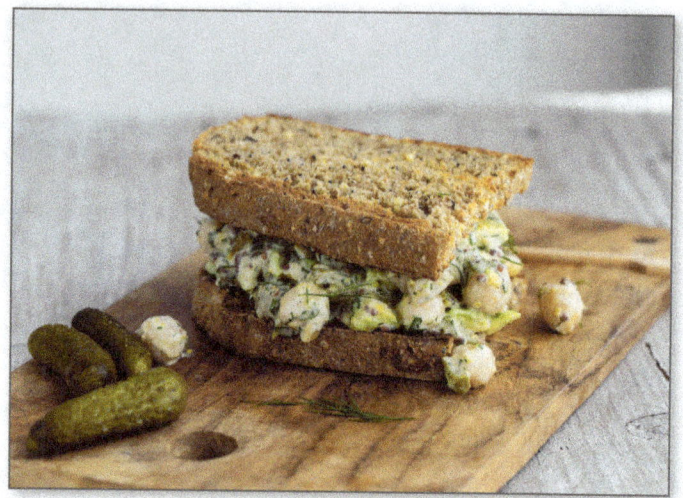

1. Place the chickpeas in a mixing bowl and mash with a fork, leaving only a few beans whole.

2. Add tahini (or mayonnaise), mustard, maple syrup, red onion, celery, pickle, capers, salt and pepper, and sunflower seeds (if using) to the mixing bowl. Mix to incorporate. Taste and adjust seasonings as needed.

3. Serve on toasted gluten-free bread or in a wrap with any other desired sandwich toppings. Delicious on crackers or as a vegetable dip.

Minimalist Baker. (n.d.). Chickpea Sunflower Sandwich. Retrieved May 18, 2023, from https://minimalistbaker.com/chickpea-sunflower-sandwich/

EASY CHICKPEA CURRY

INGREDIENTS

1 can chickpeas, drained and rinsed, or 1½-2 C cooked beans

2 C vegetable broth (chicken or water also work)

½ medium red onion, finely chopped

2 medium tomatoes, finely chopped

½ tsp cumin seeds

2 tbsp olive or canola oil

2 cloves garlic, minced

1 tbsp grated fresh ginger

1 tsp curry powder

¼ tsp red pepper flakes (optional)

¼ C plain yogurt at room temperature mixed with 2 tbsp water (sub for ½ can coconut milk if dairy free)

2 tbsp cilantro (plus more for garnish, optional)

Salt to taste

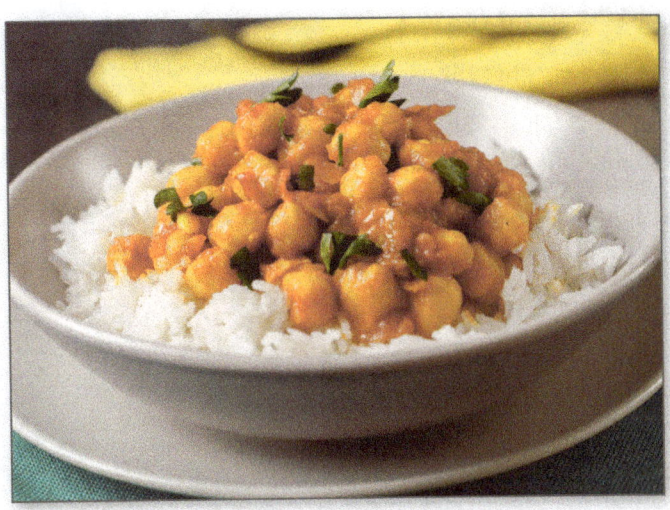

INSTRUCTIONS

1. In a wide saute pan, heat the oil over medium heat. Add the cumin seeds and let them sputter for 20 seconds, then add the tomatoes, onion, ginger and garlic. Cook until the expressed liquid evaporates and the mix is soft with a little oil on the sides, about 5 minutes.

2. Add the dried spices and saute for 1 minute.

3. Add the chickpeas and the vegetable broth. Stir to combine and bring to a boil, then reduce heat to medium and cook until mixture is saucy and thickened, about 5-7 minutes. Smash some of the chickpeas to thicken the sauce if desired.

4. Remove from heat and stir in yogurt quickly and continuously so it doesn't curdle. Add chopped cilantro. Taste and adjust salt and serve over rice or other cooked grain.

THAI PEANUT COCONUT CAULIFLOWER CURRY

INGREDIENTS

½ tbsp coconut oil

3 cloves garlic, minced

1 tbsp grated ginger

1 large carrot, sliced

3-4 C cauliflower florets (1 small head)

1 bunch green onions, diced

1 can coconut milk (lite works)

⅓ C water or vegetable broth

2 tbsp red curry paste (like Thai Kitchen brand)

2 tbsp creamy peanut butter

½ tbsp gluten-free soy sauce or coconut aminos

½ tsp turmeric

½ tsp cayenne

½ tsp salt

1 red pepper, julienned

1 can chickpeas, rinsed and drained or 1.5–2 C cooked

½ C frozen peas

Garnishes: fresh cilantro, green onion, chopped
    peanuts, fresh lime

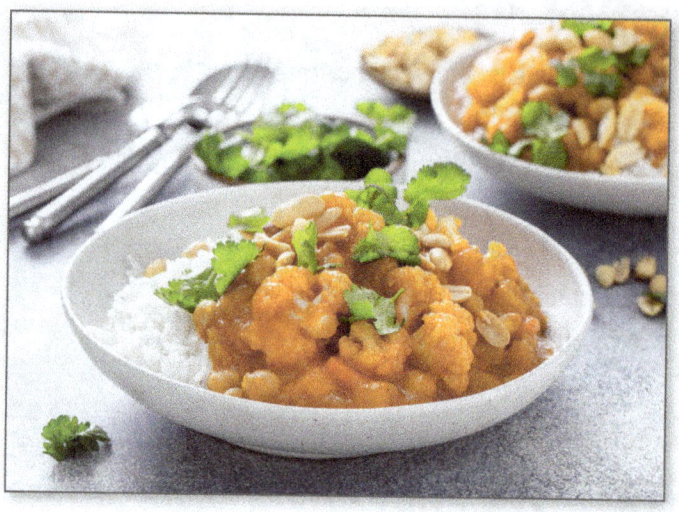

INSTRUCTIONS

1. Heat the coconut oil in a large deep skillet over medium high heat then add the garlic and ginger and cook for 30 seconds.

2. Add the cauliflower, green onion, and carrots and saute another 3-5 minutes until the cauliflower starts to brown and the onion softens.

3. Add in coconut milk, water, curry paste, peanut butter, soy sauce, cayenne, turmeric, and salt and stir to combine.

4. Mix in the bell pepper and chickpeas and simmer over medium-low heat for 10 minutes. Stir in peas and simmer another minute then taste and adjust seasonings if needed.

5. Serve over rice or quinoa and garnish with cilantro, peanuts, green onion or a squeeze of fresh lime.

CHANA SAAG

(From *Budget Bytes*)

INGREDIENTS

1 yellow onion, diced

2 cloves garlic, minced

1 tbsp grated fresh ginger

2 tbsp olive oil

1 tbsp curry powder hot or mild

1 tsp ground cumin

¾ tsp salt

1 tomato, diced

1 lb fresh or frozen chopped spinach, or kale, chard or other dark leafy green (not lettuce)

2 cans chickpeas, rinsed and drained or 3 C cooked

½ C water

1 13-oz can coconut milk

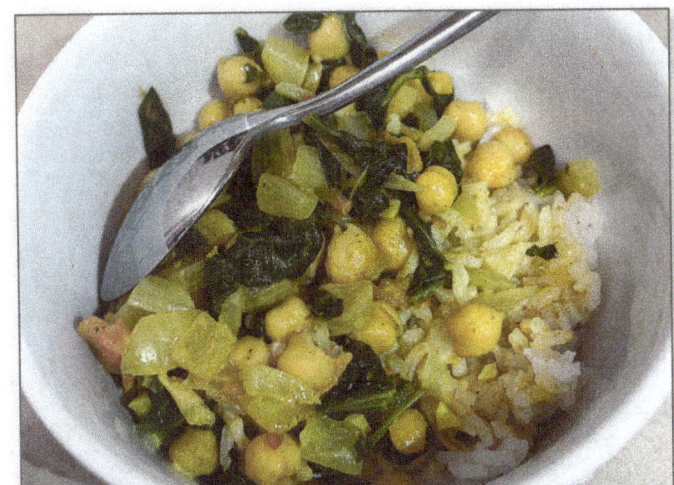

INSTRUCTIONS

1. Heat the olive oil in a large skillet over medium heat and saute the onion, garlic, and ginger for about 5 minutes until the onion is soft.

2. Add the curry powder and cumin, continue to stir and cook for about a minute. Add the diced tomato and salt and cook until the tomato has broken down, about five minutes.

3. Stir the chickpeas, spinach and half cup of water into the skillet and simmer for 5 minutes.

4. Reduce heat to medium low and add the coconut milk. If you want a thicker sauce, allow the mixture to simmer longer. You can also puree a portion of the mix if you want it smoother. Taste and add salt if needed.

5. Serve over rice or other grain, or eat with flatbread or tortilla.

Budget Bytes. (2020, February 9). Chana Saag. Retrieved May 18, 2023, from https://www.budget-bytes.com/chana-saag/

MAIN DISHES

LENTIL-A-RONI

(From *Isa Does It*)

INGREDIENTS

1 lb gluten free pasta (can also serve sauce over rice or other whole grain)

½ C cashews, soaked (sunflower seeds work great too)

1 C vegetable broth

1 tbsp olive oil

1 small yellow onion, finely chopped

1 tsp salt

3 cloves garlic, minced

2 tsp dried thyme

1 tsp italian seasoning (optional)

Pinch of black pepper

1½ C cooked brown lentils

1 (28 oz) can crushed tomatoes

1 tsp dried basil

Chopped greens (optional)

Chopped fresh basil for serving

⅛ tsp red pepper flakes (optional)

A few turns of balsamic vinegar (optional)

INSTRUCTIONS

1. Bring a large pot of salted water to a boil for the pasta and cook according to package directions. Set aside.

2. Drain cashews and blend them with the broth until very smooth. This could take 1-5 minutes depending on your blender.

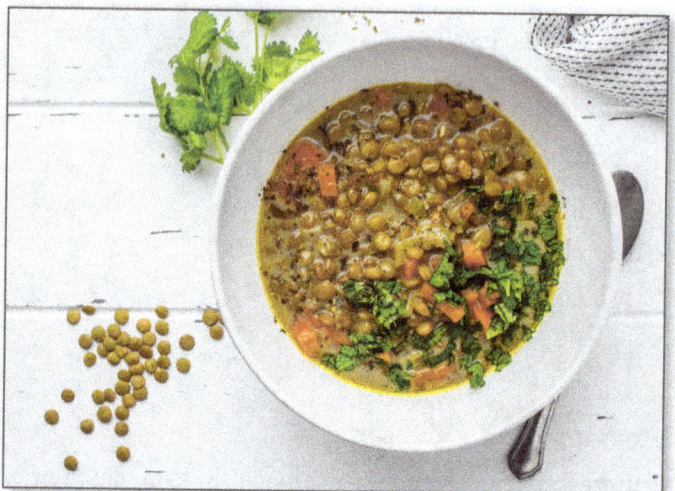

3. Preheat a large saucepan over medium heat and saute the onion with water or oil and a pinch of salt for 3ish minutes until translucent. Add the garlic and saute 30 seconds.

4. Add the thyme, remaining salt, pepper and saute 30ish seconds. Add lentils and toss to coat. Use a small masher or fork to partially mash some of the lentils.

5. Add the tomatoes and cover the pot, letting it cook for about 5 minutes. Pour in the cashew mixture and let thicken for about 3 minutes, stirring occasionally.

6. Stir in chopped greens if using. Taste for seasoning—add red pepper flakes if using. Add the pasta, toss to coat, heat through then serve! Can also just serve the sauce over pasta instead of mixing it in. Also delicious served over a baked potato, cooked grain, or vegetables.

Moskowitz, I. C. (2013). Isa Does It: Amazingly Easy, Wildly Delicious Vegan Recipes for Every Day of the Week. Little, Brown and Company.

MAIN DISHES

LENTIL "MEATBALLS"

(Adapted from *Forks over Knives*)

INGREDIENTS

1 C dry brown lentils

1¼ C water

8 oz button or bella mushrooms

1 C onion, chopped

3 cloves garlic, minced

¼ C oat flour

3 tbsp gluten-free soy sauce

2 tbsp tomato paste

1 tbsp nutritional yeast (optional)

1 tsp oregano

1 tsp onion powder

¾ tsp salt

½ tsp pepper

For serving: spaghetti sauce, gluten free pasta, fresh basil, parmesan cheese

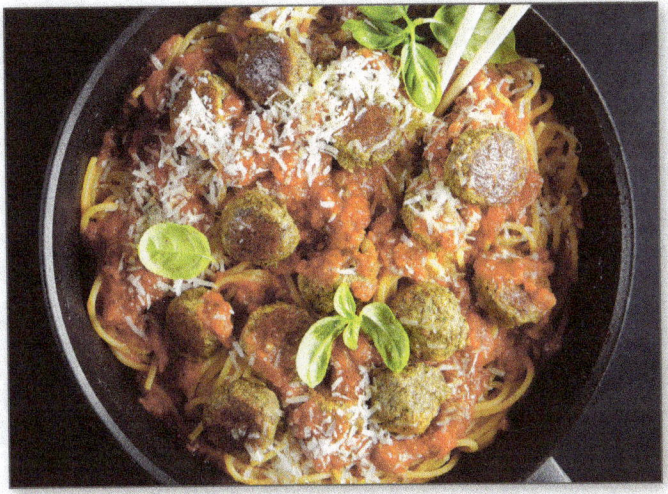

INSTRUCTIONS

1. Add the lentils and water to a large saucepan and bring to a boil. Reduce heat, cover and simmer for about 10-15 minutes (make sure to not burn the lentils).

2. Add the mushrooms, onion and garlic and cover and cook for another 15 minutes until lentils are tender.If there is excess water, cook uncovered until remaining liquid has evaporated.

3. Stir in the oat flour, soy sauce, tomato paste, nutritional yeast, oregano, onion powder, salt and pepper. Cook on low, uncovered, about 10 minutes until the liquid is absorbed and the pan is dry. Be careful not to scorch the lentils.

4. Remove from heat and allow the mixture to cool. You can do this more quickly by spreading it out in a pan.

5. Preheat an oven to 300° F and line a baking sheet with parchment paper. Scoop out 2 tbsp of mixture to form balls and place on the pan. Repeat until all the mixture is used. Bake for 45 minutes until crisp and lightly browned on the outside.

6. Serve with cooked gluten-free pasta and sauce. Garnish with chopped basil and parmesan if desired.

Thacker Wendel, D. (2019, January 24). Lentil Meatballs Marinara. Forks Over Knives. Retrieved May 18, 2023, from https://www.forksoverknives.com/recipes/vegan-baked-stuffed/lentil-meatballs-marinara/

"SAUSAGE" LENTIL GRAVY

(From *Happy Herbivore*)

INGREDIENTS

1 C cooked lentils

1 C almond or soy milk, plain (cow's milk if not dairy-free)

2 tbsp tamari or soy sauce

½ tsp rubbed sage

1 tsp dried thyme

1 tsp onion powder

1 tsp garlic powder

¼ tsp smoked paprika

1 tbsp cornstarch with 1 tbsp water

¾ tsp ground fennel

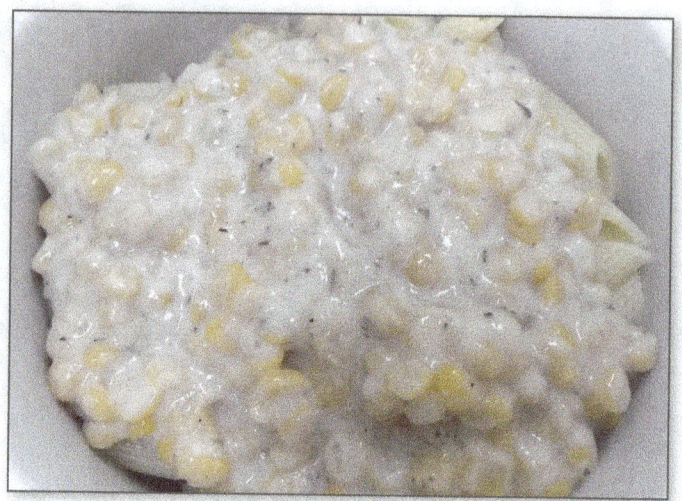

INSTRUCTIONS

1. Place cooked lentils in a skillet.

2. In a small bowl or measuring cup, combine almond milk and spices together, adding a few dashes of smoked paprika.

3. Cover and bring to a near boil.

4. Mix cornstarch (or flour) into 2 tbsp cold water to make a slurry. Stir slurry into milk and lentil mix and cook until it thickens.

5. Serve over baked, roasted, or mashed potatoes or other roasted vegetables.

Happy Herbivore. (n.d.). Vegetarian Lentil Sausage Gravy (Vegan & Soy-Free). Retrieved May 18, 2023, from https://happyherbivore.com/recipe/vegetarian-lentil-sausage-gravy-vegan-soy-free/

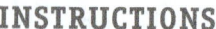
MAIN DISHES

LENTIL TACO MEAT

(From *The Conscious Plant Kitchen*)

INGREDIENTS

2 tsp Olive Oil

½ Yellow Onion diced

1¼ C Cooked Brown Lentils equivalent to 1 can 15 oz, rinsed, drained

1¼ C Cauliflower Rice fresh or frozen

1 tsp Cumin

1 tsp Salt

½ tsp Garlic Powder

½ tsp Paprika

½ tsp Oregano

¼ tsp Chili Powder

¼ C Vegetable Broth

3-4 tbsp Vegan Worcestershire Sauce or 1 tbsp of tamari sauce

½ C Tomato Paste

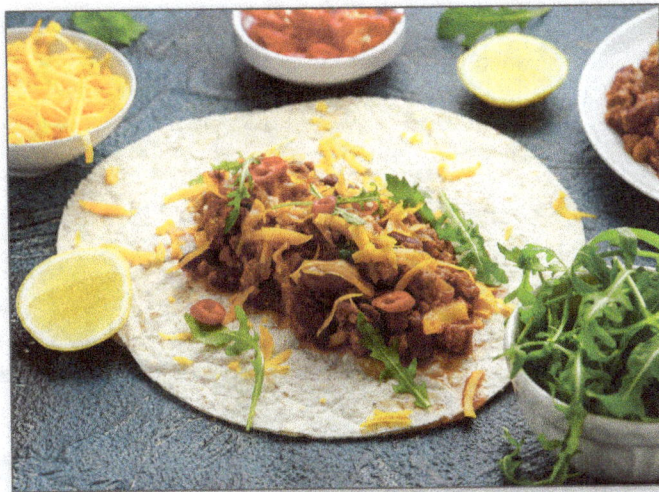

INSTRUCTIONS

1. In a large skillet or Dutch oven, heat olive oil and stir fry the onion until fragrant - about 1 minute.

2. Stir in cooked, drained, canned brown lentils and cauliflower rice and stir fry for 1 minute.

3. Stir in spices: cumin, garlic powder, paprika, oregano, salt chili powder.

4. Stir in tomato paste, vegetable broth, and vegan Worcestershire sauce.

5. Reduce heat, and simmer for 5-6 minutes or until the mixture thickens. The longer you cook the lentils, the thicker and dryer the sauce. For a smoother sauce, stop the heat after 3-4 minutes of cooking.

Claudepierre, C. (2021, June 1). Lentil Taco Meat. The Conscious Plant Kitchen. Retrieved May 18, 2023, from https://www.theconsciousplantkitchen.com/lentil-taco-meat/

LENTIL SLOPPY JOES

INGREDIENTS

1 C lentils, uncooked

3 C water

1 tbsp olive oil

1 medium onion, diced

1 medium green bell pepper, diced

3 garlic cloves, minced

2 tbsp chili powder

1½ tsp smoked paprika

1 (15 oz) can tomato sauce

2 tbsp ketchup

3 tbsp mustard

3 tbsp brown sugar

¼ tsp pepper

1 tsp salt, or to taste

INSTRUCTIONS

1. Cook the lentils by bringing the 3 C of water and 1 C lentils to a boil. Once boiling, lower heat and simmer for 18-20 minutes or until tender. Drain excess liquid and set aside.

2. Heat the olive oil in a large skillet over medium heat. Once hot, add the chopped onion, green bell pepper and garlic and sauté for 3-4 minutes.

3. Now add the chili powder and smoked paprika, and stir to coat the vegetables for about 1 minute. Add a little water if it's too dry.

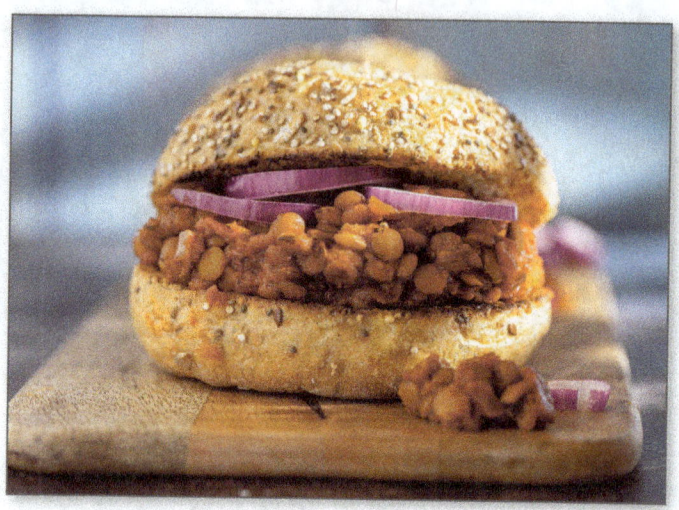

4. Next, add the tomato sauce, ketchup, mustard and maple syrup. Stir until well incorporated. Add in the cooked lentils and stir. Season with salt to taste.

5. Serve on gluten-free burger buns and top with red onions or coleslaw (see recipe below). Also great over potatoes, rice, or as a wrap filling.

QUICK COLESLAW

• 1 (1 lb) bag coleslaw mix (or 6 C shredded cabbage),

• Dressing: 1 tbsp dijon mustard, ¼ C cider vinegar, 1 tbsp sugar, ¼ C olive oil, 1 tsp celery seed, 4 diced green onions, Salt and pepper to taste

Add all dressing ingredients to a jar and shake to mix. Pour desired amount over coleslaw cabbage mix.

LENTIL STUFFED PEPPER SKILLET

INGREDIENTS

1 tbsp olive oil

1 small onion, diced

2 green pepper, chopped

½ tsp garlic powder

½ tsp salt

¼ tsp pepper

⅛ tsp smoked paprika

½ tsp italian seasoning

1 (15 oz) can tomato sauce*

1 C cooked lentils (⅓ C dry lentils boiled 25 minutes in 2 C water with 1 tsp garlic powder and 1 bay leaf, remove bay leaf and drain)

1½ C cooked brown rice

¾ C shredded mozzarella cheese (omit if dairy free)

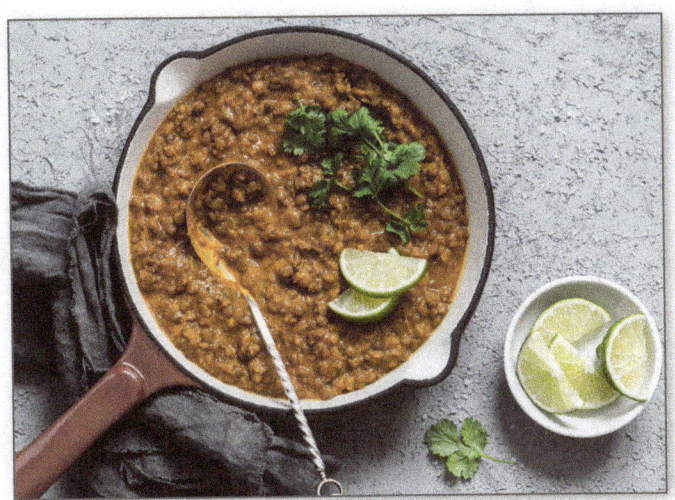

INSTRUCTIONS

1. Prepare the lentils by adding ⅓ C lentils to 2 C of water in a medium saucepan. Add 1 tsp garlic powder and 1 bay leaf. Bring to a boil then simmer, covered, for 20-25 minutes until lentils are tender. Remove bay leaf and drain. You can also use leftover cooked lentils for this recipe.

2. In a large skillet, heat oil over medium heat. Add the onion and green peppers and saute until the onions are translucent and the peppers have started to soften.

3. Add the salt, pepper, smoked paprika, Italian seasoning, tomato sauce, drained lentils and brown rice. Stir together then cover to heat through on medium low for about 3 minutes.

4. Remove lid and top with shredded mozzarella cheese, then cover again until cheese melts. Alternatively, if you are using an oven safe skillet pan you can put the whole thing in the oven under the broiler for a few minutes until the cheese is bubbly and just starts to brown.

*If you have leftover spaghetti sauce you can use it in place of the tomato sauce and Italian seasoning.

COCONUT CURRY LENTILS

INGREDIENTS

1 tbsp oil

1 diced onion

2 cloves garlic, minced

1½ tsp fresh ginger, grated or finely chopped

1 tbsp curry powder

1.5 tsp garam masala

¾ tsp turmeric

1½ C lentils (red or brown or mix)

2 (15 oz) cans crushed tomatoes (diced or pureed work as well)

4 C water (more if needed)

1 tsp salt

1 can coconut milk

Half bunch chopped cilantro

½ tsp cayenne (optional)

Additional vegetables: carrots, mushrooms, sweet potatoes, green beans, peppers, greens/cabbage etc.)

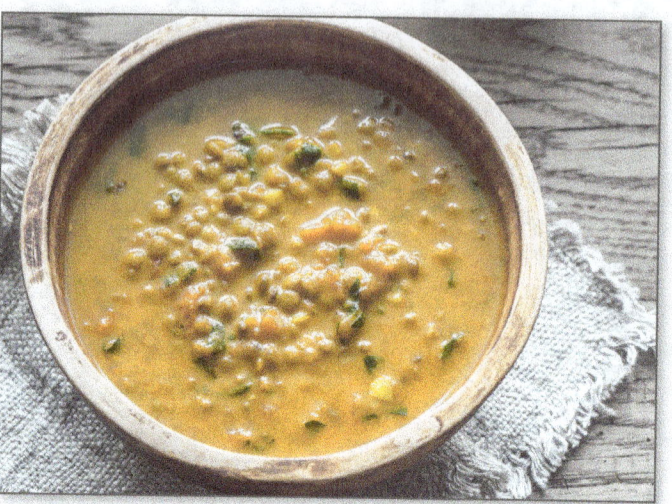

INSTRUCTIONS

1. In a large pot, saute onion until translucent (mushrooms if adding), then add spices and garlic and stir until fragrant.

2. Add water, tomatoes, lentils and any additional vegetables (save leafy greens or cabbage until the end) and simmer until lentils and vegetables are tender- about 25 minutes. Add additional water as needed.

3. Once lentils are done, stir in a can of coconut milk and cilantro and adjust seasonings if needed. Stir in leafy greens if using.

4. Serve over rice, quinoa, other whole grain, squash or vegetables, or eat as soup.

LENTIL MUSHROOM BOURGUIGNON

INGREDIENTS

1 large onion, chopped in chunks

2 cloves garlic, minced

6 carrots, diced

8 oz baby bella mushrooms, chopped (other varieties can work)

⅔ C lentils

1 quart water

1 (15 oz) can tomato sauce (can also use 1 quart pureed tomatoes and reduce water to 2 C)

½ C red wine vinegar

1 tbsp worcestershire sauce (make sure it's gluten free)

1 tsp sugar

1 tsp salt

1 tsp dry basil

1 tsp dry thyme

2 bay leaves

½ tsp pepper

1-2 tbsp cornstarch

INSTRUCTIONS

1. In a large pot, saute the onion in 1 tbsp of olive oil until it starts to soften.

2. Add the mushrooms and garlic and saute another couple minutes until the mushrooms soften.

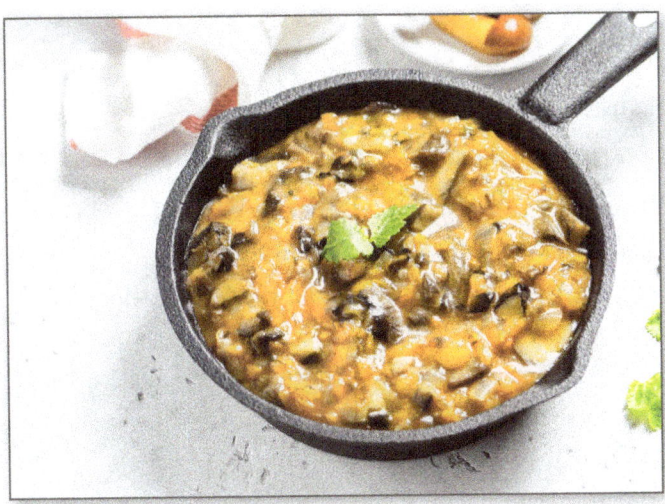

3. Add all the remaining ingredients excluding the cornstarch and stir to combine. Bring to a boil, then reduce heat, cover and simmer until the lentils and carrots are tender, about 30 minutes.

4. Combine cornstarch with a small amount of cold water to make a slurry and stir into the stew and heat until the mixture bubbles and thickens. Use more or less cornstarch depending on your preference. Can also substitute other thickeners such as arrowroot or tapioca.

5. Serve with baked or mashed potatoes.

This recipe also works great in a slow cooker—just mix all the ingredients in a crockpot besides the cornstarch and cook on high 3-4 hours or until lentils and carrots are tender.

PASTA E FAGIOLI

(From *The High-Protein Vegetarian Cookbook*)

INGREDIENTS

1 tbsp oil

1 clove garlic, minced

½ medium yellow onion, diced

1 (28 oz) can whole peeled tomatoes

1 (15 oz) can cannellini beans, rinsed and drained or
   1½ C cooked beans

1 (15 oz) can kidney beans, rinsed and drained or 1.5
   C cooked beans or lentils

¼ C sun dried tomatoes, chopped

2 tbsp tomato paste

¾ tsp sea salt

¼ tsp black pepper

1 tsp thyme

1 tsp oregano

1 tsp basil

1 tsp rosemary

2 bay leaves

1 C small gluten-free noodles (more if you plan to
   serve this over noodles)

Optional: chopped green or kalamata olives, or 1 tbsp
   capers, artichoke hearts etc for briny flavor, or
   sprinkle with parmesan cheese if not dairy-free

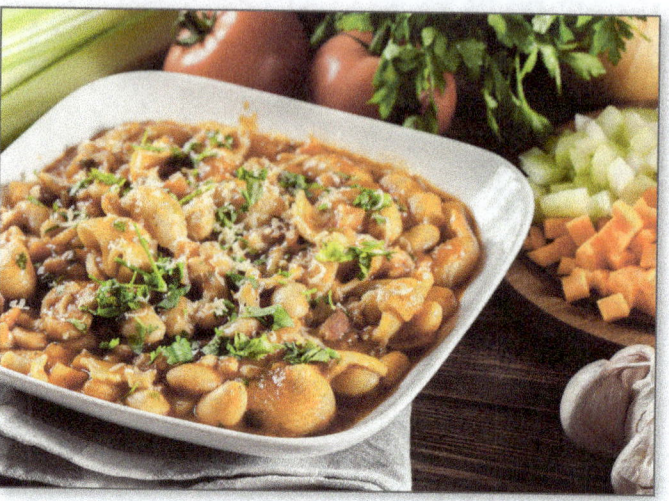

INSTRUCTIONS

1. In a large saute pan or dutch oven, saute garlic for 30
   seconds in oil, add the onion and cook until softened.

2. Pour in tomatoes and use a spoon to break them apart a
   bit. Add beans and sun dried tomatoes, tomato paste, and
   seasonings. Simmer 20 minutes

3. Cook noodles according to the package.

4. Once the bean mixture is done simmering, remove the bay
   leaves then puree 3 C of the mixture and add it back in.
   Stir in any optional ingredients such as olives, capers or
   artichoke hearts and heat a few more minutes. Add the
   noodles to the mix or serve over noodles.

Parker, K., & Smith, K. (2012). The High-Protein Vegetarian Cookbook: Hearty Dishes That Even Carnivores Will Love. W.
W. Norton & Company.

MAIN DISHES

DOUBLE BEAN BURGERS (OR TACO FILLING OR SALAD TOPPING)

(Adapted from *The High- Protein Vegetarian Cookbook*)

INGREDIENTS

2 tbsp ground flaxseed mixed with 6 tbsp warm water

1 can black beans, rinsed, drained, patted dry*

1 can kidney beans, rinsed, drained, patted dry

1 tbsp tamari sauce

2 cloves garlic, minced

1 small onion or shallot, diced

½ C old-fashioned oats

½ C unsalted pepitas or pumpkin seeds (sunflower seeds work as well, or omit)

½ tsp dry oregano

½ tsp paprika

½ tsp chili powder

¼ tsp ground cumin

3 tbsp chopped cilantro

½ tsp pepper

Salt to taste (½ tsp)

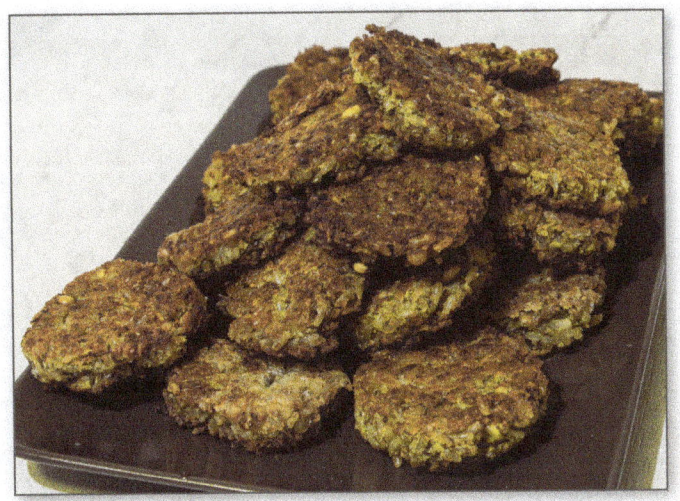

INSTRUCTIONS

1. Combine flaxseed and water, mix with a fork and let sit for 5 minutes.

2. Pour the beans in a bowl and mash well with a fork. Mix in tamari, garlic, onion, oats, pepitas, and spices. Taste and adjust seasonings.

3. Pour in the flax mixture, mix well and refrigerate for 30 minutes.

4. Preheat oven to 350° F.

5. Scoop out ½ C mixture and form into patties on parchment lined baking sheets. Bake for 15 minutes on each side and serve on a gluten-free bun or in a wrap.

Leftover patties are also good crumbled on salad or served as taco meat. Alternatively you can mix the ingredients excluding the flax and heat through and serve in tortillas or on salads.

*Note: works great with many different bean combos—just use about 3 C of drained beans or lentils total.

PROTEIN POWERHOUSE VEGGIE BURGERS

(Adapted from *The High- Protein Vegetarian Cookbook*)

INGREDIENTS

4 C water

1 C dry lentils

½ C water water mixed with 3 tbsp flaxseed meal

2 cans black beans, rinsed, drained, patted dry (or 3 C cooked beans)

1 C cooked quinoa

½ C oats processed into flour (blend rolled oats in a blender until fine)

3 cloves garlic, minced

½ red onion, minced

1 red pepper finely chopped

½ C walnuts, chopped

1 tbsp ground cumin

½ tsp cayenne

1 tsp sriracha or hot sauce

1 tsp salt

½ tsp black pepper

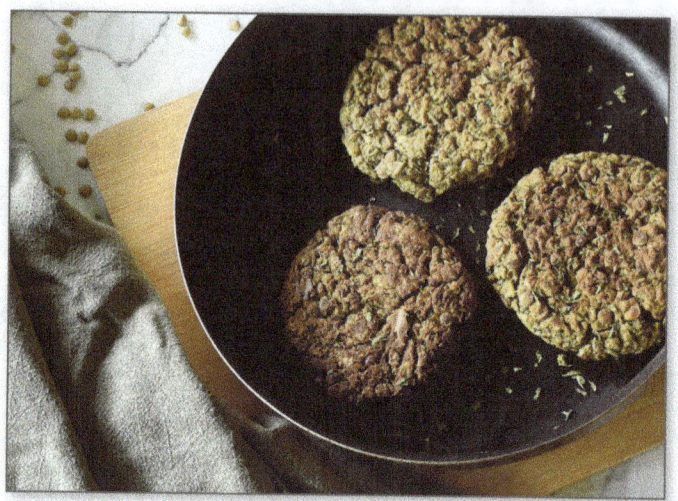

INSTRUCTIONS

1. Bring 4 C of water and 1 C of lentils to a boil in a saucepan, reduce heat and simmer for 20 minutes until lentils are tender. Drain water and pat dry with a paper towel.

2. Combine ground flax and warm water and let sit for 10 minutes to thicken.

3. Puree the lentils with 1 can of black beans (An immersion blender in a bowl works great for this or you can use a blender or your hands). Pour the puree into a large bowl with the remaining ingredients and adjust spices to your liking if necessary.

4. Refrigerate mixture 1 hour to make it easier to form patties.

5. Preheat oven to 375° F.

6. To form patties grab a handful of the mixture and form into a ball. It will be a bit sticky. Drop it onto a parchment-lined sheet and press down lightly with your fingers to flatten. Repeat to form about 11 patties. Bake for 12 minutes on one side and then flip and bake for 12 minutes on the other side.

7. Serve with hamburger toppings on a gluten free bun, or crumble and use in a wrap or as a salad topping.

TAMALE PIE

INGREDIENTS

Filling:

1 diced onion

1 bell pepper any color, diced

3 cloves garlic, minced

1 can beans—any kind, or 1½ C cooked

1 can drained corn, or 1½ C frozen

1 (15 oz) can diced tomatoes

1 (8 oz) can tomato sauce, or 1 C of salsa

2 tsp ground cumin

1 tbsp chili powder

¾ tsp salt

1 (4 oz) can mild green chilis (optional)

1 C shredded cheese (optional)

Topping:

¾ C cornmeal (regular or whole grain),

2 C water or broth (if using broth omit the salt)

¾ tsp salt

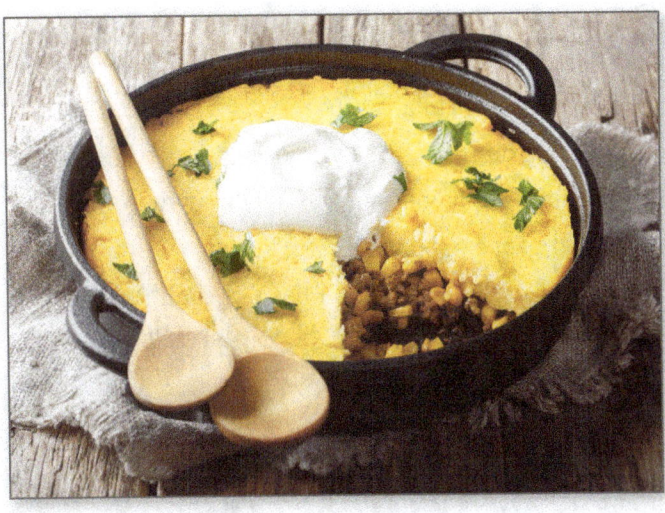

INSTRUCTIONS

1. In a large oven-safe skillet, saute onion, peppers, and garlic for a few minutes then add the remaining filling ingredients (excluding the cheese). Simmer for 15 minutes, uncovered, stirring as needed. Remove from heat and stir in the cheese. If not using an oven safe skillet then transfer the filling to a baking dish.

2. Preheat oven to 350° F.

3. Add topping ingredients to a saucepan and stir over medium-low heat until the mixture is thick. Using a large spoon, spoon the cooked topping over the filling and spread in an even layer.

4. Bake in the preheated oven for 30 minutes then let cool. It will thicken as it cools.

5. Serve with cheese, sour cream, cilantro, avocado, and tomatoes if desired.

VEGGIE BLACK BEAN ENCHILADAS

(Adapted from *Cookie and Kate*)

INGREDIENTS

2 C homemade enchilada sauce

2 tbsp olive oil

1 C chopped red onion (about 1 small red onion)

1 red bell pepper, chopped

1 bunch of broccoli or 1 small head of cauliflower (about 1 lb), florets removed and sliced into small, bite-sized pieces

1 tsp ground cumin

¼ tsp ground cinnamon

5 to 6 oz baby spinach (about 5 C, packed)

1 can (15 oz) black beans, drained and rinsed, or 1½ C cooked black beans

1 C shredded Monterey Jack cheese, divided

½ tsp salt, to taste

Freshly ground black pepper, to taste

8 Gluten-free tortillas

Handful of chopped cilantro, for garnishing

Homemade Enchilada Sauce:

3 tbsp olive oil

3 tbsp flour (whole wheat flour, all-purpose flour and gluten-free flour blends all work!)

1 tbsp ground chili powder (scale back if you're sensitive to spice or using particularly spicy chili powder)

1 tsp ground cumin

½ tsp garlic powder

¼ tsp dried oregano

¼ tsp salt, to taste

Pinch of cinnamon (optional but recommended)

2 tbsp tomato paste

2 C vegetable broth

1 tsp apple cider vinegar or distilled white vinegar

Freshly ground black pepper, to taste

1. Measure the dry ingredients (the flour, chili powder, cumin, garlic powder, oregano, salt and optional cinnamon) into a small bowl and place it near the stove. Place the tomato paste and broth near the stove as well.

2. In a medium-sized pot over medium heat, warm the oil until it's hot enough that a light sprinkle of the flour/spice mixture sizzles on contact. Be patient and don't step away from the stove!

3. Pour in the flour and spice mixture. While whisking constantly, cook until fragrant and slightly deepened in color, about 1 minute. Whisk the tomato paste into the mixture, then slowly pour in the broth while whisking constantly to remove any lumps.

4. Raise heat to medium-high and bring the mixture to a simmer, then reduce heat as necessary to maintain a gentle simmer. Cook, whisking often, for about 5 to 7 minutes, until the sauce has thickened a bit and a spoon encounters some resistance as you stir it. (The sauce will thicken some more as it cools.)

5. Remove from heat, then whisk in the vinegar and season to taste with a generous amount of freshly ground black pepper. Add more salt, if necessary.

INSTRUCTIONS

1. Preheat oven to 400° F with one rack in the middle of the oven and one in the upper third. Lightly grease a 9 by 13-inch pan with olive oil or cooking spray.

2. In a large skillet over medium heat, warm the olive oil until simmering. Add the onions and a pinch of salt. Cook, stirring often, until the onions are tender and translucent, about 5 to 7 minutes. Add the broccoli and bell pepper, stir, and reduce heat to medium-low. Cover the skillet. Cook, stirring occasionally, for about 8 to 9 minutes, or until the broccoli is brighter green and just starting to turn golden on the edges.

3. Add the cumin and cinnamon to the skillet and cook until fragrant, about 30 seconds. Add the spinach, a few handfuls at a time, stirring until it has reduced in size. Repeat with remaining spinach and cook until all of the spinach has wilted.

4. Transfer the contents of the pan to a medium mixing bowl. Add the drained beans, ¼ C cheese and a drizzle of enchilada sauce (about 2 tbsp). Season with ½ tsp salt and some freshly ground black pepper, to taste.

5. Assemble the enchiladas: Pour ¼ C enchilada sauce into your prepared pan and tilt it from side to side until the bottom of the pan is evenly coated. To assemble your first enchilada, spread ½ C filling mixture down the middle of a tortilla, then snugly wrap the left side over and then the right, to make a wrap. Place it seam side

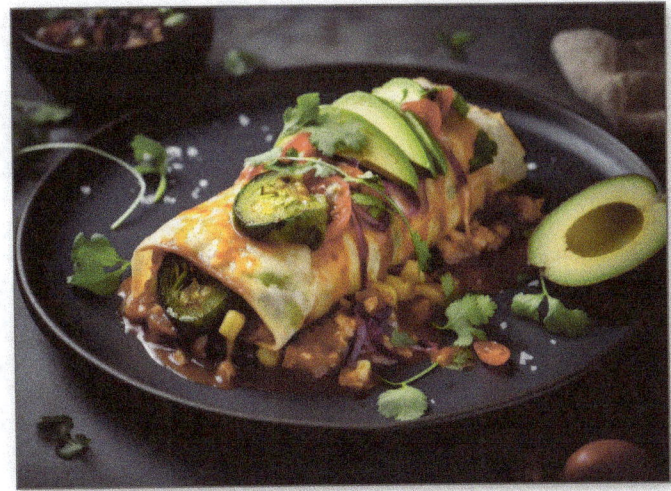

down against the edge of your pan. Repeat with remaining tortillas and filling.

6. Drizzle the remaining enchilada sauce evenly over the enchiladas, leaving the tips of the enchiladas bare. Sprinkle the remaining shredded cheese evenly over the enchiladas.

7. Bake, uncovered, on the middle rack for 20 minutes. If the cheese on top isn't golden enough for your liking, carefully transfer the enchiladas to the upper rack of the oven and bake for an additional 3 to 6 minutes, until sufficiently golden and bubbly.

8. Remove from oven and let the enchiladas rest for 10 minutes (they're super hot!). Before serving, sprinkle chopped cilantro down the center of the enchiladas. Serve immediately.

Cookie and Kate. (n.d.). Vegetarian Enchiladas Recipe. Retrieved May 18, 2023, from https://cookieandkate.com/vegetarian-enchiladas-recipe/

EASY LENTIL SHEPHERD'S PIE (VEGETARIAN)

(Adapted from *Spend With Pennies*)

INGREDIENTS

1 C brown lentils or green lentils

3-4 C vegetable broth or beef broth if not making vegetarian

2 tsp olive oil

½ C onion chopped

1 C chopped mushrooms about 4 oz

1 carrot chopped

1 rib celery chopped

½ C frozen peas defrosted

½ tbsp GF flour

2 tsp Worcestershire sauce (use vegetarian Worcestershire sauce if desired)

3 tbsp tomato paste

2 tbsp parsley chopped

salt & pepper to taste

2½ C mashed potatoes

INSTRUCTIONS

1. Preheat oven to 400° F.

2. Combine lentils and 3 C broth in a saucepan and bring to a boil. Reduce heat to a simmer and cover. Cook for 20-25 minutes or until lentils are tender.

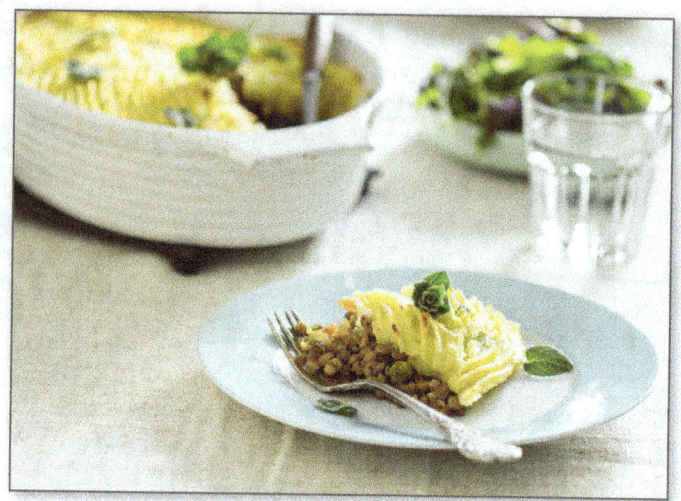

3. Meanwhile, cook onion, mushrooms, carrot, and celery in olive oil over medium heat until onion and carrot are softened. Stir in flour and cook 1 minute more.

4. Add lentils (and their broth), Worcestershire sauce, and tomato paste. Stir in peas and simmer uncovered for 10 minutes adding more broth as needed to create a sauce. Stir in parsley and season with salt & pepper to taste.

5. Spoon lentil mixture into a deep-dish pie plate. Top with mashed potatoes and bake 20-25 minutes or until potatoes are browned.

MAIN DISHES

TUSCAN WHITE BEAN SKILLET RECIPE

INGREDIENTS

2 tbsp olive oil, divided

8 oz brown mushrooms, sliced

1 large onion, diced

3 cloves garlic, minced

½ C drained and chopped oil-packed sun dried tomatoes

2 (14.5 oz) cans fire-roasted diced tomatoes (regular works if its all you have on hand)

3 C cooked Cannellini beans, or 2 cans rinsed and drained (can sub other type of white or kidney beans)

1 can quartered artichoke hearts, rinsed

½ tsp salt

½ tsp pepper

1 tsp oregano

½ tsp thyme

1 tsp sugar

Parsley for garnish

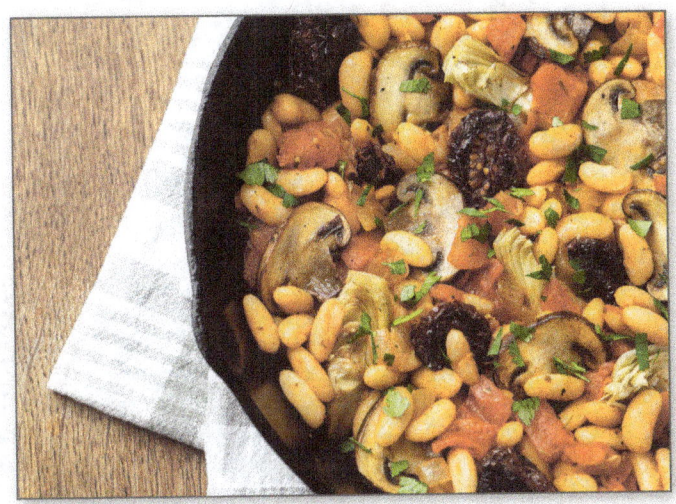

MAIN DISHES

INSTRUCTIONS

1. Heat a tbsp of oil in a large skillet over medium high heat. Add a single layer of mushrooms to the pan and brown 1-2 minutes on each side, cook in batches if needed and transfer to a bowl.

2. Add another tbsp of oil to the pan and saute the onions till they start to brown then add the garlic and sun dried tomatoes and saute another 2 minutes until fragrant and soft.

3. Add the tomatoes, beans, artichoke hearts, salt, pepper, oregano, thyme and sugar. Reduce the heat to medium, cover and cook for 10 minutes. Next add the mushrooms back to the pan and continue to cook until heated through.

4. Garnish with chopped parsley and serve over cooked grain, gluten free noodles, gluten free flatbread, or winter squash.

CHILI SKILLET

INGREDIENTS

1 tbsp oil

1 medium onion, minced

1 green pepper, chopped

2 cloves garlic, minced

1 lb ground beef

4 tsp chili powder

1 C tomato juice

1 can kidney beans undrained, or 1½ cooked beans
   and extra ½ C water

1 tsp oregano

1 tsp salt

½ C uncooked quinoa, white rice or other quick cooking whole grain like buckwheat

1 C frozen corn

1 small can (2.25 oz) chopped black olives, drained

1 C shredded cheese if not dairy free

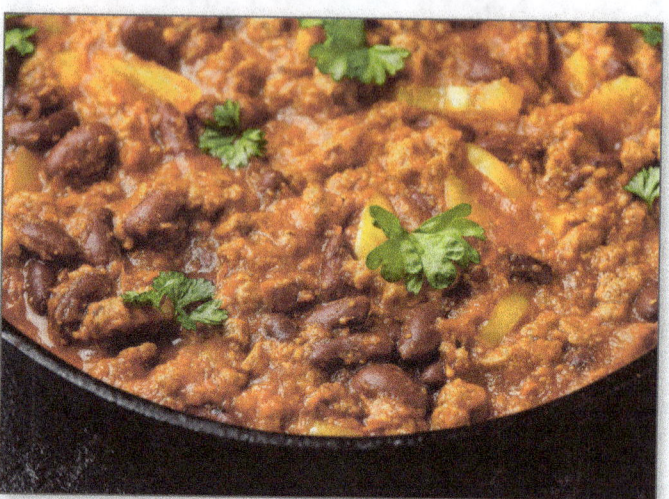

INSTRUCTIONS

1. In a large skillet or dutch oven, heat oil over medium heat and briefly saute onion, green pepper and garlic. Push to one side.

2. Add ground beef and saute until no longer pink. Stir in chili powder and cook 30 seconds.

3. Add tomato sauce, undrained kidney beans, oregano, salt and quinoa (or rice). Stir and bring to a boil. Cover pot and simmer for 25 minutes.

4. Stir in corn and olives. Cover and cook for 5 minutes. Sprinkle cheese on top and cover long enough to melt.

QUINOA PIZZA BITES

(From *USU Extension*)

INGREDIENTS

2 C cooked quinoa

2 Large Eggs

½ C Chopped Onion

1 C Shredded Mozzarella Cheese

2 tsp Minced Garlic

2 tsp Dried Basil

1 C Chopped Pepperoni Slices

½ tsp Salt

½ tsp Paprika

1 tsp Dried Crushed Oregano

Pizza Sauce (for dipping)

INSTRUCTIONS

Preheat the oven to 350° F. Mix all ingredients except the pizza sauce in a medium mixing bowl. Distribute the mixture in a greased mini muffin tin (or use a cookie scoop to form the bites on a cookie sheet) filling each cup to the top and gently pressing to compact. Bake the bites for 15-20 minutes.

Utah State University Extension. (n.d.). Recipes. Retrieved May 22, 2023, from https://extension.usu.edu/nutrition/recipes/index

PUMPKIN ROLL

(From USU Extension)

INGREDIENTS

Roll

¾ C GF 1-to-1 Baking Flour (containing xanthan gum)

¾ C Sugar

¾ tsp Salt

1 tsp Baking Soda

¾ tsp Cinnamon

3 eggs

⅔ C Canned Pumpkin

Powdered Sugar for Rolling

Filling

8 oz Cream Cheese (room temp.)

1 tbsp Butter, Melted

1 tsp Vanilla

1 C Powdered Sugar

INSTRUCTIONS

1. Preheat the oven to 350° F. Grease a 15 X 10" jelly roll pan. Cut parchment paper to fit the bottom of the pan leaving an inch overhanging on each short side. Lightly grease the parchment paper and sides of the jelly roll pan.

2. In a medium mixing bowl, combine the GF flour, sugar, salt, baking soda, and cinnamon whisking to combine. Add the eggs and canned pumpkin mixing until smooth.

3. Pour the mixture over the parchment paper and spread until even using a spatula. Bake for 16-18 minutes,

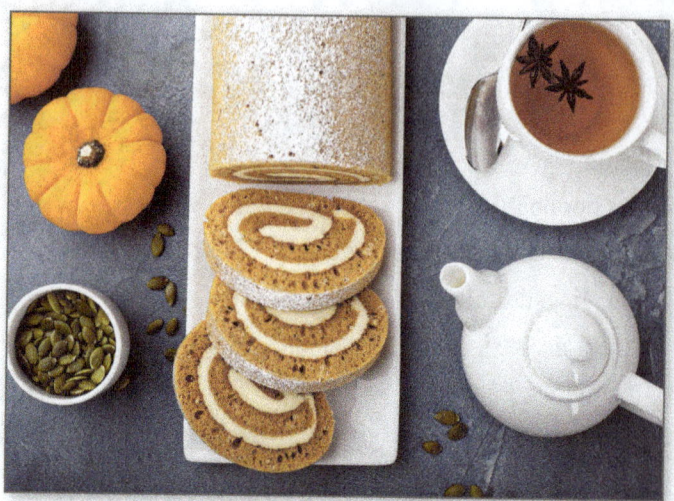

when the edges pull away from the sides of the pan and the center is done.

4. Lay a large tea towel on the countertop and dust with a thick layer of powdered sugar all over the towel. When the cake comes out of the oven, turn the pan upside down on the sugar laden towel so the parchment paper is on top. Carefully peel the parchment paper off. Starting at the long end, roll the pumpkin cake up with the towel to cool.

5. While the roll cools, make the filling. Using a hand or stand mixer whip the cream cheese, butter, vanilla, and powdered sugar together until light and creamy. When the roll is cool, unroll and carefully spread an even layer of the filling across the cake. Roll the cake up without the towel, tightly wrap in plastic and refrigerate for an hour before serving. The roll will be good in the refrigerator for up to 2 days.

HOMEMADE RANCH DRESSING (GF, DF)

(From *USU Extension*)

INGREDIENTS

1 C Mayonnaise

2-4 tbsp Almond Milk

2 tsp Red Wine Vinegar

2 tsp Dried Dill

2 tsp Onion Powder

½ tsp Dried Thyme

½ tsp Garlic Powder

½ tsp Salt

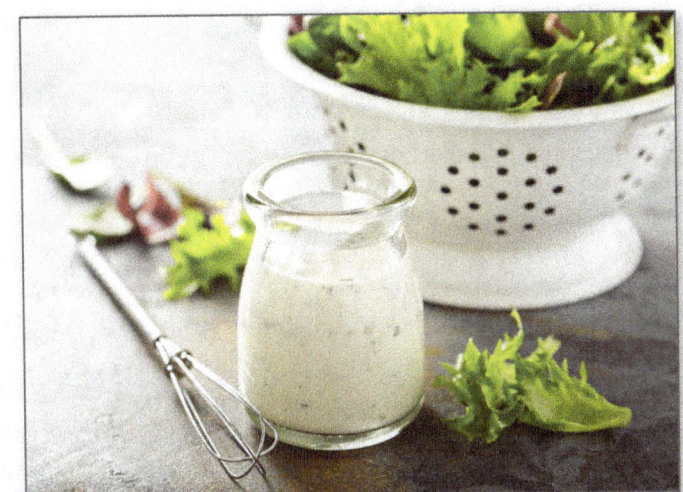

INSTRUCTIONS

Combine all ingredients and mix well. Use almond milk to obtain the desired thickness.

POPPED SORGHUM

(From *Bob's Red Mill*)

INGREDIENTS

¼ C Sorghum Grain

Toppings and Spices as desired

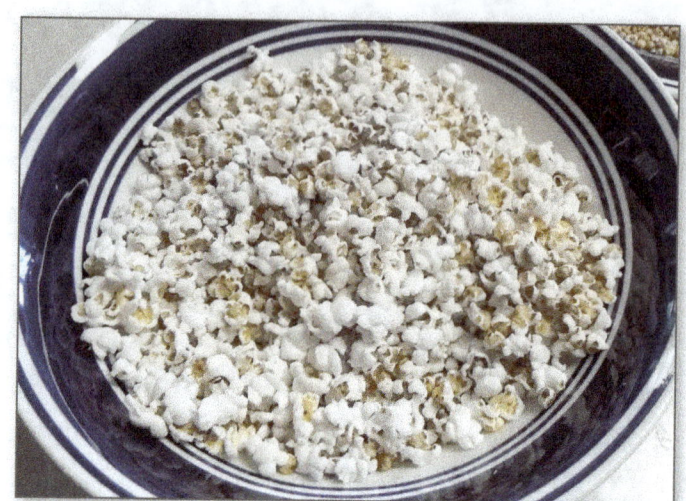

INSTRUCTIONS

Stovetop:

1. Heat a pot with a tight-fitting lid over medium heat. When the pan is hot, add the sorghum grains and cover with a lid. Cook, shaking pot often without removing the lid until the sorghum grains begin to pop. Once the popping begins, shake the pot continuously with the lid in place.

2. When ⅔ of the grains have popped, remove from heat and pour out the popped grains; return unpopped grains to heat and continue as above until most grains have popped. Remove from heat when there is more than 10 seconds between pops. Season with toppings as desired.

Microwave:

1. Place sorghum grains in a clean small brown paper bag. Fold top down to close and place folded side down in the microwave. Heat on high for about 2 minutes (varies depending on microwave's strength).

2. After 2 minutes, remove the bag from the microwave and pour off the popped grains. Return unpopped grains to the microwave and continue popping in 30 second intervals. Remove from the microwave when there is more than 5 seconds between pops. Season with toppings as desired.

Bob's Red Mill. (n.d.). How to Make Popped Sorghum. Retrieved May 18, 2023, from https://www.bobsredmill.com/recipes/how-to-make/popped-sorghum/

DESSERTS & SNACKS

POPPED SORGHUM PEANUT BUTTER BALLS

(From *Sorghum Checkoff*)

INGREDIENTS

½ C whole grain sorghum

½ tsp cinnamon

1 tbsp peanut flour

¾ C fresh ground peanut butter

½ C mini chocolate chips

½ C chopped salted peanuts

2 oz 70% dark chocolate

1 tbsp coconut oil

INSTRUCTIONS

1. Pop sorghum using the microwave or stovetop (see pg 234). When the sorghum has popped, pour onto a parchment lined baking sheet to cool.

2. In a bowl add the cinnamon, peanut butter, chocolate chips and peanuts and mix together. Add the sorghum to this mixture a little at a time and stir until well combined.

3. Cover the bowl and place it in the freezer for 10-15 minutes until the batter is not sticky and on the firm side.

4. While the popped sorghum mixture is in the freezer place water in the bottom of a double boiler over medium heat. Place the coconut oil and dark chocolate on the top of the double boiler, stirring occasionally until melted and remove the pan from the heat.

5. Remove the popped sorghum mixture from the freezer and use a 2 tbsp scooper to scoop the mixture on the parchment lined baking sheet. Alternatively, you can form the popped sorghum balls with your hands. Spraying your hands with cooking oil can help with the stickiness.

6. Transfer the melted chocolate to a zip-top sandwich bag, squeezing the chocolate down towards one of the bottom corners and snip the corner. Drizzle chocolate over each Popped Sorghum Peanut Butter Ball.

7. Refrigerate for a minimum of 15 minutes so the chocolate sets before serving. They can be stored in an airtight container in the refrigerator for several days or in the freezer for a few weeks.

Sorghum Checkoff. (n.d.). Popped Sorghum Peanut Butter Balls. Retrieved May 18, 2023, from https://www.sorghumcheckoff.com/recipes/popped-sorghum-peanut-butter-balls/

DESSERTS & SNACKS

POPPED SORGHUM SNACK BALLS

(From *My Quiet Kitchen*)

INGREDIENTS

¼ C Sorghum Grain

1 C Rolled Oats

¼ C Brown Rice Syrup (Or Corn Syrup)

2 tbsp Maple Syrup

¼ C Tahini

½ tsp Salt

3-4 tbsp Sesame Seeds

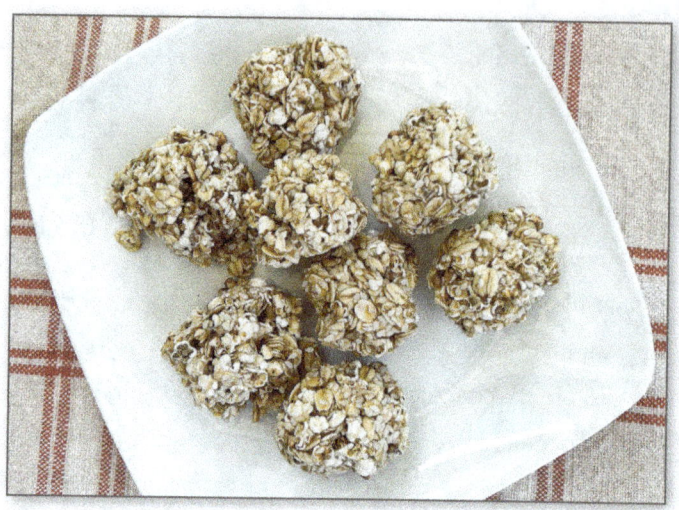

INSTRUCTIONS

1. Pop Sorghum (see pg 234).

2. In a large bowl combine the popped sorghum and rolled oats.

3. In a small bowl combine the tahini, brown rice syrup, maple syrup, and salt. Warm slightly in the microwave (about 15 seconds). Alternatively, these three ingredients can be warmed in a small pot on the stove.

4. Pour tahini mixture onto the oats and sorghum, stirring to combine. Add the sesame seeds and continue to stir until everything is well incorporated.

5. Barely wet your palms (to prevent sticking). Scoop about 1½ tbsp of the mixture into one hand and squeeze tightly; roll the mixture in your hands to form a smooth ball.

My Quiet Kitchen. (2021, May 10). Popped Sorghum Balls. Retrieved May 18, 2023, from https://myquietkitchen.com/popped-sorghum-balls/

GRAHAM CRACKERS

INGREDIENTS

½ C Melted Butter

3 tbsp Honey or Molasses

¼ C Brown Sugar

1 tsp Baking Powder

1½ C Jaylee's 100% Whole Grain Flour (pg 248-249)

3 tbsp Water

1 tsp Vanilla

½ tsp Salt

1½ tsp Cinnamon

½ tsp Baking Soda

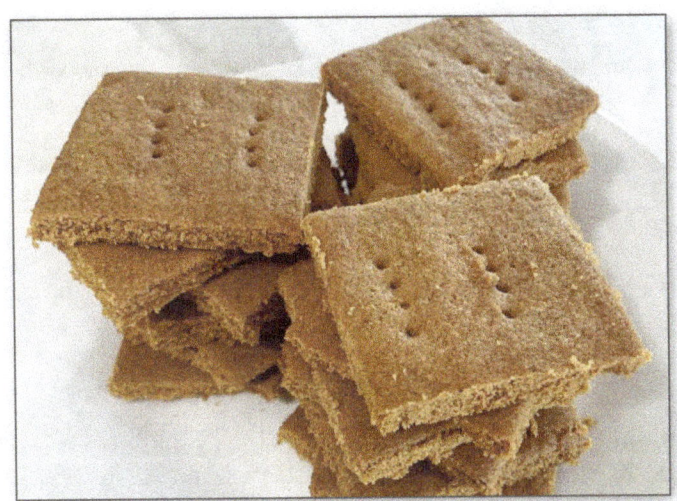

INSTRUCTIONS

Mix all ingredients until well combined. Place dough between two sheets of parchment paper the size of a large baking pan. Roll dough to edges of the paper. Remove top sheet and place on pan. Score with a pizza cutter and prick with a fork in the desired pattern. Bake at 325° F for 15-17 minutes. Cool sheet on a rack.

CRISPY CHICKPEAS

INGREDIENTS

2 cans chickpeas, drained and rinsed (or 3 C cooked)

2 tbsp olive oil

½ tsp salt (1 tsp is using cooked beans with no salt)

2 tsp spices or fresh herbs*

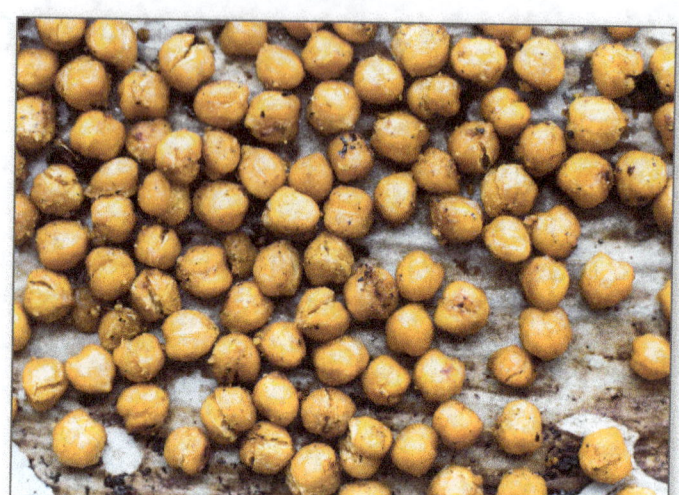

INSTRUCTIONS

1. Preheat the oven to 375° F.

2. Drain and rinse the chickpeas then pat dry with a paper towel and allow to air dry for a couple minutes.

3. In a medium bowl, toss the chickpeas with the salt and olive oil and whatever other spices you are using and then spread out on a baking sheet. Use parchment paper to make clean up easy.

4. Roast the chickpeas for 25-30 minutes for chickpeas that are crispy on the outside but still soft in the middle or 45-60 minutes for chickpeas that are crispier. Stir or shake the pan every 10-15 minutes so it roasts evenly.

5. These are a great garnish for hummus, adding to a salad, wrap or grain bowl, or just for eating as a snack.

Variations: feel free to experiment with your own combinations

- Spicy: ½ tsp each chili powder, pepper, cumin, and smoked paprika
- Rosemary garlic: 1 tsp garlic powder and 1½ tsp freshly chopped rosemary
- Cinnamon sugar: 1 tbsp sugar, 1 tsp cinnamon, reduce salt to ¼ tsp
- Curry: 1½ tsp curry powder, ¼ tsp pepper
- Italian: 2 tsp Italian seasoning
- Barbeque: 2 tsp maple syrup, ½ tsp smoked paprika, ½ tsp chili powder, ½ tsp garlic powder, ¼ tsp pepper

SIMPLE HUMMUS

INGREDIENTS

1 can garbanzo beans, drain and reserve liquid (1½ C cooked beans)

2 tbsp olive oil

2 tbsp tahini (can omit if you don't have it on hand or substitute with 2 tbsp of sesame seeds—just puree longer)

½ tsp salt

Juice from 1 medium lemon (about 2 tbsp)

1 clove garlic, chopped

¼ tsp cumin

2-4 tbsp water (or reserved liquid from beans)

Olive oil for serving

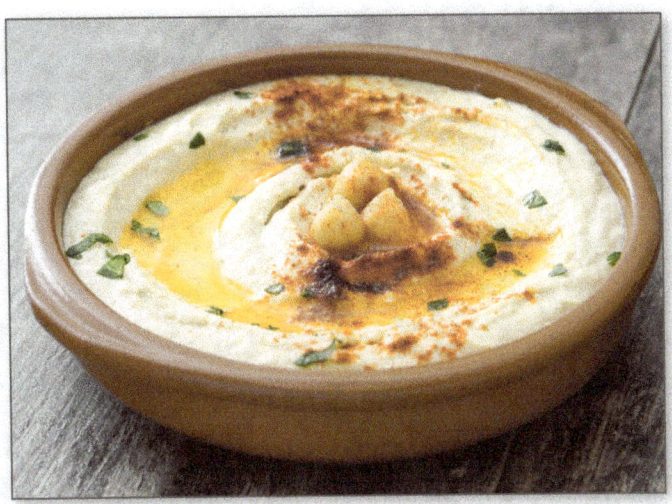

INSTRUCTIONS

Add all the ingredients to a food processor except the extra water and oil. Puree until smooth adding water(or reserved liquid) as needed. Tastes best if made ahead of time and flavors have time to blend. Drizzle with extra olive oil when serving if desired.

Variations:

- Smoky and Spicy—Add ¼ tsp crushed red pepper and ⅛ tsp smoked paprika.

- Roasted red pepper—add ¾ C jarred roasted red pepper and a shake of cayenne pepper. Reduce added water.

- Roasted garlic—roast a head of garlic and add all the roasted cloves to the hummus. To roast garlic- preheat the oven to 400° F. Remove the excess papery peels from a head of garlic and cut off the top part of the head to expose all the cloves. Place the head on a piece of foil large enough to wrap the head, and then drizzle with 1 tbsp of olive oil. Wrap the garlic up in the foil and roast in the oven for 35 minutes.

- Cilantro lime—use lime juice in place of lemon juice and add 1 C loose cilantro leaves and a few grates of lime zest.

- Black bean—use black beans instead of garbanzo beans and add ¼ tsp smoked paprika and ¼ tsp cayenne.

ZUCCHINI CAKE

INGREDIENTS

1½ cup sugar

¾ cup oil

2 Eggs

2 cups grated zucchini

2 teaspoons vanilla

2 ½ C Flour

¼ C Cocoa

½ tsp. Salt

1 tsp. Baking Soda

¾ tsp. Xanthan Gum (omit if flour blend contains)

½ C Buttermilk

Optional—1½ c chocolate chips

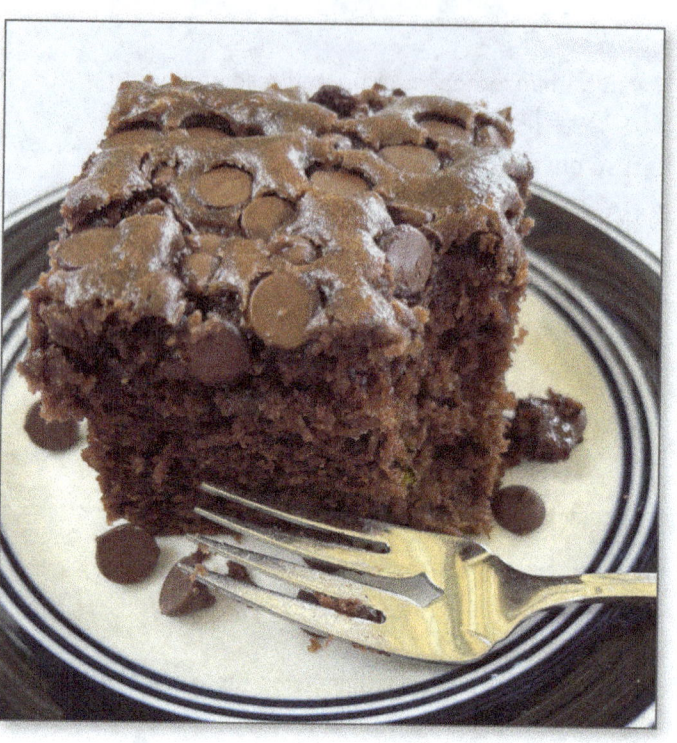

INSTRUCTIONS

In a large mixing bowl cream sugar and oil together well.
Add eggs and beat. Add zucchini. Mix dry ingredients
together then mix into the zucchini mixture . Add buttermilk and beat well. Pour into a sprayed or
greased 9x13 inch pan, sprinkle top with chocolate chips and bake at 325° F for 40-45 minutes.

Tips: If testing with a toothpick, avoid poking close to a chocolate chip. If cake edges look dry,
brush lightly with water immediately after removing from the oven.

APPLE CAKE

INGREDIENTS

1½ cups sugar

¾ cup oil

2 eggs

2 cups grated apple (no need to peel before grating)

2¾ cups flour

1 teaspoon salt

1 teaspoon baking soda

1½ teaspoon cinnamon

⅛ teaspoon ginger

¾ teaspoon xanthan gum (omit if flour blend
    contains)

½ cup buttermilk

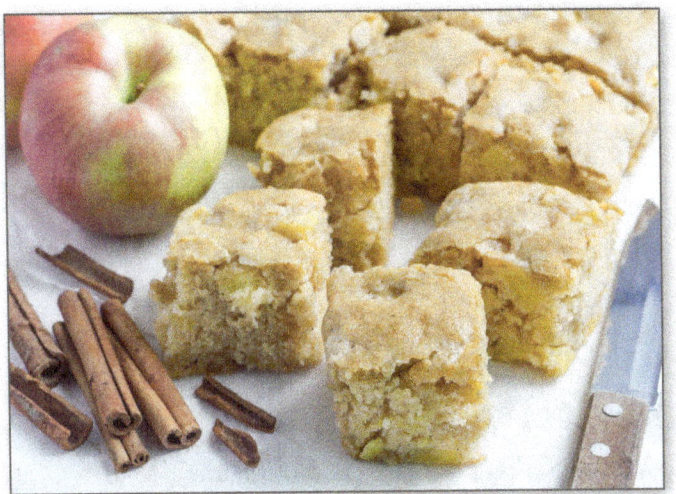

INSTRUCTIONS

In a large mixing bowl cream sugar and oil together well. Add eggs and beat. Add apple.
Mix dry ingredients together then stir into apple mixture. Add buttermilk and whip well.
Pour into a greased or sprayed 9x13 inch pan and bake at 325° F for 40-45 minutes.

   Note: This is the same base recipe as the Zucchini Cake on page 250 and is
adaptable to other fruits and vegetables. I have used pears and carrots with success.

NO-BAKE OATMEAL COOKIES

INGREDIENTS

½ C butter

½ C milk

2 C sugar

3 tbsp cocoa

3 C quick oats

½ C peanut butter

1 tsp vanilla extract

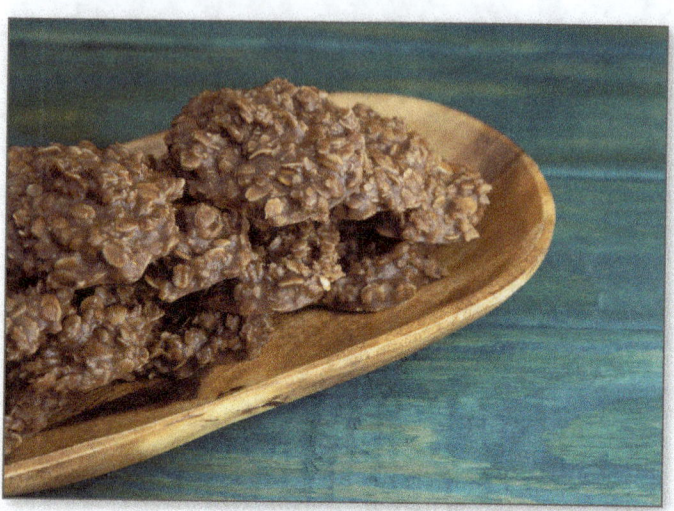

INSTRUCTIONS

Melt butter (or substitute) in a saucepan over medium heat, then add milk, sugar and cocoa. Bring the mixture to a steady boil, and boil steadily for 90-120 seconds. Remove from heat and stir in oats, peanut butter and vanilla extract. Allow mixture to cool a few minutes then scoop 2 tbsp portions onto a cookie sheet and cool until hardened.

BEST BROWNIES

INGREDIENTS

123 g Flour (1 C)

288 g Sugar (1½ C)

3 g Baking Powder (1 tsp)

5 g Salt (3/4 tsp)

38 g Cocoa (⅓ C)

3 g Xanthan (¾ tsp)—omit if flour blend contains xanthan

¼ C Butter or Oil

2 Eggs, Beaten

1 tsp Vanilla Extract

3 Tbsp—More may be needed depending on flour blend

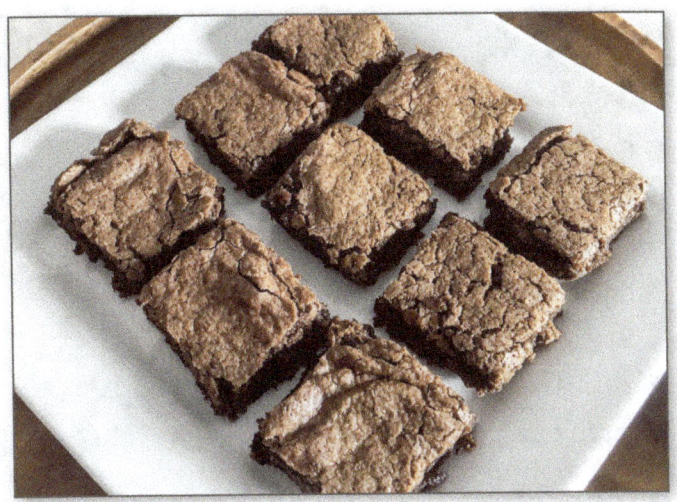

INSTRUCTIONS

Preheat the oven to 350° F. Grease an 8-inch square pan. Combine melted butter or oil, eggs, vanilla, and brownie mix. Beat until smooth. Extra beating produces a crispy top and gooey center. Pour into the prepared pan. Bake for 35-40 minutes, until a toothpick comes out clean. Cut into 2-inch bars when cool. Makes 16 brownies.

DESSERTS & SNACKS

CHOCOLATE MILLET PUDDING

(Adapted from *Grain Power: Over 100 Delicious Gluten-Free Ancient Grains & Superblend Recipes*)

INGREDIENTS

1¼ C water

½ C millet seeds

¼ C milk of choice

⅓ C white sugar

3 tbsp unsweetened cocoa powder

¼ tsp cinnamon

Pinch of salt

Whipped cream (optional)

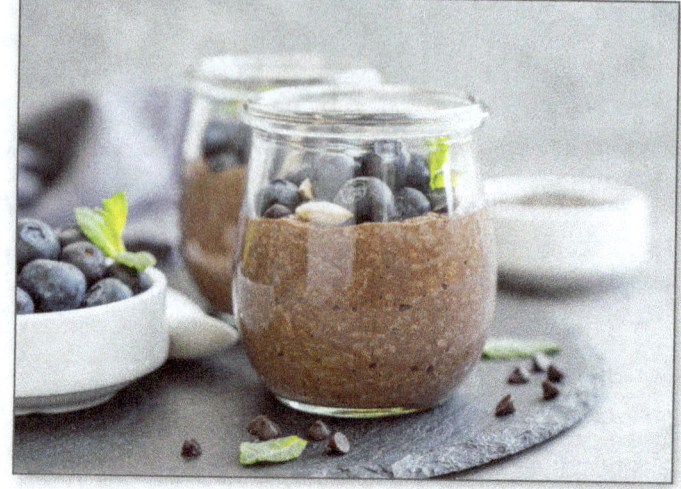

INSTRUCTIONS

Combine the water and millet in a medium saucepan. Bring to a boil then reduce to a simmer. Cover and simmer for 25 minutes until all water is absorbed. Remove the lid and fluff with a fork. Set aside and allow to cool.

Blend cooked millet, milk, sugar, cocoa, cinnamon and salt in a blender or food processor until smooth. Mixture should be very thick, but if it is not completely smooth or too thick add a little more milk. Scoop into four serving dishes and chill for 1 hour or overnight. Garnish with whipped cream just before serving.

Add 1-2 tbsp peanut butter when blending.

Mexican version: add a pinch of cayenne pepper when blending.

Top with fresh bananas, strawberries, or other fruit and whipped cream.

Sprinkle with coconut and slivered almonds.

Green, P., & Hemming, C. (2014). Grain Power: Over 100 Delicious Gluten-Free Ancient Grains & Superblend Recipes. Penguin Random House.

DESSERTS & SNACKS

BASIC FOOD STORAGE FLOUR

White Rice	1.0 Part	11.11%
Sorghum	4.0 Parts	44.44%
Teff	4.0 Parts	44.44%

Combine grains to be ground and mix. Grind on a fine setting to create the desired flour.

I developed this recipe with long term preparedness in mind. The thought was to include a minimal number of grains that tasted good, stored well, and had a good nutrient profile. That is why sorghum and teff are included. White rice is included because many people already have this in storage and it adds starch. I prefer the lighter texture of flours with added starch. With this in mind you could add sweet or sticky rice to add a larger percentage of starch or replace or partially replace all the white rice with a starch like tapioca.

You must add xanthan or other gum at the recipe level.

JAYLEE'S 100% WHOLE GRAIN FLOUR

This is a delicious and wonderfully nutritious gluten-free flour that is especially good in bread, muffins and pancakes. The whole grain flavor also pairs especially well with cinnamon, peanut, honey and banana.

BREADS

FLOUR BLEND

1 C (139g) Millet Flour

1⅓ C (199g) Brown Rice Flour

3½ C (432g) Sorghum Flour

2/3 C (106g) Teff Flour

¼ C (37g) Buckwheat Flour

⅛ C (15g) Quinoa Flour

1 tbsp (12g) Xanthan Gum* (omit if you prefer to add at the recipe level)

1 tbsp (12g) Psyllium Husk Powder* (omit if you prefer to add at the recipe level)

INSTRUCTIONS

Combine all flours and mix well until blended. Add xanthan and psyllium if desired. Store in an airtight container in a cool, dry place.

*For xanthan only flour, double the xanthan and omit the psyllium. Many recipes like cakes and cookies are better without psyllium.

*Psyllium is an excellent addition to breads and will increase rise and shelf life, however it can make other baked goods dry. Omit the psyllium and double xanthan or increase the liquid in your recipe to overcome this problem.

HOME MILLED 100% WHOLE GRAIN FLOUR

This is a delicious and wonderfully nutritious gluten-free flour that is especially good in bread, muffins and pancakes. The whole grain flavor also pairs well with cinnamon, peanut, honey, and banana.

GRAIN BLEND

1⅓ C (284g) Millet

2 C (398g) Brown Rice

4 C + 2 tbsp (785g) Sorghum

½ C + 3 tbsp (142g) Teff

¼ C + 1 tbsp (57g) Buckwheat

2 tbsp (28g) Quinoa

1 tbsp (12g) Xanthan Gum* (omit if you prefer to add at the recipe level)

1 tbsp (12g) Psyllium Husk Powder* (omit if you prefer to add at the recipe level)

INSTRUCTIONS

Combine the grains and mix until they are evenly distributed. **Caution: Do not add xanthan and psyllium before milling. This will damage your mill.** Add grains to the mill hopper and grind on the fine setting. Add xanthan and psyllium if desired. Store in an airtight container in a cool place.

*For xanthan only flour, double the xanthan and omit the psyllium. Many recipes especially cakes and cookies are better without psyllium.

*Psyllium is an excellent addition to breads and muffins and will increase rise and shelf life, however it can make other baked goods dry. Omit the psyllium and double the xanthan or increase the liquid in your recipe to overcome this problem.

Note: Grain/flour proportions are forgiving but gum levels are not. For this reason, we prefer to measure grains in cups and then add xanthan and psyllium at the recipe level. You can also weigh grains and use the weights included in the recipe.

JAYLEE'S ALL-PURPOSE, WHOLE GRAIN FLOUR

This flour is a delicious compromise between the tasty nutrition of a 100% whole grain flour and the fluffy texture of starchy flours.

BREADS

FLOUR BLEND

1 C (139g) Millet Flour

1⅓ C (199g) Brown Rice Flour

3½ C (432g) Sorghum Flour

⅔ C (106g) Teff Flour

¼ C (37g) Buckwheat Flour

⅛ C (15g) Quinoa Flour

1¾ C (221g) Tapioca Starch

2½ tsp (10g) Xanthan Gum* (omit if you prefer to add at recipe level)

2½ tsp (10g) Psyllium Husk Powder* (omit if you prefer to add at recipe level)

INSTRUCTIONS

Combine all flours and starch and mix well until blended. Add xanthan and psyllium if desired. Store in an airtight container in a cool, dry place.

*For xanthan only flour, double the xanthan and omit the psyllium. Many recipes like cakes and cookies are better without psyllium.

*Psyllium is an excellent addition to breads and muffins and will increase rise and shelf life, however it can make other baked goods dry. Omit the psyllium and double the xanthan or increase the liquid in your recipe to overcome this problem.

HOME MILLED ALL-PURPOSE FLOUR

This flour is a delicious compromise between the tasty nutrition of a 100% whole grain flour and the fluffy texture of starchy flours.

GRAIN BLEND

½ C + 2 Tbsp (139g) Millet

1 C (199g) Brown Rice

2⅔ C (432g) Sorghum

½ C (106g) Teff

¼ C (37g) Buckwheat

⅛ C (15g) Quinoa

1¾ C (221g) Tapioca Starch

2⅔ tsp (10g) Xanthan Gum* (omit if you prefer adding at the recipe level)

2⅔ tsp (10g) Psyllium Husk Powder*(omit if you prefer adding at the recipe level)

INSTRUCTIONS

Combine grains and mix until the grains are evenly distributed. **Caution: Do not add tapioca, xanthan and psyllium before milling. This will damage your mill.** Add grains to mill hopper and grind on the fine setting. Mix the flour with the tapioca starch and add xanthan and psyllium if desired. Store in an airtight container in a cool place.

*For xanthan only flour, double the xanthan and omit the psyllium. Many recipes especially cakes and cookies are better without psyllium.

*Psyllium is an excellent addition to breads and will increase rise and shelf life, however it can make other baked goods dry. Omit the psyllium and double xanthan or increase the liquid in your recipe to overcome this problem.

Note: Grain/flour proportions are forgiving but gum levels are not. For this reason, we prefer to measure grains in cups and then add xanthan and psyllium at the recipe level. You can also weigh grains and use the weights included in the recipe.

TREE STREET GRAINS BREAD

BREADS

This is an easy and delicious recipe for 100% whole grain breads. It was developed by the former owner of Tree Street Grains, Dave Cobia, for use with his 9 grain flour blend which is now available through Vivian's Live Again or use Jaylee's 100% whole grain flour.

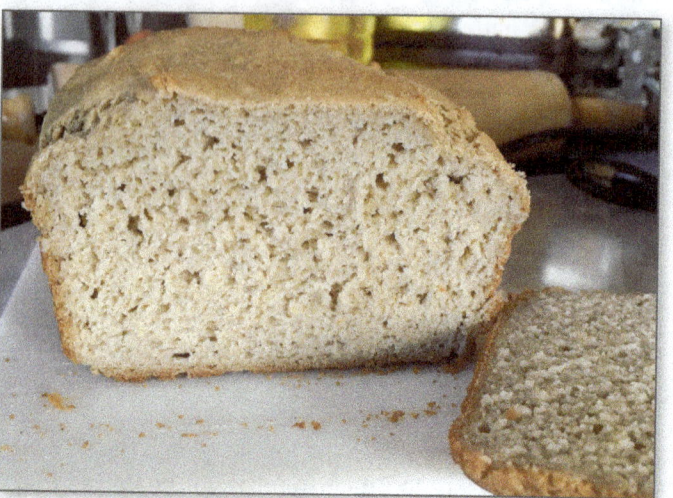

INGREDIENTS

1½ C Warm Milk*

2 Eggs

¼ C Sugar

¾ tsp Salt

2½ C Jaylee's 100% Whole Grain Gluten Free Flour (pg. 246)

1½ tbsp Dry Active Yeast

1¼ tsp Xanthan Gum (Omit xanthan and psyllium if already found in the chosen flour blend)

1¼ tsp Psyllium Husk

INSTRUCTIONS

Combine all ingredients and mix on medium speed for 6 minutes. Pour/spoon into a greased 9"x5" loaf pan. Smooth the top of the bread dough and allow to rise about ½" from the top of the pan. Do not let dough rise to the top of the pan prior to baking. Bake at 325° F for about 50 minutes.

*Milk can be replaced with water or non-dairy milk.

*Powdered milk may also be blended with the flour and liquid replaced with warm water. Use ¼ C milk powder for each cup of liquid or ¼ C plus 2 tbsp milk powder in this recipe.

NO-FAIL BREAD

COMBINE THE FOLLOWING DRY INGREDIENTS AND MIX WELL:

2¼ C GF Flour

2 tbsp Sugar

1 tbsp Yeast

2 tsp Baking Powder

¼ tsp Salt

1 tsp Xanthan Gum (omit if flour contains)

1 tsp Psyllium Husk

Add:

1¼ C Water

2 tbsp oil

2 eggs

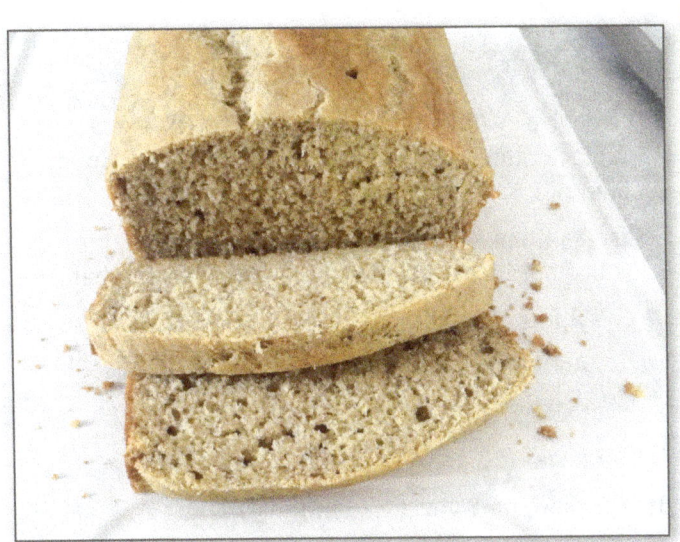

INSTRUCTIONS

Stir dry ingredients to combine. Then add wet ingredients and beat on high for 3-4 minutes. Place batter in a greased 8.5"x4.5" loaf pan (the Pyrex size). Allow to rise about 1/2 inch from the top of the pan. Do not let batter rise to the top of the pan before baking. Bake at 350° F for 55 minutes or until internal temperature reaches 200-205° F. Place a sheet of foil lightly on top of the loaf halfway through baking to prevent over browning. Remove from oven and allow to cool. Remove from pan and cut when completely cooled.

ARTISAN BREAD

(From *Gluten-Free Artisan Bread in Five Minutes a Day*)

INGREDIENTS

6½ C Jaylee's Whole Grain Flour (990 g) **OR** 1½ C Tapioca Starch and 5 C Jaylee's Whole Grain Flour Blend

3 tbsp Xanthan Gum - Omit xanthan and psyllium if your flour blend already contains those ingredients.

¼ C Psyllium Husk

1 tbsp Active Dry Yeast (10 g)

1 tbsp Salt (17 g)

2 tbsp Sugar (30 g) - Optional

3¾ C Lukewarm Water (100F) (850 g)

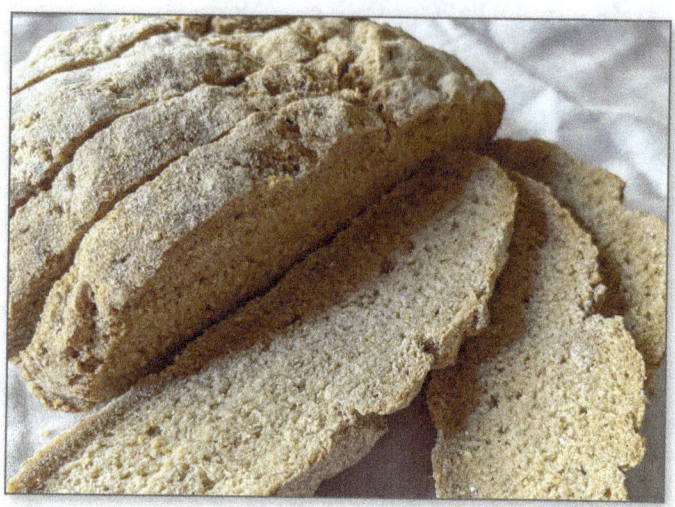

INSTRUCTIONS

Whisk together the flour, yeast, salt, and sugar (if using) in a 5-6 quart bowl or not airtight food container.

Add the water and mix with a spoon or a heavy-duty stand mixer and the paddle attachment. Mix slowly at first, then increase the speed to medium high and mix until very smooth for about 2 minutes if using a mixer. If hand-mixing, it will take longer.

Let the dough rise at room temperature for roughly 2 hours. Cover with a lid that fits the container, but leave it cracked. After this first 2 hour period, the dough can be refrigerated for 10 days or can be baked immediately.

To bake, pull off a 1-pound ball of dough. Use a pizza peel prepared by liberally sprinkling with cornmeal or by using parchment paper. Pat the dough into shape and use wet fingers to smooth. Allow the dough to rest for 60 minutes loosely covered in plastic wrap or in an overturned bowl.

Preheat a baking stone to 450° F for 20-30 minutes and place an empty metal broiler tray for holding water on a lower shelf in the oven.

Dust the top of the loaf with flour and slash a ½ inch deep decoration on the top of the loaf with a wet serrated knife.

Slide the loaf onto the preheated stone placing the peel a few inches beyond where you want the loaf to land. Carefully pull the peel from underneath the loaf and quickly but carefully pour 1 C hot water in the metal broiler tray and close the door to trap the steam. Bake for 45 minutes or until the crust is browned and firm to the touch. Allow the loaf to cool completely on a wire rack for best results.

This recipe will make 4 1-pound loaves.

Note: When ¼ tapioca starch/flour, ¾ Jaylee's Whole Grain Flour was used to make the above Artisan Bread, the resulting bread had a higher rise and better texture.

Hertzberg, J., & François, Z. (2014). Gluten-Free Artisan Bread in Five Minutes a Day. St. Martin's Press.

CHICKPEA WHITE BREAD

This recipe is a favorite for several reasons. It has a fabulous texture and enough structure to make rolls on a cookie sheet rather than muffin pans. It is also very nutritious with the chickpea flour which adds folate and is a great middle ground between whole grain and white bread.

INGREDIENTS

1½ C (152.5 g) Chickpea/Garbanzo Bean Flour

1 C (152.5 g) Teff Flour*

¼ C (29 g) Sorghum Flour

½ C (80 g) Tapioca Starch

2 tbsp (23 g) Sugar

1½ tsp (7 g) Salt

1½ tsp (7 g) Psyllium Husk Powder

1¼ tsp (5 g) Xanthan Gum

1½ tbsp (15 g) Yeast

¼ C (47 g) Oil

2 C (469 g) Water

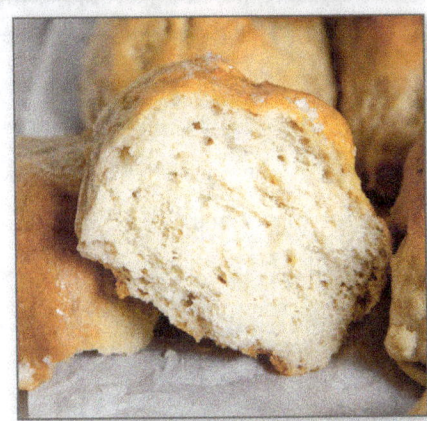

INSTRUCTIONS

Mix dry ingredients. Add wet ingredients and beat on high for 2-3 minutes. Dough should look smooth. Spoon into a greased 9x5 loaf pan and shape with wet fingers. Let dough to rise to ½ inch below the top of the pan. Preheat oven to 350° F and bake for 55-60 minutes or until internal temperature reaches 200-205° F. For a lighter crust lay a lightly greased foil on top of the loaf during baking.

For rolls: form dough with an ice cream scoop dipped in water or with wet fingers. Place on a greased cookie sheet. Allow to rise about 15 minutes and bake at 350° F for 20 minutes.

*Use ivory teff for a more white bread flavor. Brown teff has a more whole grain flavor.

OAT TORTILLAS

BREADS

INGREDIENTS

2 C rolled oats

1½ C water (might need an extra ½ C)

½ tsp salt

Cooking spray

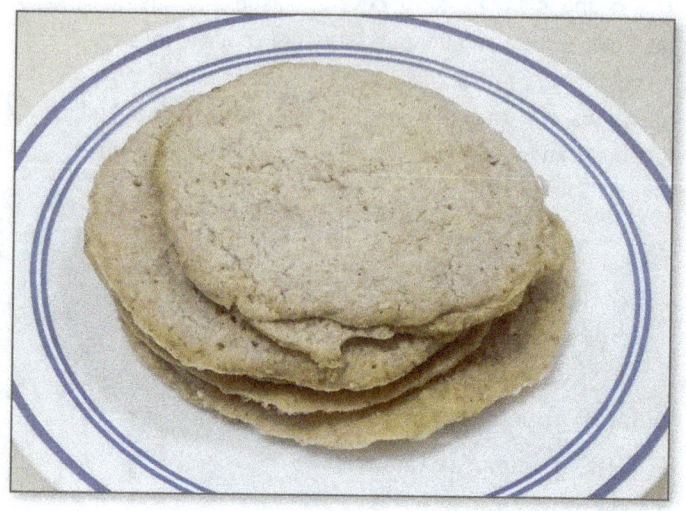

INSTRUCTIONS

1. Add all the ingredients to the jar of a blender and let soak for about 5 minutes.

2. Blend the mixture until smooth- it should be a little bit runnier than pancake batter. Add extra water if needed.

3. Preheat a non-stick skillet over medium low heat and coat with cooking spray.

4. Pour ¼ C of batter into the heated skillet and spread it around into a thin layer with the back of a spoon or measuring cup if needed.

5. Cook until the wrap is bubbly on top then flip and cook for another couple minutes.

6. Repeat steps 4 and 5 until you've used all the mix. Be sure to spray the pan each time before adding more batter.

7. Use in place of tortillas or as a wrap.

LENTIL FLATBREAD

INGREDIENTS

1 C split red lentils

2 C water

½ tsp salt

Cooking spray

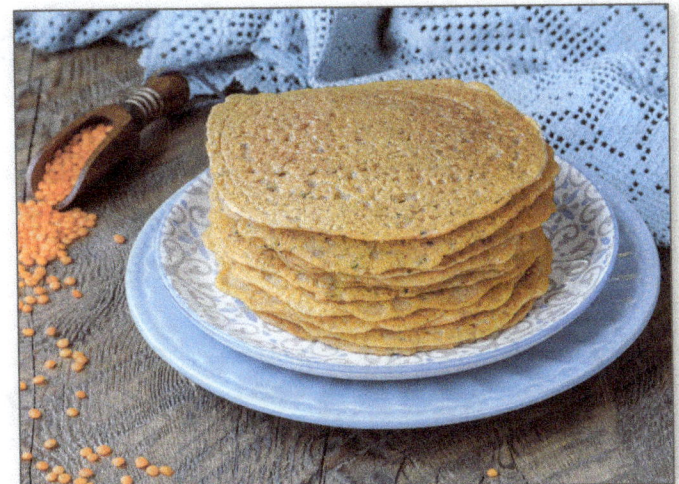

INSTRUCTIONS

1. Rinse the lentils in a strainer under running water then put in the blender with 2 C fresh water and allow the lentils to soak for at least 15 minutes (or overnight).

2. Blend the lentils and water for about a minute until the mixture is smooth and let rest for 15 minutes. Add the salt and mix again.

3. Preheat a non-stick skillet over medium low heat and coat with cooking spray.

4. Pour ¼ C of batter into the heated skillet and spread it around into a thin layer with the back of a spoon or measuring cup.

5. Cook 2-3 minutes on each side and then cool on a rack.

6. Repeat steps 4 and 5 until you've used all the mix and be sure to spray the pan each time before adding more batter.

7. Use in place of tortillas or as a wrap.

Feel free to add extra seasonings (1-2 tsp) to the batter after blending such as garlic powder, onion powder, curry powder, Italian seasoning, cinnamon and raisins, etc.

This recipe also works with regular brown lentils—just soak them for at least a couple of hours.

If your wrap seems gooey try reducing the heat and cooking it longer and also be sure not to skip spreading the batter into a thin layer after adding it to the pan.

The mixture will stick to pans pretty easily so a non-stick pan and cooking spray are essential. A good seasoned cast iron skillet with cooking spray works as well.

SOUP OR SAUCE (SOS) MIX
A REPLACEMENT FOR CANNED CREAM SOUPS

(From *USU Extension*)

INGREDIENTS

2 C Powdered Non-fat Dry Milk

¾ C Cornstarch

¼ C Instant Chicken Bouillon (Regular or Low Sodium)

1-2 tbsp Dried Onion Flake

1-2 tsp Italian Seasoning (Optional)

INSTRUCTIONS

The above recipe is equal to 9 cans (10.5 oz) of cream soup. Combine all ingredients in a resealable plastic bag and mix well. Store in a closed plastic bag or an air-tight container until use. This mix does not need to be refrigerated.

For 1 can of cream soup:

Combine ⅓ C mix and 1 ¼ C cold water. Whisk until blended. Cook and stir on a stove top or in the microwave until thickened. Add the thickened mixture to casseroles as you would a can of soup.

Utah State University Extension. (n.d.). Recipes. Retrieved May 22, 2023, from https://extension.usu.edu/nutrition/recipes/index

MIXES

ALFREDO SAUCE

(From *USU Extension*)

INGREDIENTS

⅓ C SOS Mix

1¼ C Cold Water

¼ C Parmesan Cheese

½ C Sour Cream

⅛ tsp Black Pepper

¼ tsp Garlic Powder

INSTRUCTIONS

In a small bowl, combine all ingredients, mix well and cook until thick. Serve the sauce over cooked gluten-free noodles or on pizza.

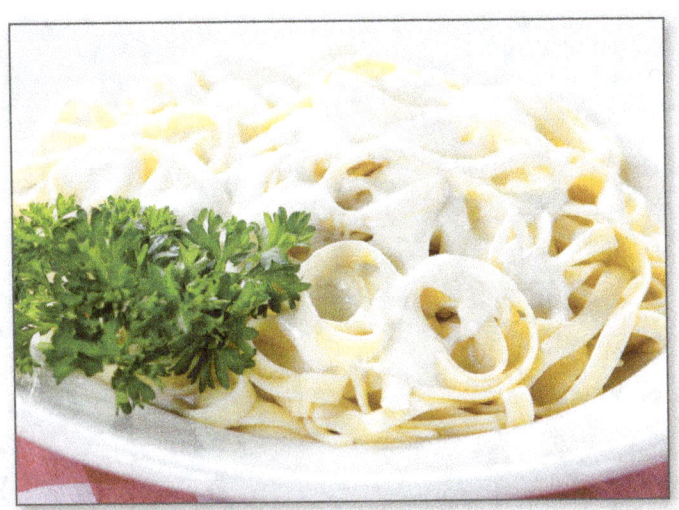

CHICKEN ENCHILADA CASSEROLE

(From *USU Extension*)

INGREDIENTS

1 pkg Corn Tortillas

1 lb Cooked, Diced, or Shredded Chicken

1 tbsp Vegetable Oil

1 Onion, Chopped

1 Can Green Chilies, Chopped

1 C SOS Mix

4 C Water

¾ C Shredded Cheddar Cheese

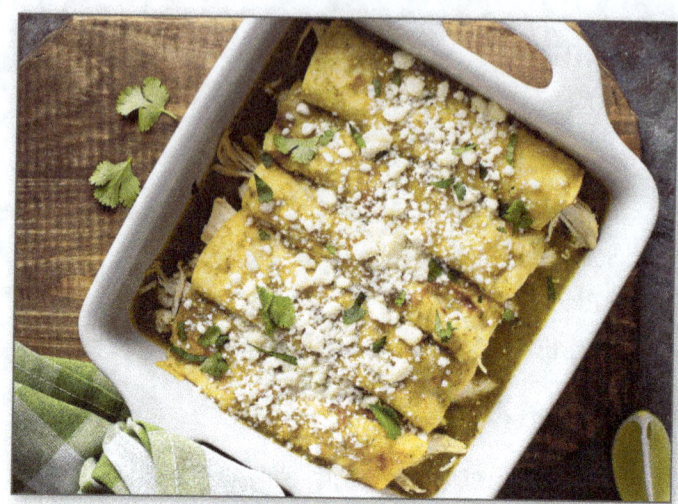

INSTRUCTIONS

Make the sauce by combining the dry sauce mix and water. Cook and stir on the stovetop or microwave until thickened. Sauté the onion and green chilies in the oil; add sauce and simmer for 15 minutes.

Cut tortillas in quarters and use them to line the bottom of the casserole dish. (Spray the dish with non-stick spray prior to putting in ingredients). Spread the sauce over the tortillas. Add a layer of chicken, a layer of sauce, and sprinkle with cheese. Repeat. Bake at 350° F for 20 minutes. Additional tortillas may be heated and served with the casserole. If crisp tortillas are preferred, allow the sauce to chill before using.

BROWNIE MIX

(Adapted from *Make-A-Mix: 306 recipes to save time and money*)

INGREDIENTS

492 g Flour (4 C)

1152 g Sugar (5¾ C)

20 g Salt (1 tbsp)

12 g (1 tbsp + 1 tsp) Baking Powder

152 g (⅓ C) Cocoa

12 g Xanthan (1 tbsp)—Omit if flour blend contains xanthan

INSTRUCTIONS

Combine all ingredients in a large bowl and stir with a wire whisk until evenly distributed. Store in an air-tight container. Makes about 10 cups Brownie Mix or 4 batches. Use within 10-12 weeks.

Note: This recipe is very good with Jaylee's Blend flour or 100% Whole Grain Flour. When made with white gf flour these were slightly fluffier. Most commercial all-purpose type gluten-free flours have a higher percentage of xanthan than we wrote this recipe for. If you eat the white flour brownies warm you may detect a slight gumminess.

Eliason, K., Harvard, A., & Westover, B. (1993). Make-A-Mix: 306 recipes to save time and money. ISBN 1-55561-073-0.

EASY BROWNIES

(Adapted from *Make-A-Mix* cookbook)

INGREDIENTS

460 g (2¼ C) Brownie Mix

¼ C Butter or Oil

2 Eggs, Beaten

1 tsp Vanilla Extract

3 tbsp Water—More may be needed depending on flour blend

INSTRUCTIONS

Preheat the oven to 350° F. Grease an 8-inch square pan. Combine melted butter or oil, eggs, vanilla, water, and brownie mix. Beat until smooth. Extra beating produces a crispy top and gooey center. Pour into the prepared pan. Bake for 30-35 minutes, until a toothpick comes out clean. Cut into 2-inch bars when cool. Makes 16 brownies.

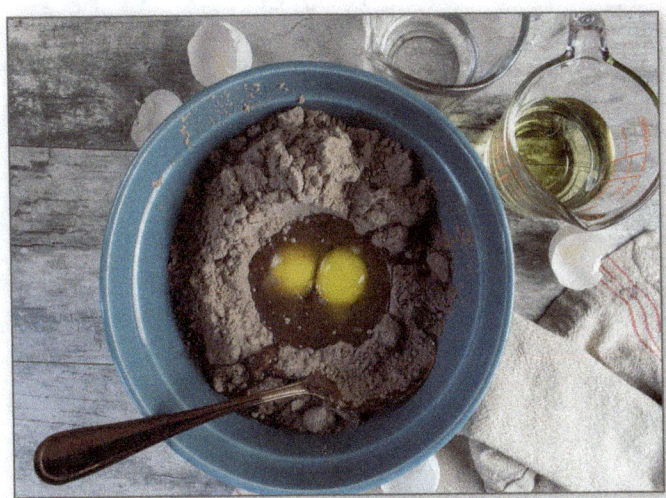

VANILLA PUDDING & PIE FILLING MIX

(From *Make-A-Mix: 306 recipes to save time and money*)

INGREDIENTS

2⅓ C Granulated Sugar

1¾ C Cornstarch

¾ tsp Salt

INSTRUCTIONS

Combine all ingredients in a large bowl. Stir with a wire whisk until blended. Pour in a tight-fitting container and store in a cool dry place. Use within six months. Makes about 4 cups of mix.

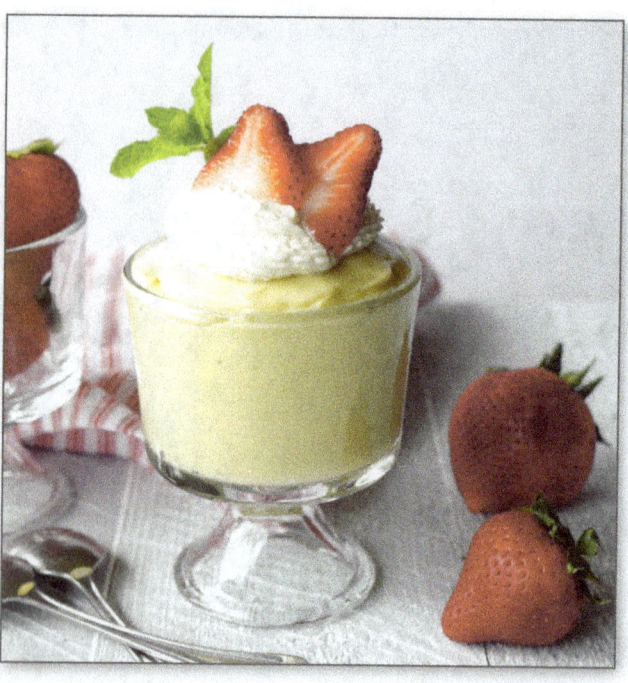

CREAMY VANILLA PUDDING

(*Make-A-Mix*)

INGREDIENTS

2 Egg Yolks

⅔ C Vanilla Pudding & Pie Filling Mix

2¾ C Milk of choice

2 tbsp Butter or Margarine

1½ tsp Vanilla Extract

INSTRUCTIONS

In a medium bowl, beat egg yolks; set aside. In a medium saucepan, combine pudding mix and milk. Cook and stir over medium heat until the mixture thickens and begins to bubble. Stirring vigorously, pour about half of the hot mixture into the beaten egg yolks. Stir egg-yolk mixture into the remaining hot mixture. Cook and stir 1 minute longer.

Remove mixture from heat. Stir in the butter or margarine and vanilla until blended. Pour the cooked pudding into 6 dessert cups or bowls. Cover with plastic wrap and refrigerate for 1 hour. Makes 6 servings.

CHOCOLATE PUDDING MIX

INGREDIENTS

4 C Sugar

¾ C Cocoa Powder

1 C Cornstarch

1 tsp Salt

INSTRUCTIONS

Mix all ingredients until combined. Makes about 6 cups pudding mix. Store in an airtight container.

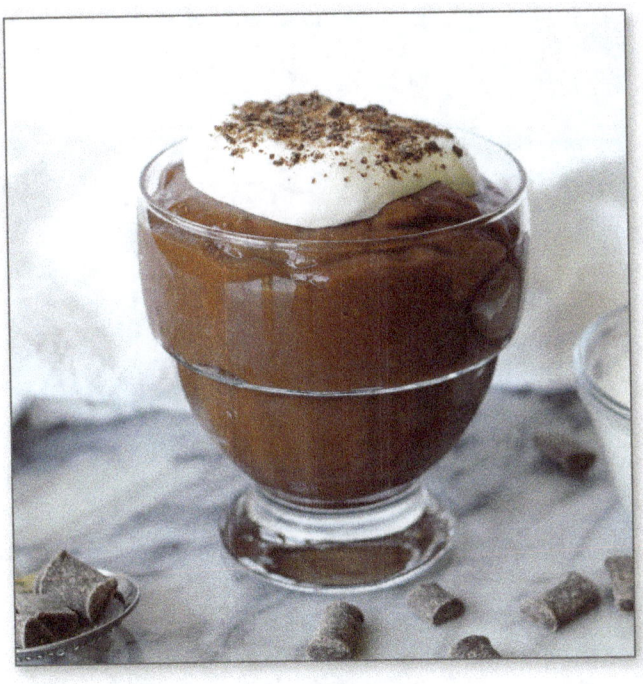

CHOCOLATE PUDDING

INGREDIENTS

1⅓ C Chocolate Pudding Mix

2 C Milk of choice

3 Egg Yolks

2 tbsp Butter or Margarine

1½ tsp Vanilla

INSTRUCTIONS

In a large saucepan combine chocolate pudding mix, milk, egg yolks, and butter. Heat on medium heat stirring consistently until the mixture boils. Boil for about a minute. Remove from heat and add vanilla. Pour into a glass bowl and cover with plastic wrap barely touching the top of the pudding to prevent a skin from forming. Place in the refrigerator to cool.

If desired, the pudding can be used as pie filling. Pour pudding in a pre-baked pie shell and cover pudding in the same manner with plastic wrap. Place pudding in the refrigerator to cool.

ALL-PURPOSE CAKE MIX

(From Make-A-Mix: 306 recipes to save time and money)

INGREDIENTS

5 C GF Flour with Xanthan Gum*

3⅛ C Sugar

½ C Cornstarch

2½ tbsp Baking Powder

1½ tsp Salt

*Add 3½ tsp Xanthan if flour blend does not contain. This may need to be adjusted depending on flour blend.

INSTRUCTIONS

Mix until well combined. Makes approximately 9 cups of mix.

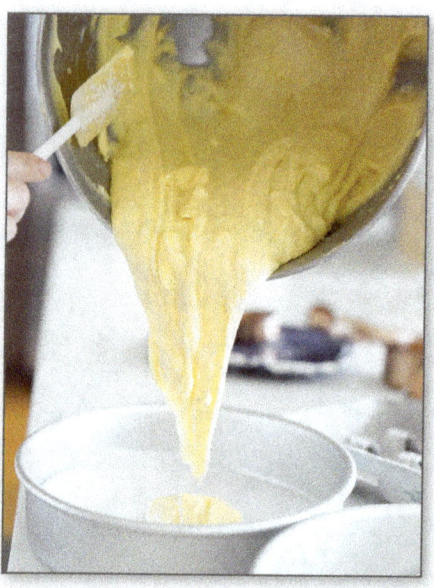

YELLOW CAKE

INGREDIENTS

2½ C All-Purpose Cake Mix

½ C + 2 tbsp Milk

½ tsp Vanilla

2 Eggs

½ C + 2 tbsp Shortening/Oil

INSTRUCTIONS

Preheat oven to 350° F. Mix the shortening and cake dry cake mix together. Add the eggs, milk, and vanilla and whip for two minutes. Bake for 30-45 minutes or until a toothpick poked in the center comes out clean. To prevent the top of the cake from becoming too brown, cover with aluminum foil for the last 15 minutes of baking.

MIXES

MUFFIN MIX

(From *Make-A-Mix: 306 recipes to save time and money*)

INGREDIENTS

8 C GF Flour

3 C Sugar

3 tbsp Baking Powder

2 tsp Salt

2 tsp Ground Cinnamon

2 tsp Ground Nutmeg

1 tbsp + 1 tsp Xanthan (16 g) Omit if using a flour blend containing xanthan

1 tbsp + 1 tsp Psyllium (16 g) Omit if using a flour blend containing xanthan/psyllium

INSTRUCTIONS

Combine all ingredients in a large bowl and mix well. Place in an airtight container and store in a cool dry place. Use within 6-8 months. Makes about 11½ cups of mix.

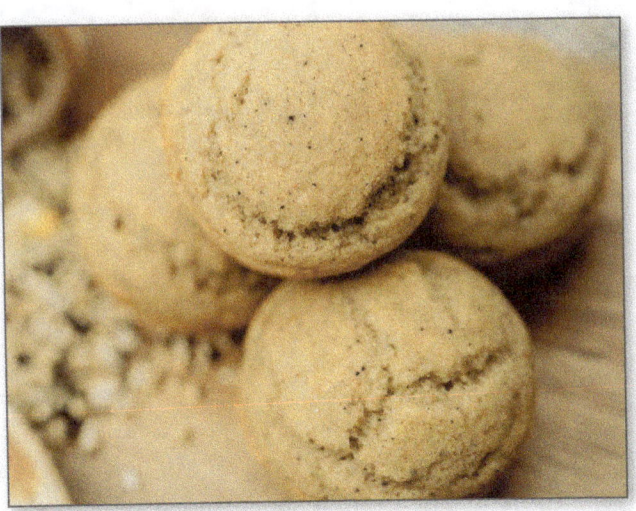

MELT-IN-YOUR-MOUTH MUFFINS

(From *Make-A-Mix: 306 recipes to save time and money*)

INGREDIENTS

2¾ C Muffin Mix

1 Egg, Beaten

1 C Milk

½ C Butter or Oil

INSTRUCTIONS

Preheat the oven to 400° F. Spray muffin pans with vegetable cooking spray. Combine egg, milk, and butter or oil in a medium mixing bowl. Add muffin mix and mix well. Fill the prepared muffin tins ¾ full. Bake for 18-20 Minutes, until golden brown. Makes 10 large muffins.

Variations:

Cornmeal Muffins: Decrease muffin mix to 2 ¼ C and add ½ C cornmeal.

Dried Fruit Muffins: Add 1 C chopped dried fruit (cherries, peaches, blueberries, pineapple, strawberries) to liquid ingredients. Add 1 tsp vanilla.

Banana Muffins: Mash 1 banana (1/2 C) and add to liquid ingredients. Add 1 tsp vanilla.

Blueberry Muffins: Fold in 1 C fresh or frozen blueberries into the basic muffin batter just before filling the muffin tins. Add 1 tsp vanilla.

PANCAKE MIX

INGREDIENTS

4 C GF Flour*

¼ C Baking Powder

¼ C Sugar

2 tsp Salt

1 tsp Xanthan if flour does not include

INSTRUCTIONS

Combine all ingredients well and place in an air-tight container. Store in a cool dry place and use within 6 months. Makes about 4½ C of mix.

*Note: The level of xanthan will greatly effect the texture of pancakes. Some commercial flours which include xanthan produce rubbery pancakes. This can be corrected by using flour without xanthan and adding xanthan to your preference.

PANCAKES

INGREDIENTS

1 C Pancake Mix

1 Egg

¾ C Milk

1 tsp Vanilla

2 tbsp Oil

INSTRUCTIONS

Preheat the griddle to 375° F or frying pan on medium heat.

Combine and mix all ingredients until well incorporated.

Cook on the griddle until bubbles form and pop. Flip and bake for another 30 seconds - 1 minute.

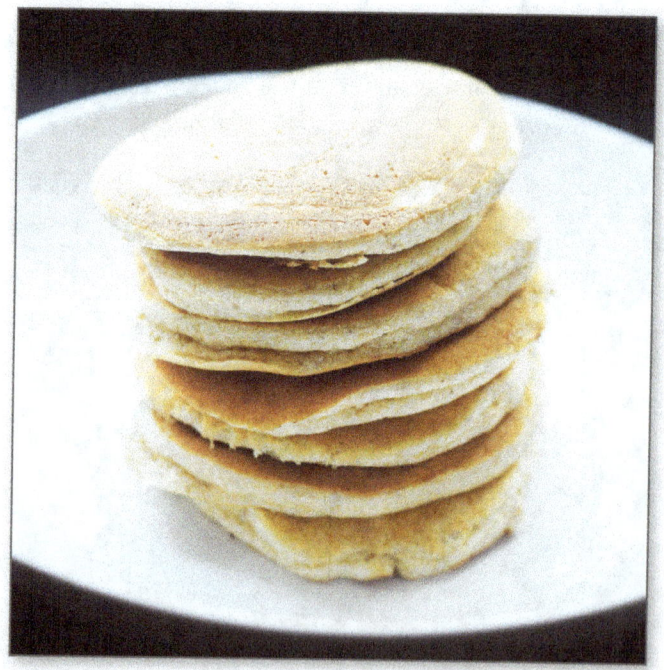

MEET LAURA HUFFMAN

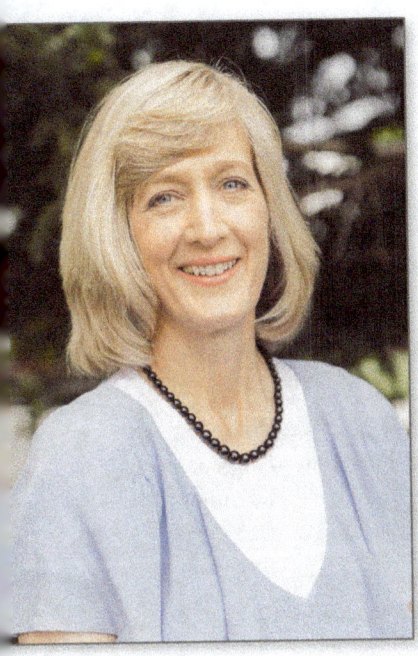

PEOPLE OFTEN AS-SUME that I or some-one in my family is glu-ten-free because I own a gluten-free mix compa-ny. Actually, no one in my family lives gluten-free. However, I have several nephews who are aller-gic to peanuts and soy. Besides that, no one has a problem with food, aside from overeating it, especially around the holidays!

The first glu-ten-free person I knew was a friend from church named Helene, who has Celiac disease. I had known about gluten from child-hood because of my mom's impromptu lessons on bread making. Still, I had no idea it was a problem for any-one. As I spent time with Helene and asked questions, I learned that gluten-free food is often expensive, poor tasting, and low in nutrients. I also learned that being gluten-free makes people feel excluded on social occa-sions where food is involved.

As my friend explained her problems with a glu-ten-free diet, I thought, "There's got to be a better way to eat." Those thoughts lingered with me for a long time. I began reading books about being gluten-free, learning medical implications, looking at websites, and attending gluten-free cooking classes.

I never dreamed this initial curiosity of the glu-ten-free world would lead me to build a business - I just wanted to help my friends eat better for less money and feel included at social functions. A woman in a glu-ten-free cooking class I attended complained she was robbed of her ability to cook when celiac disease elimi-nated canned cream soups. I told her how to make her own mix. Later I made a dairy-free version for a local summer camp. Remembering how happy I made the woman from the class helped me see I should start a business and share my ideas with other struggling fam-ilies.

Since then, I've met hundreds of gluten-free peo-ple who voiced the many difficulties and challenges of a gluten-free diet. I've shared and continue to share my ideas for adapting recipes, resolving recipe failures, sav-ing money, and food storage with many members of the gluten-free community.

Although this was helpful, I was only reaching one person at a time. I wanted to reach more people be-cause I see a great need in the gluten-free community and decided to write this book. No one should have to work that hard to eat, and the food should DEFINITELY NOT taste bad.

I continue to work on my business and share my gluten-free food information and products with the world.

Visit me on the web

https://viviansliveagain.com

IG: https://www.instagram.com/viviansliveagain/

FB: https://www.facebook.com/WheatFreeNutrition

ADDITIONAL RESOURCES

Websites, Books, and Further Reading

24 Carrot Life. (2014, November 12). Coconut Buckwheat Granola. Retrieved May 18, 2023, from https://24carrotlife.com/2014/11/12/coconut-buckwheat-granola/

American Celiac Disease Alliance. (n.d.). Retrieved May 3, 2023 from http://www.americanceliacsociety.org/index.html

Andress, E. L., & Harrison, J. A. (2006). Freezing Vegetables. National Center for Home Food Preservation, University of Georgia. Retrieved May 10, 2023, from https://nchfp.uga.edu/publications/uga/uga_freeze_veg.pdf

Becker, S. (2016). The Essential Home-Ground Flour Book. Robert Rose. ISBN 978-0-7788-0534-2.

Beyond Celiac. (n.d.). Celiac disease. Retrieved April 30, 2023, from https://www.beyondceliac.org/celiac-disease/

Bob's Red Mill. (n.d.). How to Make Popped Sorghum. Retrieved May 18, 2023, from https://www.bobsredmill.com/recipes/how-to-make/popped-sorghum/

Bon Appétit. (2014, January 27). Herbed Brown Rice Mujadarra. Retrieved May 18, 2023, from https://www.bonappetit.com/recipe/herbed-brown-rice-mujadarra

Budget Bytes. (2020, February 9). Chana Saag. Retrieved May 18, 2023, from https://www.budgetbytes.com/chana-saag/

Budget Bytes. (2019, September 7). Easy Rosemary Garlic White Bean Soup. Retrieved May 18, 2023, from https://www.budgetbytes.com/easy-rosemary-garlic-white-bean-soup/

Canadian Celiac Association. (n.d.). About celiac disease. Retrieved April 30, 2023, from https://www.celiac.ca/about-celiac-disease/

Celiac Community Foundation of Northern California. (n.d.). About celiac disease. Retrieved April 30, 2023, from https://celiaccommunity.org/about-celiac-disease/

Celiac Disease Foundation. (n.d.). Retrieved May 3, 2023 from https://celiac.org/

Celiac Support Organization. (n.d.). Retrieved May 3, 2023 from http://celiacsupportorganisation.com/

Claudepierre, C. (2021, June 1). Lentil Taco Meat. The Conscious Plant Kitchen. Retrieved May 18, 2023, from https://www.theconsciousplantkitchen.com/lentil-taco-meat/

Cookie and Kate. (n.d.). Best Quinoa Salad Recipe. Retrieved May 18, 2023, from https://cookieandkate.com/best-quinoa-salad-recipe/

Cookie and Kate. (n.d.). Crispy Falafel Recipe. Retrieved May 18, 2023, from https://cookieandkate.com/crispy-falafel-recipe/

Cookie and Kate. (n.d.). Easy Refried Beans Recipe. Retrieved May 18, 2023, from https://cookieandkate.com/easy-refried-beans-recipe/print/28453/

Cookie and Kate. (n.d.). Mujaddara Recipe. Retrieved May 18, 2023, from https://cookieandkate.com/mujaddara-recipe/

Cookie and Kate. (n.d.). Thai Peanut Quinoa Salad Recipe. Retrieved May 18, 2023, from https://cookieandkate.com/thai-peanut-quinoa-salad-recipe/

Cookie and Kate. (n.d.). Vegetarian Enchiladas Recipe. Retrieved May 18, 2023, from https://cookieandkate.com/vegetarian-enchiladas-recipe/

Eliason, K., Harvard, A., & Westover, B. (1993). Make-A-Mix: 306 recipes to save time and money. ISBN 1-55561-073-0.

Fav Family Recipes. (n.d.). Food Storage Tips: Where to Store Food. Retrieved May 6, 2023, from https://www.favfamilyrecipes.com/food-storage-tips-where-to-store-food/#:~:text=Store%20food%20in%20a%20cool,will%20protect%20food%20from%20moisture.

Federal Emergency Management Agency. (2004). Food and Water in an Emergency. https://www.fema.gov/pdf/library/f&web.pdf

Full of Plants (n.d.). Retrieved May 18, 2023. https://fullof-plants.com.

Gardening Know How. (n.d.). Search results. Retrieved May 2, 2023, from https://www.gardeningknowhow.com/extension-search

Generation GF. (n.d.). Kids with Celiac Disease. Retrieved May 18, 2023, from https://gluten.org/community/kids/#:~:text=What%20is%20Generation%20GF%3F,your%20kids%20covered%20from%20A%2D

Gimme Some Oven. (n.d.). Fried Rice Recipe. Retrieved May 18, 2023, from https://www.gimmesomeoven.com/fried-rice-recipe/

GFF Magazine. (n.d.). Retrieved May 3, 2023 from https://gffmag.com/recipes/

gfJules. (n.d.). Retrieved May 3, 2023 from https://gfjules.com/recipes/

Gluten-Free Living. (n.d.). Retrieved from https://www.glutenfreeliving.com/

Gluten-Free on a Shoestring. (n.d.). Retrieved May 3, 2023 from https://glutenfreeonashoestring.com/

Gluten Intolerance Group. (n.d.). About gluten intolerance. Retrieved April 30, 2023, from https://gluten.org/about-gluten-intolerance/

Grant, B. L. (n.d.). How Many Vegetables per Person per Year? Gardening Know How. Retrieved May 10, 2023, from https://www.gardeningknowhow.com/edible/vegetables/vgen/how-many-vegetables-per-person-per-year.htm

Green, P., & Hemming, C. (2014). Grain Power: Over 100 Delicious Gluten-Free Ancient Grains & Superblend Recipes. Penguin Random House.

Happy Herbivore. (n.d.). Vegetarian Lentil Sausage Gravy (Vegan & Soy-Free). Retrieved May 18, 2023, from https://happyherbivore.com/recipe/vegetarian-lentil-sausage-gravy-vegan-soy-free/

Hertzberg, J., & François, Z. (2014). Gluten-Free Artisan Bread in Five Minutes a Day. St. Martin's Press.

Hunn, N. (2013). Gluten-Free on a Shoestring Bakes Bread: Biscuits, Bagels, Buns, and More. Da Capo Lifelong Books.

Iowa Girl Eats. (n.d.). Retrieved May 3, 2023 from https://iowagirleats.com/recipes/

James, S. (2017, June 1). Cooking at home tonight? It's most likely cheaper and healthier, UW study finds. Retrieved May 4, 2023, from https://sph.washington.edu/news-events/news/cooking-home-tonight-its-most-likely-cheaper-and-healthier-uw-study-finds

Krishnamurthy, K. (2017). A review of the methods available for estimating shelf life of ambient processed food products. Critical Reviews in Food Science and Nutrition, 57(3), 438-450. https://doi.org/10.1080/10408398.2013.858086

Krissoff, L. (2012). Whole Grains for a New Generation: Light Dishes, Hearty Meals, Sweet Treats, and Sundry Snacks for the Everyday Cook. Stewart, Tabori & Chang.

Luther, D. (2015). The Prepper's Water Survival Guide. ISBN 978-1-61243-448-3.

Making Thyme for Health. (n.d.). One-Pot African Peanut Stew. Retrieved May 18, 2023, from https://www.makingthymeforhealth.com/one-pot-african-peanut-stew/

Minimalist Baker. (n.d.). Chickpea Sunflower Sandwich. Retrieved May 18, 2023, from https://minimalistbaker.com/chickpea-sunflower-sandwich/

Moskowitz, I. C. (2013). Isa Does It: Amazingly Easy, Wildly Delicious Vegan Recipes for Every Day of the Week. Little, Brown and Company.

MySymptoms. (n.d.). Retrieved May 3, 2023, from https://www.mysymptoms.net/

My Quiet Kitchen. (2021, May 10). Popped Sorghum Balls. Retrieved May 18, 2023, from https://myquietkitchen.com/popped-sorghum-balls/

National Celiac Association. (n.d.). About celiac disease. Retrieved April 30, 2023, from https://nationalceliac.org/about-celiac-disease/

Parker, K., & Smith, K. (2012). The High-Protein Vegetarian Cookbook: Hearty Dishes That Even Carnivores Will Love. W. W. Norton & Company.

ProvidentLiving.com. (n.d.). Food storage calculator. Retrieved May 4, 2023, from https://providentliving.com/preparedness/food-storage/foodcalc/

Ready.gov. (n.d.). Ready.gov. https://www.ready.gov/

Salsbury, B. (1995). Preparedness Principles: The Complete Personal Preparedness Resource Guide for Any Emergency Situation. Gold Leaf Press. ISBN 0-88290-806-5.

Sorghum Checkoff. (n.d.). Popped Sorghum Peanut Butter Balls. Retrieved May 18, 2023, from https://www.sorghumcheckoff.com/recipes/popped-sorghum-peanut-butter-balls/

Simple Veganista. (n.d.). Healthy Baked Beans (Instant Pot). Retrieved May 18, 2023, from https://simple-veganista.com/healthy-baked-beans-instant-pot/

Simply Gluten Free. (n.d.). Retrieved May 3, 2023, from https://simplygluten-free.com/

Simply Quinoa. (2018, August 30). Mexican Quinoa Stuffed Sweet Potatoes. Retrieved May 18, 2023, from https://www.simplyquinoa.com/mexican-quinoa-stuffed-sweet-potatoes/

Spend With Pennies. (2022, March 21). Chickpea Salad. Retrieved May 18, 2023, from https://www.spendwithpennies.com/chickpea-salad/

Spend With Pennies. (2020, March 16). Easy Lentil Shepherd's Pie (Vegetarian). Retrieved May 18, 2023, from https://www.spendwithpennies.com/easy-lentil-shepherds-pie-vegetarian/#wprm-recipe-container-179900

Spokin. (n.d.). Allergy-Friendly Recipes. Retrieved May 3, 2023 from https://www.spokin.com/food-allergy-friendly-recipes

Spoonful. (n.d.). Retrieved May 3, 2023, from https://spoonfulapp.com/

Square Foot Gardening. (n.d.). Square Foot Gardening. Retrieved May 13, 2023, from https://squarefootgardening.org/

StillTasty. (n.d.). Food Storage - How Long Can You Keep...? Retrieved May 2, 2023, from https://www.stilltasty.com//Fooditems/food_storage_info

Thacker Wendel, D. (2019, January 24). Lentil Meatballs Marinara. Forks Over Knives. Retrieved May 18, 2023, from https://www.forksoverknives.com/recipes/vegan-baked-stuffed/lentil-meatballs-marinara/

The Church of Jesus Christ of Latter-day Saints. (n.d.). Longer-term food supply. Retrieved May 3, 2023, from https://www.churchofjesuschrist.org/topics/food-storage/longer-term-food-supply?lang=eng#2.

The Church of Jesus Christ of Latter-day Saints. (n.d.). Provident Living. https://providentliving.churchofjesuschrist.org/?lang=eng. Retrieved May 10, 2023.

The Provident Prepper. (n.d.). Packaging dry foods in plastic bottles for long-term food storage. Retrieved May 12, 2023, from https://theprovidentprepper.org/packaging-dry-foods-in-plastic-bottles-for-long-term-food-storage/

U.S. Department of Health & Human Services. (n.d.). Food safety in disaster or emergency. Retrieved May 2, 2023, from https://www.foodsafety.gov/keep-food-safe/food-safety-in-disaster-or-emergency

University of Minnesota Extension. (n.d.). How to freeze fruit for the best flavor. Retrieved May 2, 2023, from https://extension.umn.edu/preserving-and-preparing/how-freeze-fruit-best-flavor#apricots-425261

Utah State University Extension. (n.d.). Food Storage: Preserving and preparing. Retrieved May 2, 2023, from https://extension.usu.edu/preserve-the-harvest/files/Food-Storage-Booklet.pdf

Utah State University Extension. (n.d.). Gardening basics. Retrieved May 9, 2023, from https://extension.usu.edu/yardandgarden/gardening-basics

Utah State University Extension. (n.d.). Recipes. Retrieved May 22, 2023, from https://extension.usu.edu/nutrition/recipes/index

Wageningen Seed Science Centre. (n.d.). Low oxygen seed storage. Retrieved May 2, 2023, from https://www.wur.nl/en/research-results/projects-and-programmes/wageningen-seed-science-centre-1/research-topics-projects/research-topics-wssc/seed-technology/low-oxygen-seed-storage.htm

Wells, S. (2023, February 8). Black Bean Soup. Our Best Bites. Retrieved May 18, 2023, from https://ourbestbites.com/black-bean-soup/

Podcasts and Videos

A Canadian Celiac Podcast. (n.d.). [Audio podcast]. Retrieved May 3, 2023 from https://acanadianceliacpodcast.libsyn.com/

Back Pack Hack. (2016, September 30). DIY Emergency 100 Hour Candles [Video]. YouTube. https://www.youtube.com/watch?v=fCgsbiTdnDA

Gluten Free Baking Show. (n.d.). [Audio podcast]. Retrieved May 3, 2023 from https://www.gfbakingshow.com/

Gluten-Free News. (n.d.). [Audio podcast]. Retrieved May 3, 2023 from https://podcasts.apple.com/us/podcast/gluten-free-news/id1474822074

Gluten-Free You and Me. (n.d.). [Audio podcast]. Retrieved May 3, 2023 from https://podcasts.apple.com/us/podcast/gluten-free-you-me/id1466183042

Oh Crumbs Podcast. (n.d.). [Audio podcast]. Retrieved May 3, 2023 from https://theglutenfreeblogger.com/oh-crumbs-podcast-episodes/

The Celiac Project Podcast. (n.d.). [Audio podcast]. Retrieved May 3, 2023 from https://celiacprojectpodcast.libsyn.com/

Travel Gluten Free Podcast. (n.d.). [Audio podcast]. Retrieved May 3, 2023 from https://www.travelglutenfreepodcast.com/

Online Shopping and Coupons

Alpine Food Storage. (n.d.). Home page. Retrieved May 5, 2023, from https://www.alpinefoodstorage.com

Azure Standard. (n.d.). Drop point locator. Retrieved Month Day, Year, from https://www.azurestandard.com/drop-point-locator/

CouponBirds. (n.d.). Retrieved May 3, 2023, from https://www.couponbirds.com/

Find Me Gluten Free. (n.d.). Retrieved May 3, 2023, from https://www.findmeglutenfree.com/

Find Me Gluten Free Products. (n.d.). Shipping now. Retrieved May 3, 2023, from https://www.findmeglutenfree.com/products/brands/shipping-now

Gluten Free Mall. (n.d.). Retrieved May 3, 2023, from https://glutenfreemall.com/

Gluten Free Palace. (n.d.). Retrieved May 3, 2023, from https://www.glutenfreepalace.com/

Finke, J. (n.d.). Find Gluten-Free Coupons & Deals. Good For You Gluten Free. Retrieved May 3, 2023, from https://www.goodforyouglutenfree.com/find-gluten-free-coupons-deals/

Join Honey. (n.d.). Retrieved May 3, 2023, from https://www.joinhoney.com/

Nulife Market. (n.d.). Home page. Retrieved May 1, 2023 from https://nulifemarket.com/

Teff Company. (n.d.). Home. Retrieved May 5, 2023, from https://teffco.com/

The Gluten-Free Shoppe. (n.d.). Retrieved May 3, 2023, from https://theglutenfreeshoppe.com/

The Gluten-Free Prairie. (n.d.). Home. Retrieved May 3, 2023, from https://www.glutenfreeprairie.com/

The Krazy Coupon Lady. (n.d.). Retrieved May 3, 2023, from https://thekrazycouponlady.com

The Nut Garden. (n.d.). Retrieved May 5, 2023, from https://www.thenutgarden.com/

WebstaurantStore. (n.d.). Gluten-free foods. Retrieved May 1, 2023, from https://www.webstaurantstore.com/57613/gluten-free-foods.html

INDEX

Spread the Word about
THE GLUTEN-FREE PANTRY

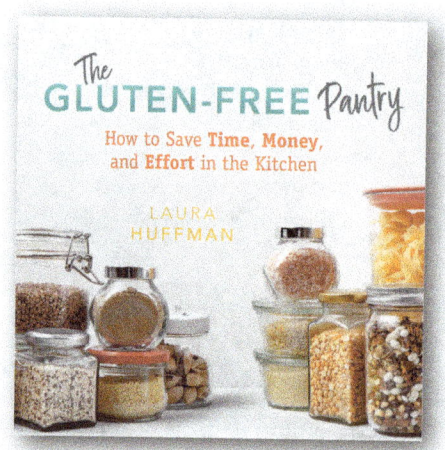

THANK YOU FOR READING MY BOOK!

Do you know someone who is new to eating gluten-free, emergency preparedness, provident living, or would simply like to save money on their grocery bill?

Share my handy little book with a friend today and spread the word about making gluten free living easier.

I'd appreciate it if you'd leave a review on Amazon letting me know what you liked about the book and what you thought of my book. Leaving a review lets others see my book and helps me get seen on Amazon.

Laura Huffman

www.ingramcontent.com/pod-product-compliance
Lightning Source LLC
Chambersburg PA
CBHW080838120626
46553CB00009B/2473